CLINICAL MANAGEMENT OF SPEECH DISORDERS

Donald E. Mowrer
James L. Case
Arizona State University

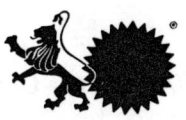

AN ASPEN PUBLICATION®
Aspen Systems Corporation
Rockville, Maryland
London
1982

Library of Congress Cataloging in Publication Data

Mowrer, Donald E.
Clinical management of speech disorders.

Includes bibliographies and index.
1. Speech therapy.   I. Case, James L.
II. Title.
RC423.M618   616.85′506   81-19050
ISBN: 0-89443-393-8   AACR2

Copyright © 1982 Aspen Systems Corporation

All rights reserved. This book, or parts thereof, may not be reproduced in any form or by any means, electronic or mechanical, including photocopy, recording, or any information storage and retrieval system now known or to be invented, without written permission from the publisher, except in the case of brief quotations embodied in critical articles or reviews. For information, address Aspen Systems Corporation, 1600 Research Boulevard, Rockville, Maryland 20850.

Library of Congress Catalog Card Number: 81-19050
ISBN: 0-89443-393-8

Printed in the United States of America

1 2 3 4 5

Table of Contents

Preface vii

SECTION I—ARTICULATION DISORDERS 1

  Chapter 1—The Classification and Development of Articulation .. 3

      Classification of Speech Sounds 4
      The Speech-Producing Mechanism 9
      Description of Speech Sounds 11
      The Development of Articulation 17

  Chapter 2—Assessing Articulation Skills 31

      Types of Articulation Tests 31
      Features of Articulation Tests 34
      Description of Specific Articulation Tests 36
      Tests Related to Articulation Ability 46
      Summary 49

  Chapter 3—The Treatment of Articulation Disorders 51

      Preliminary Considerations 51
      Procedures for Evoking Consonant Sounds 59
      Incorporating the Target Sound in Words and
         Phrases 74
      Using the Target Sound in Connected Speech 77
      Using the Target Sound at the Automatic Speech
         Level 77

Motivation 82
Behavioral Objectives 84
Example of Child with Multiple Articulation
    Errors 86
Execution of Therapy Procedures 93
Evaluation of Progress 98

SECTION II—VOICE DISORDERS 101

Chapter 4—Voice Therapy in the School System 103

Medical Evaluation and Referral Processes 104
Screening and Identification Processes 106
Parameters of Voice 108
Specific Disorders of Voice 117
Disorders of Resonance 140
Summary 153

**Chapter 5—Psychogenic and Neurogenic Voice Disorders in
    Adults** 157

Psychogenic Voice Disorder 158
Specific Techniques of Therapy 164
Summary of Psychogenic Voice Disorder 169
Spasmodic (Spastic) Dysphonia 170
Summary of Spasmodic (Spastic) Dysphonia 174
Neurogenic Voice Disorder 174
Miscellaneous Neurogenic Voice Disorders 181
Summary of Neurogenic Voice Disorder 182

Chapter 6—Vocal Abuse in Adults 185

Contact Ulcers 185
Summary of Contact Ulcers 194
Vocal Nodules in Adults 194
Summary of Abuses 204
Pitch Evaluation in Vocal Nodules 204
Vocal Quality in Persons with Vocal Nodules 205
Therapy for Vocal Nodules 207
Case Example of Vocal Nodules with Serious
    Complications 208
Summary 209

Chapter 7—Alaryngeal Phonation Therapy **211**

    Surgical Aspects of Laryngectomy 211
    Role of the SLP in Laryngectomy Rehabilitation .. 213
    Extrinsic Methods of Alaryngeal Phonation 213
    Intrinsic Methods of Alaryngeal Phonation 216
    Methods of Producing Esophageal Speech 217
    Summary of Methods of Alaryngeal Phonation 220
    Rehabilitation of Laryngectomized Persons 220
    Goal of Functional Esophageal Speech 231
    Case of Example of Alaryngeal Phonation 232
    Radiation without Surgery 233
    Phonation from Shunt Reconstruction 233
    Summary 234

SECTION III—FLUENCY DISORDERS **237**

  Chapter 8—Defining and Assessing Stuttering Behavior **239**

    Defining Stuttering 239
    Causes of Stuttering 242
    Assessing Stuttering Behaviors 249
    Summary 257

  Chapter 9—Treatment Procedures for Stutterers **261**

    Overview of Therapy Goals 262
    Attending to Moment of Stuttering 264
    Attending to Fluent Speech 269
    Summary 283

Index **287**

Preface

Those who work in the helping professions search constantly for practical information that can aid them in providing more effective services. There are numerous texts describing how services should be provided that have been studied by students enrolled in speech/language pathology courses. However, the rule seems to be that theoretical models seldom can be applied to the real world. The ideal situation never seems to exist.

What the authors attempt in this book is to bridge the gap between theory and practice by illustrating through case studies how to manage the communication difficulty of individuals with articulation, voice, or fluency disorders. Although it is assumed that the reader is academically competent in speech/language pathology, a brief review of essential information in each of the three areas is presented. This introduction also serves to familiarize other professionals with the fundamental information necessary to understand basic treatment procedures.

The major emphasis of this book is on updating the speech/language pathologist in knowledge of procedures that can be used to change speech behaviors. The three areas analyzed—articulation, voice, and fluency—were selected because they represent a large portion of the caseload these pathologists usually treat. The authors decided the language area was too broad to be covered in this book. Consequently, it is not included.

The three chapters in Section I deal with articulation disorders. Chapter 1, a review of speech sounds, describes how they are classified and produced and how they become part of a child's developing phonological system.

Chapter 2 discusses how articulation skills are assessed, using a variety of measurement techniques. This chapter provides a comprehensive summary of articulation tests—not only the familiar ones that are used frequently but also some of the newer instruments designed to measure special features of phonological processes.

Chapter 3, the final and longest of the section, deals exclusively with the treatment of articulation disorders. Criteria for selecting the target sound are provided, followed by a detailed explanation of procedures used to evoke eight of the most commonly misarticulated sounds. Motivational factors and the use of behavioral objectives in a behavior therapy model are discussed in relation to the use of accountability in communication disorders. The treatment method focuses on coarticulation activities that move rapidly into conversational speech patterns. In the last section of this chapter, a case study of a child who has a multiple articulation problem is presented, illustrating the step-by-step process used in remediating the disorder. This therapy format can be generalized to many functional articulation problems that speech/language pathologists encounter so frequently.

Section II focuses on problems relating to voice disorders. Chapter 4 provides practical information to facilitate the identification and management of typical types of voice disorders found in the school system. Problems of screening, medical referral, teacher support, and management considerations for disorders of pitch, vocal abuse, and abnormal resonance are discussed.

Chapter 5 presents practical techniques of managing adult voice disorders caused by psychogenic or neurogenic factors. Only the common disorders are covered. References are included for the many less common but clinically significant psychogenic and neurogenic disorders.

In Chapter 6, common forms of, and problems in, vocal abuse by adults are covered in extensive clinical detail. Practical management techniques for vocal nodules and contact ulcers are described.

Chapter 7 deals with voice disorders resulting from laryngeal amputation because of cancer or trauma. The more common methods of alaryngeal communication management such as electrolarynges and esophageal speech are detailed.

Each voice chapter contains case examples of how specific techniques of evaluation and treatment are applied. The philosophy here is practical and applicable, with the hope of avoiding sacrificing basic principles of voice science.

Section III deals with fluency disorders, more commonly called stuttering. Chapter 8 includes a working definition of stuttering based upon events that can be observed and counted objectively, followed by discussion of possible causes. Finally, details of procedures for assessing stuttering are presented to assist the speech/language pathologist in evaluating and planning therapy.

Chapter 9 emphasizes treatment procedures. Three procedures—those of Van Riper, Webster, and Mowrer—are described and data on each method are provided.

Dr. Mowrer was responsible for the chapters on articulation and fluency disorders, and Dr. Case wrote the section on voice disorders.

The authors hope this book provides practicing speech/language pathologists and other professionals who work on communication-related problems with practical procedures they can use as guidelines for their own therapies.

Donald E. Mowrer
James L. Case
January 1982

Section I
Articulation Disorders

Chapter 1

The Classification and Development of Articulation

The study and treatment of articulation disorders—particularly the orderly process in which articulation skills are acquired—is one of the more fascinating areas in speech pathology. Only now are experts discovering some of the laws that operate as children learn a phonological system. Many more laws have yet to be found but a basic order governing the acquisition of speech sounds seems to be emerging.

Another factor is that principles of behavior therapy can be used successfully in modifying articulation skills. It is highly rewarding to see significant changes brought about by using well-established procedures.

Observing young toddlers coping with the complex articulatory movements required to speak words intelligibly is one of the most intriguing events adults witness as children mature. Learning articulation skills involves a growth process of continuous change until the phonological system is mastered. Parents see their children progress through the various stages of articulation development without realizing how difficult this process is to master. Most parents simply expect their children to talk as they expect them to walk. They pay little attention to the subtle shifts that occur during periods of sound change when their child progresses from saying *fum* to *thumb* or from *tee* to *tree*. The young child's ability to pronounce speech sounds seems to emerge as a developmental process closely akin to others such as learning to eat, walk, draw, play, and follow directions. To the casual observer it just seems to happen.

While this development may appear to be typical of most children as they learn articulatory skills, it is not necessarily true for all. It is known that 5 to 10 percent of school-aged children have communication problems and most of them have difficulty pronouncing sounds (Byrne & Shervanian, 1977, p. 5). Children who misarticulate sounds often are ridiculed, misunderstood, and frustrated when communicating with others.

Many children overcome problems in articulating sounds even without special attention but there is no way of knowing the long-term effects of frustration they experience during the learning process. Rather than allow these children to struggle on their own, experts can provide valuable guidance that should help speed up the sound-learning process. This section on articulation focuses on the nature of this guidance and information that speech therapists and special educators must know to provide it. A repertoire of techniques is outlined that will help speech/language pathologists (SLPs) aid both children and adults who wish to learn to articulate sounds correctly.

In many instances, parents can take sole responsibility for providing instructions to help their child learn to articulate correctly. In other instances, classroom teachers may perform the function. In still other cases, the skills of a speech/language pathologist are required to conduct a thorough diagnosis of the problem, after which a suitable treatment plan can be developed and executed. In some instances, the services of other professionals such as physicians, psychologists, social workers, or orthodontists may be required to help diagnose or treat speech problems.

Before specific remedial techniques that can be used to help individuals learn correct articulation are presented, several important factors relating to sound production are discussed.

CLASSIFICATION OF SPEECH SOUNDS

Sounds are divided into two major groups: consonants and vowels. The airstream is restricted either partly or totally during consonant production but faces practically no restraints in vowel sounds. Consonant sounds are misarticulated more frequently than are vowels.

Consonants

Throughout this text, sounds are enclosed by brackets or slash marks— by brackets [ ] when they represent sounds as they actually are spoken and by slash marks / / when they denote sounds not as they are spoken but simply as theoretical versions. While most consonants are represented using their alphabet letter equivalent, some sounds require the use of special symbols.

The instrument used to represent sounds is the International Phonetic Alphabet (IPA). The symbols are shown in Exhibit 1-1. The TH sound in the word *thumb,* for example, is written using the symbol / θ / to indicate it is a voiceless sound. The TH sound in the word *them* is voiced so it is represented by a different symbol / ð /. The sound of the SH in the word

Exhibit 1-1 Classification of English Consonant Sounds According to Manner and Place of Production

Manner of articulation		Place of articulation						
		Bilabial	Labiodental	Dental	Alveolar	Palatal	Velar	Glottal
Stops	VL	p (pit)			t (tick)		k (kit)	ʔ (button)
	V	b (bit)			d (dig)		g (get)	
Fricatives	VL		f (fit)	θ (thin)	s (sit)	ʃ (shoe)		h (hit)
	V		v (vat)	ð (them)	z (zip)	ʒ (measure)		
Affricatives	VL					tʃ (chair)		
	V					dʒ (jew)		
Nasals	V	m (mit)			n (not)		ŋ (sing)	
Liquids	V				l (lip)	r (rat)		
Glides	V	w (win)				y (yet)		

shoe is written as / ʃ /, the S in *measure* is / ʒ /, the CH in *chair* is / tʃ /, the J in *jewel* is / dʒ /, the NG in *sing* is / ŋ /, and the voiced H in *ahead* is / ɦ /. When the vocal cords are closed abruptly, a glottal stop sound is produced that is represented by the symbol / ʔ /. It often is substituted for the T sound in words such as *mountain* or *button*.

Aside from these few special symbols, the other consonant sounds are represented with familiar letters. G is /g/, K is /k/, F is /f/, D is /d/, and so on. The sound enclosed by slash marks or brackets is not pronounced like the alphabet letter equivalent. /s/ is pronounced like the S in the word *soap* not as the ES vowel-consonant combination. /k/ is produced as a voiceless sound, not as *kay* with the accompanying vowel sound. /b/ is not *bee* but becomes *buh*. The exhibit shows the key words for correct pronunciation of these phonetic sounds.

Most classification systems divide English consonant sounds into two major divisions according to the place where they are produced and the manner in which the airstream is modified. This classification system also is shown in Exhibit 1-1.

Place of Articulation

The place of articulation is defined in terms of the point where there is maximum constriction or stoppage of the airstream. While the tongue plays a major role in this during the production of many sounds, some are created by a constriction of other parts of the oral region. For example, /p/ is produced by action of the lips contacting each other (bilabial sounds) and /w/ by a partial closure and rounding of the lips. For sounds made by the lips and teeth (labiodental), the bottom teeth and upper lip meet to produce /f/ and /v/. The glottal stop / ʔ /, and the fricatives /h/ and / ɦ / do not require tongue movement; instead, they are produced by modifying the airstream at the vocal cords. The tongue plays a major role in the production of all of the other sounds. Alveolar sounds /t, d, l, n, s, z/ are formed as the tip of the tongue nearly touches the alveolar gum ridge just behind the upper front teeth. As Exhibit 1-1 shows, six consonants are produced at this point. The /s/ and /z/ formed there are two of the sounds misarticulated most frequently.

The blade of the tongue moves slightly backward close to the roof of the mouth (hard palate) to produce the palatal sounds. These sounds, / ʃ , tʃ , dʒ , ʒ , r/, especially the /r/, also are among those most frequently misarticulated. The tongue is involved directly in the production of 17 English consonant sounds but not for the remaining eight. It is interesting to note that the tongue of one man was surgically removed yet he learned to articulate intelligibly by using compensatory movements (Goldstein, 1940). Such cases are exceptions, not the rule.

Manner of Articulation

The manner of articulation can be divided into two classifications: one consists of voiced and unvoiced sounds, the other is related more closely to the way the airstream is influenced. They are grouped together, also as shown in Exhibit 1-1. The sonorant sounds, that is, nasals, liquids, and glides, all are voiced sounds; obstruents, or stops, fricatives, and affricatives, are divided into pairs of voiced and voiceless sounds called cognates.

When a *stop* consonant is produced, the airstream or air pressure is blocked completely, then released suddenly. Four of these sounds are voiceless, three are voiced. Since they literally explode as they are released in certain positions in words they often are referred to as *plosives*.

Ten sounds comprise the *fricatives*, so named because they are produced as a result of the friction of the airstream as it rushes through a restricted passageway. The /s/ and /z/ sounds and the palatals / ʃ / and / ʒ / also are called *sibilants* because of the hissing sound they make. Half of the fricatives are voiced, half unvoiced.

When a stop is combined with a fricative, the new sound is called an *affricative*. This sound is produced when the airstream is first stopped, then slowly released with friction as when /t/ and / ʃ / are combined to form /tʃ /. The two affricative sounds, / dʒ / and /tʃ /, also are called sibilants because of their hissing quality.

There is much less constriction of the airstream when *nasal, liquid*, and *glide* sounds are produced. The chief characteristic of the nasals is that they are produced or resonated in the nasal cavity since the airstream is blocked from passing through the oral cavity.

The liquid sound /l/ is produced quite differently from others. The tongue tip completely restricts the airstream, forcing air to emerge past the two sides of the tongue in a lateral direction. /l/ is the only sound in the English language produced by a lateral airstream.

The other liquid sound, /r/, also is unique in that it occurs only in the initial position of a syllable or within a cluster such as /dr/, /tr/, /fr/, /str/, and the like. /r/ acts as a syllable releaser. The vowel-like / ɚ / is a different sound that usually occurs at the end of a syllable in such words as *her, mother*, or *turn* or in a few initial syllable positions as in *earth* or *early*. / ɚ / or its stressed counterpart / ɝ / is always a syllable arrestor. It is called a post vocalic sound.

Finally, the least constricted sounds, /w/ and /j/, comprise the *glides*. /w/ and /j/ are referred to as *semivowels* since they share similar features with vowel sounds, depending upon whether they initiate or terminate a syllable.

Vowels

Children master vowel production by the time they are 3 years old but do not cope fully with consonants until they are 6 to 8 (Irwin, 1947, 1948). Occasionally, some have difficulty producing vowels but in most cases, consonants are the stumbling points.

Vowel sounds are classified along two dimensions, each reflecting the position of the tongue within the oral cavity. The position and shape of the tongue play the major role in determining the type of vowel sound produced. The classification system for all 12 English vowel sounds is shown in Exhibit 1-2. Vowels are characterized by a voiced airstream that is relatively unrestricted as it passes through the oral cavity.

The first dimension of the vowel classification system deals with the position of the tongue as high in the mouth, in the midline, or low. Thus, the /i/ sound in *feet* requires the tongue be in a high position near the hard palate. The /æ/ in *bat* is produced with the tongue in a downward position. The positional variations can be understood better by saying each vowel in the series from the high /i/ to the low /æ/. The jaw drops down slightly each time a speaker changes from one vowel to another that is produced by a lower tongue position.

Exhibit 1-2 Classification of English Vowel Sounds According to High-Low and Front-Back Position of Tongue in Oral Cavity

	FRONT	CENTER	BACK
HIGH	i (feet) I (sit)		u (moon) U (book) o (boat)
MIDDLE	e (bake) ɛ (set)	ɚ (mother) ɜ (hurt) ə (sofa) ʌ (put)	ɔ (law)
LOW	æ (man)		a (father)

Classification and Development of Articulation

The second dimension divides the mouth into front, midline, and back as to where the tongue is positioned. For example, the /æ/ in *bat* requires the tongue to be positioned in the front of the mouth, the /ə/ in *sofa* is produced in the midsection, and the /ɔ/ in *bought* is produced when the tongue is in the back. Thus, both tongue position and tongue shape are key factors in determining the nature of the vowel sound.

When two vowels are produced together, they may form a sound called a *diphthong*. Diphthongs are special types of vowels in the same way that affricative sounds are special types of consonants. The five diphthongs in English are /ai/ in *high*, /aʊ/ in *house*, /eɪ/ in *day*, /oʊ/ in *coat*, and /ɔɪ/ in *oil*.

Vowels also differ according the their *length* (the amount of time they are prolonged), their *pitch*, and the amount of *tension* present in the oral region while they are being spoken.

THE SPEECH-PRODUCING MECHANISM

Location of Important Areas

The location of the regions of the head and neck important to speech production is shown in Figure 1-1. Pressure exerted by the muscles of the rib cage provides the power to force air upward through the larynx. This airstream passes through the opening at the vocal cords. It is at the vocal cords that outgoing air can be transformed into sound by their vibratory action (opening and closing). This rapid vibratory action of the vocal cords produces the voicing to produce such sounds as /b/, /g/, /z/, /r/, and all vowel sounds. If the cords do not vibrate, air passes through them to produce the voiceless sounds such as /s/, /f/, /ʃ/, /k/, and so on.

From the pharynx, the air can travel in one of two directions: out through either (1) the oral cavity when the *velum* is moved back and upward against the rear wall of the pharynx or (2) the nasal cavity of the *dorsum* or back part of the tongue is pushed up against the rear of the hard palate. This blocks the air from entering the mouth.

If the airstream travels through the oral cavity, it passes over the tongue or, in the case of the /l/, around its sides. Four sections of the tongue are identified because each plays an important role in the articulation of specific sounds: the *tip*, the *blade*, the *center*, and the *dorsum*. Along the palate or roof of the mouth are three important areas: (1) the movable *velum* at the rear of the hard palate, (2) the *hard palate*, which is the bony shelf separating the oral and nasal cavities, and (3) the *alveolar ridge* that forms the inside gumline of the upper front teeth in the forwardmost area of the hard palate.

Figure 1-1 Key Head and Neck Areas in Speech Production

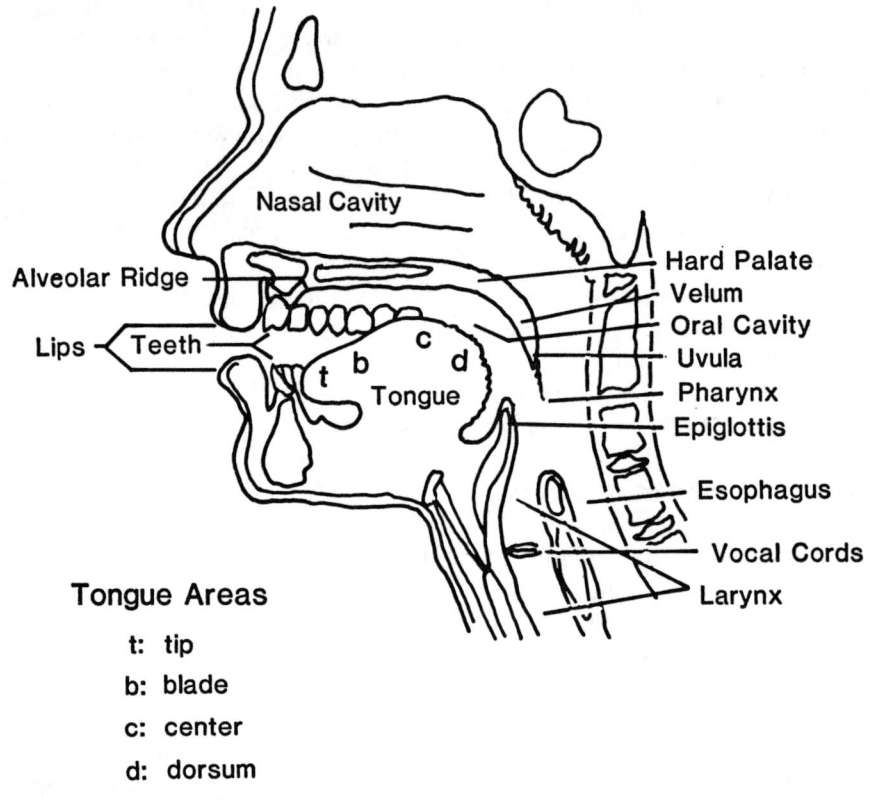

Finally, the *teeth* and *lips* form the most forward section of the *articulators*. Their position can be changed by lowering or raising the *mandible* or jaw. The entire muscle system that moves the articulators is far too complex to be discussed here. These muscles play an important role in the production of speech sounds. If they do not function correctly because of either atrophy or lack of control, severe articulation problems can and do develop.

Function of the Articulators

The major portion of the sound required for speech is produced by the vibratory action of the vocal cords housed in the *larynx*. The action of the vocal cords determines the basic pitch of the sound. Pitch also is changed by the *resonators* after the sound travels upward and out of the oral or nasal cavities. Pitch inflection information is important in transmitting meaning to speech.

After the airstream passes through the vocal cords, it can be modified by the resonators and/or the articulators. The resonators consist of the tubes, passageways, and cavities in the pharynx, nasal, and oral chambers. As the term suggests, resonators strengthen or amplify sounds as they pass through the cavity. Some characteristics of the sound may be reduced while others remain unchanged. Resonation contributes to the *quality* of the sound. Differences among the different vowel sounds are created by the resonation of air in chambers created by the tongue as it is shaped into various positions. These positions create different cavity shapes that resonate various frequencies, resulting in different vowel sounds.

These articulators (vocal cords, velum, hard palate, alveolar ridge, teeth, lips, mandible, and tongue) all play important roles in the formation of discrete vowel or consonant sounds.

The velum, jaw, lips, and tongue are the movable parts that can create airstream changes by forming an obstruction or constricting it at fixed points—the teeth, alveolar ridge, and hard palate. The alveolar ridge is one of the most important points where the tongue makes contact or near contact for the production of /n, l, t, d, s, z/. The lips are instrumental in producing /m, p, b/ and, in conjunction with the lower teeth, /f, v/. Lip-rounding plays a role in the formation of many vowels and diphthongs as well as the voiced and voiceless /w/ sounds.

The center and blade portions of the tongue move close to the hard palate to produce affricative sounds / dʒ , tʃ , ʃ , ʒ /. The dorsum of the tongue touches the rear of the hard palate and is released to produce /k, g/.

DESCRIPTION OF SPEECH SOUNDS

Segmental Phonemes

When an infant utters sounds that have no meaning and are not used for communicating a message, they are called *phones*. When sounds are used in a consistent manner to communicate messages to others, they are called *phonemes*. For example, the word *pig* contains three phonemes, /p/, /ɪ/, and /g/. By changing one of the phonemes, the word acquires a new meaning. If the /p/ is changed to /f/, the result is *fig;* if the phoneme /r/ is used instead of /p/, *rig* emerges. Therefore, when a sound change results in a meaning change, the sounds that are altered are called phonemes. All of the sounds listed in Exhibits 1-1 and 1-2 are phonemes.

A phoneme may include a group of several sounds that differ from each other only slightly. There can be many variations in a way a sound is pronounced. If these variations do not change the meaning of the word, they are considered as being members of the same phoneme family. For example: a speaker pronounces the word *keep* slowly and listens to the sound of the /k/. The person then says *cope* and finds a difference in the sounds of the two /k/s. The /k/ in *keep* is produced in a forward position in the mouth because of the influence of the front high /i/ vowel whereas the /k/ in *cope* is produced in a low back position because of anticipation of the back /o/ vowel. The /k/ sound used in *keep* can be substituted for the /k/ in *cope* and the meaning of the word does not change even though slightly different sounds are being used. These different /k/ sounds are called *allophones* and belong to the /k/ phoneme group of sounds. The three sounds of /t/ in the words *stop, tap,* and *boat* also are different sounds but since they can be interchanged without altering the meaning of the word, they are called allophones of the /t/ phoneme. Although /t/ and /d/ sound similar, they are different phonemes because if one sound is substituted for another as in *tack* and *pack,* they signal different meanings.

Young children soon learn to ignore certain differences among sounds (allophones) and attend to the features that change meaning (phonemes). Most adults who have learned English as a second language find it difficult to distinguish between some allophones of English. For example, those who learned Spanish as a first language often cannot discriminate between the English /s/ and /z/ because these sounds exist as allophones in their native language. Teaching English as a second language involves helping such individuals learn to make these critical sound discriminations.

Distinctive Features

Individual sounds are classified using a different system that involves describing each one according to acoustic, mode, and place features (Chomsky & Halle, 1968). For example, /p/ can be described as: voiceless, consonant, produced in the front of the mouth, stop, and formed by closing the lips and opening them suddenly to release the air pressure. On the other hand, /z/ is classified as: voiced, consonant, produced at the alveolar ridge, a continuant, and produced by air turbulence rushing through a small opening. Both sounds can be described in terms of several different features.

The unique set of factors that describes one sound and makes it distinct from all others is called its *distinctive features*. The sounds /p/ and /b/ differ on only one feature—voicing; all their other features are the same.

The presence of a feature is indicated by a + sign, its absence by a − sign. /p/ is indicated using a − voice feature while /b/ is a + voice. /s/ is listed as a + continuant and /p/ as a − continuant.

Although several different kinds of feature systems have been proposed, one that is cited commonly in the literature is shown in Exhibit 1-3 (McReynolds & Huston, 1971). The first seven features pertain to the type of obstruction in the oral cavity. These are the acoustic features that are related to manner of sound production. The last five features deal with where the sound is produced or where the tongue is positioned. These refer to place of production.

Table 1-1 shows the features of four sounds. For each sound, some features are the same while others are different.

Suprasegmental Phonemes

Suprasegmental phonemes that contribute chiefly to the prosodic features of sounds also give meaning to speech sounds. Meaning can be conveyed by the way the speaker pauses between words or accents words. The following anecdote illustrates how suprasegmental phonemes contribute to meaning:

A young man asked a woman acquaintance to go to a movie. On the way home, he was a little too amorous with his embraces and the woman responded harshly, "Don't! Stop!" The young man got the message and eased off. He dated the woman several more times and they grew to like each other very much. While parked outside her house one evening, he again got carried away embracing her tenderly. As he backed off, she said pleadingly, "Don't stop."

The phonemes in the "Don't stop" messages are the same in both instances but the meanings are completely opposite because of the way they are spoken. The tone of voice, stress on certain words, and placement of pausing are important determinants of meaning. These prosodic features of speech provide much information.

Stress, pitch, and juncture comprise the major prosodic features of speech. *Stress* deals with where the accent is placed on syllables. The meaning of some words in English is determined solely by where the accent is placed. Words such as *personal* and *personnel* acquire different meanings depending on whether the stress is on the first or last syllable. Stress patterns change as suffixes are added. The second syllable is stressed in *define*, the third syllable in *definition*. Speakers of English must learn several different stress patterns because the language contains words from many different languages, each using different types of stress patterns.

Exhibit 1-3 Features Used to Classify English Consonant and Vowel Sounds

1. *Vocalic.* Constriction in the oral cavity cannot be greater than that required for the /i/ and /ʊ/. The vocal cords must be approximate to cause voicing. /i/, /u/, /e/, /o/, /r/, /l/, /æ/, /ʌ/, and /ʊ/.

2. *Consonantal.* Narrow constriction in the vocal tract. /r/, /l/, /p/, /b/, /f/, /v/, /ð/, /θ/, /tʃ/, /k/, /g/, /m/, /t/, /d/, /dʒ/, /n/, /s/, /z/, /ʃ/, /ʒ/, and /ŋ/.

3. *Rounded.* The lip orifice is narrowed. /u/, /o/, /w/, /ɔ/, /ʊ/, and /ʃ/.

4. *Nasal.* The velum is lowered to allow the air to be directed through the nose. /m/, /n/, and /ŋ/.

5. *Continuant.* A partial obstruction to the air flow in the vocal tract. /l/, /r/, /f/, /v/, /θ/, /ð/, /s/, /z/, /ʃ/, /ʒ/, and /h/.

6. *Voiced.* The vocal folds approximate to cause voicing. /r/, /l/, /b/, /d/, /v/, /g/, /z/, /m/, /n/, /ð/, /ʒ/, /dʒ/, and /ŋ/.

7. *Strident.* Noisiness produced when air is passed over a rough surface at the necessary rate of flow and angle of incidence. /f/, /v/, /s/, /z/, /ʃ/, /tʃ/, /ʒ/, and /dʒ/.

8. *Coronal.* The blade of the tongue is raised from the neutral position. /r/, /l/, /t/, /d/, /θ/, /ð/, /n/, /s/, /z/, /ʃ/, /tʃ/, /ʒ/, and /dʒ/.

9. *High.* The body of the tongue is raised above the neutral position. /i/, /u/, /w/, /ʊ/, /j/, /tʃ/, /dʒ/, /k/, /g/, /ʃ/, /ʒ/, and /ŋ/.

10. *Low.* The body of the tongue is lowered below the neutral position. / /, /u/, /h/, and /ʊ/.

11. *Back.* The body of the tongue is retracted from the neutral position. /u/, /ʌ/, /o/, /ɔ/, /w/, /k/, /g/, /ŋ/, and /ʊ/.

12. *Anterior.* Sounds produced in the front region of the mouth in front of where /ʃ/ is produced. /l/, /p/, /b/, /f/, /v/, /m/, /t/, /θ/, /d/, /ð/, /n/, /s/, and /z/.

Source: Reprinted from "A Distinctive Feature Analysis of Children's Misarticulation Training," by L. McReynolds and K. Huston by permission of *Journal of Speech and Hearing Disorders*, 36, no. 2, pp. 155–168, © 1971.

Table 1-1 Classification of 4 Sounds by 12 Distinctive Features

FEATURE	SOUND /s/ /i/ /g/ /l/				FEATURE	SOUND /s/ /i/ /g/ /l/			
Vocalic	+	−	−	−	Strident	−	+	−	−
Consonantal	−	+	+	+	Coronal	−	+	−	+
Rounded	−	−	−	−	High	+	−	+	−
Nasal	−	−	−	−	Low	−	−	−	−
Continuous	+	+	−	+	Back	=	−	+	−
Voiced	+	−	+	+	Anterior	+	+	−	+

The *pitch* used when saying words and sentences also affects meaning. For example, different intonations of the simple expression "Is that so" can mean "I'm quite annoyed about it," "Don't threaten me," "I'm glad to hear that," or "Did it really happen?"

Finally, *juncture*—the separation, pausation, or termination of a syllable—provides meaning cues. Juncture is defined as oral punctuation. It indicates where commas, semicolons, and interjections are placed. Juncture refers to pauses between words and syllables as well as where syllables are separated. For example, whether a speaker means "an ice man" or "a nice man" is determined by whether there is a slight pause after the word *a* or after the word *an*.

Coarticulation

So far, this discussion has covered how the segmental features (consonants and vowels) are written and classified and how the suprasegmental features of stress, pitch, and juncture affect the meaning of spoken words and sentences. There is one more important factor that affects articulation: *coarticulation*. An interesting thing happens to sounds when certain words are spoken in rapid succession. The separate words *did* and *you* when spoken as separate, distinct words are pronounced as [dɪd] and [ju]. But when spoken carelessly as a phrase, *did you,* in rapid succession, it sounds like dɪd ʒu. The words *hit* and *you* blend together to form hɪt ʃu. Thus, when words are spoken rapidly—that is, when they are coarticulated—some of the sounds are altered and are said to be *assimilated* or affected by neighboring sounds.

Sound Changes Due to Assimilation

One of the reasons sounds change when spoken together is because certain combinations are difficult to articulate. The word *think* is an example. At first glance, it might be guessed that it is pronounced as *thin* with a *k* added at the end as [θ ɪnk]. But upon closer inspection, it is discovered that the /n/ is made in the front of the mouth, the /k/ sound in the back. The /k/ sound exerts an influence upon the /n/, literally pulling it backward to an /ŋ/. *Think* actually is spoken as [θ ɪ ŋk], not [θ ɪnk]. In this case, the second sound, /k/, affects the first sound /n/. This same kind of change occurs in the phrase *this shovel*. The /s/ sound in the word *this* is absorbed into the /ʃ/ sound in *shovel*. The resulting pronunciation is *thishovel* written as [θɪʃ:vəl] where the /ʃ/ sound is slightly prolonged. (The use of the colon after /ʃ/ means the previous sound is prolonged.)

The first sound can affect the second, as in the case of *passed*. Since /s/ is a voiceless sound, this voicelessness affects the *ed* suffix so instead of saying *passed* ([pæ sd]), people say *past* ([pæ st]).

Assimilation is found in vowels as well. Usually only a slight vowel change occurs, such as using *git* ([gɪt]) for *get* ([g ɛ t]), or *tint* ([tɪnt]) for *tent* ([t ɛ nt]). In these cases, the vowel /ɪ/ that is located in a position slightly higher in the mouth than /ɛ/ is used as a substitute.

Syllable Changes Due to Assimilation

Even as sounds are changed by assimilation so, too, are syllables. Such cases are marked by consonant omissions and additions. For example, the /ə/ in *about* may be omitted and pronounced as *bout* ([baʊt]) or the /ə/ is omitted in *history*, resulting in a pronunciation *histry* ([hɪstrɪ]). An /ə/ sound may be added to *athlete* to give [æθəlit] instead of the correct pronunciation [æθlit]. Sometimes letters are reversed, as in the case of *pertty* ([pɝti]) for *pretty* ([prɪti]). Young children can be heard to say *efalent* for *elephant* or *bicasle* for *bicycle*. These demonstrate sound changes by assimilation.

Syllabic revisions such as the ones cited here represent ways people change syllable structures while speaking. It is important to realize that sounds produced in the context of speaking several words together differ greatly from saying single words or simply isolated sounds. This must be taken into account when teaching articulation skills.

THE DEVELOPMENT OF ARTICULATION

Speech is a learned behavior. Learning a language is not like learning how to crawl or walk in the sense that a child acquires the skill as part of a maturational process. Although some linguists maintain that humans have a built-in propensity facilitating language development (McNeill, 1970), the studies of young children reared in isolated environments apart from human contact reveal that they acquire only a simple communication system composed of grunt-like sounds (Brown, 1958). Also, it is known that children who have severe hearing losses from birth do not develop intelligible speech unless they receive special training (Murai, 1961). But when the speech development of normal children reared in a social environment is examined, some common milestones of growth can be observed among them regardless of the language to which they are exposed.

The discussion now turns to the development of articulation skills. Children pass through the series of sound-learning stages from birth through 8 years of age during the development of articulation skills.

The Reflexive Period

The neonate's first articulatory gesture consists of reflexive crying. It is physically impossible for the newborn infant to produce anything like the sounds made by older children and adults (Lieberman, 1968). The infant's tongue is too large, the oral cavity too small, and the larynx too short to produce more than just a few sounds. But during the reflexive oral activities that occur while feeding and crying, the muscles of the oral and respiratory system strengthen and develop.

Within the first month or so, most infants develop different kinds of cry patterns that signal different emotional states (Fourcin, 1978). These cry patterns could hardly be considered a language system. Most of the sounds produced during this two-month period are the front vowels /ε, ɪ, ʌ/ (Irwin, 1948). Vowels outnumber consonants in frequency of production 4.5 to 1. The back consonants /h/ and /ʔ/ comprise most of the consonant sounds. Of course, the infant also produces many lip-smacking, gurgling, and click type sounds not used in adult phonology. However, of the sounds that can be recognized as being close approximations of those made by adults, front vowels and back consonants clearly are in the majority (Irwin, 1947, 1948).

Near the end of the first month, infants gain better control over pitch and loudness variations in their cry. This control enables them to use the cry sound as a more effective communicative device. Some linguists believe that pitch control is the forerunner of phonemic development that occurs near the age of 1 year (Fourcin, 1978). Pitch control may mark the beginning of sound contrasts that are so important to the development of articulation. It also has been shown that infants can discriminate between sounds that others produce. In one experiment, infants as young as one month old could detect the difference in voicing between the contrastive sounds of /ba/ and /pa/ (Eimas, Siqueland, Jusczyk, and Vigorito, 1971).

Cooing

When infants are two to four months old, they show signs of producing a variety of sounds when they seem to be in a satisfied state. These sounds do not appear to be like the reflexive ones produced earlier. While vowels still outnumber consonants, the ratio has changed to 3.6 vowels to 1 consonant (Irwin & Chen, 1946). Front vowels and back consonants still predominate as the chief types of sounds produced.

The infant shows signs of recognizing the mother's voice and imitates some of the pitch change patterns she uses (Fourcin, 1978). There appears to be no attempt to use specific sounds themselves as meaningful communication.

Babbling

It is during this stage of sound development from four to eight months that the first significant developments in articulation occur. The infant now makes deliberate attempts to produce sounds and syllables, not as a means of communicating but more for self-stimulation and pleasure. Several syllables may be connected as the infant appears to play with the sound-producing mechanism.

More pitch change patterns are added. It has been found that infants of this age use up to seven different pitch change contours, depending upon the environmental conditions (Delack & Fowlow, 1978). This ability to respond differentially seems to be the basis for making sound contrasts when first words are spoken.

In addition to the increased number of pitch contrasts during this period, many more sounds, especially consonants, are produced. The vowel-consonant ratio has dropped to 2.8 to 1 and almost all consonants have been produced at least a few times.

While some authorities maintain that sounds the infant produces while babbling play no role in future sound development (Perkins, 1977), most linguists now feel that such experiences are the key factor that assists them in learning to use sounds in word attempts (Oller, Weiman, Doyle, & Ross, 1976). Deaf children babble very little, if at all. The same is true with infants who have normal hearing but are diagnosed as receptive aphasics (Mowrer, 1950; Myklebust, 1957).

It has been found that the types of sounds infants use while babbling are quite similar to those used by children near the age of 1, when they begin saying their first words (Oller et al., 1976). Here are a few examples:

1. Consonant clusters seldom are used during babbling and appear late in the speech of children as they use words.
2. Consonants usually are found in the initial position followed by a vowel (CV) and occur less frequently in the final vowel-consonant (VC) position during babbling. The omission of final consonants is common among young children when they begin saying words.
3. Initial stops outnumber initial fricatives 10:1. Stops frequently are substituted for initial fricatives when children begin using words.
4. Glides are more prevalent than liquids. When words are first attempted, it is common for glides to be substituted for liquids.
5. Almost all initial plosive sounds are unaspirated. Again, this is also a common practice among young children when they first attempt word production.

A relationship exists between the types of sounds or sound combinations produced during babbling and the types used as the child first attempts word productions, especially between the ages of 1 and 2. This suggests that babbling plays an important preparatory function to the type of sounds that will be produced when the child begins saying words.

It could be said that the phonological inadequacies of children who are between 1 and 2 years of age are merely reflections of the experiences they had in producing sounds at the babbling stage. If this is true, then it would seem that the experiences children have during the babbling stage may determine in part the success of later articulation.

Word Approximations

What are recognized as the first true words usually appear between the child's eighth and twelfth months (Darley & Winitz, 1961). Parents may not recognize some of these early attempts as true words since in sound structure they often do not resemble what adults say. Nevertheless, most children use certain sound combinations to express certain ideas or concepts. Some of the more familiar sound combinations are *bye-bye, mama, papa, doggie, more,* and *no.*

This stage of development is marked by the conscious control of articulatory movements in the consistent production of certain sound patterns recognized as words. Of course, many of the child's utterances still fall under the category of babbling but these sounds now can be classified under the three types of utterances called lalling, echolalia, and jargon.

Utterances classified as *lalling* include those whose articulatory movements are controlled voluntarily. The child does not attempt to use these as forms of communication. They are viewed as simple repetitions of the child's own vocalizations.

Echolalia includes vocalizations that are imitations of sound stimuli others produce. The child merely echos back what is heard, again making no attempt to communicate anything meaningful during echolalic vocalizations.

The child's endless stream of inflected vocalizations in which pitch, stress, and loudness patterns that resemble adult sentences can be detected is called *jargon*. It almost sounds as though the child is having a self-conversation. Yet it is not possible to detect any recognizable words from these vocal ramblings because the sound combinations do not correspond to adult usages.

The prosodic or suprasegmental features of the child's utterances reveal rather consistent use of declaratives, questions, and emphatics (Menyuk & Bernholtz, 1969). The prosodic elements of the child's system are mastered before the phonetic elements.

In summary, it can be concluded that the first year of life sets the stage for the emergence of the phonemic system that develops more fully between the ages of 1 and 4. First is the reflexive vocal period during which the infant develops the oral musculature needed to articulate sounds. Second is a period of the infant's awareness of sounds and the prosodic features plus some limited practice in sound production. Third comes increasing practice in sound production that further develops articulatory movement patterns. Fourth is the use of prosodic features and some true words as communicative tools that terminate the first year of articulation development. By this time, the child has had a great deal of practice producing most of the sounds used in the adult phonological system. But a strange thing happens after this time as the child begins to communicate using words.

Sound Development between 1 and 4 Years

It becomes easier to analyze the development of articulation skills after the child passes the first year. The child can be asked to repeat words, or attempts to say words can be simply observed and what sounds are used or not used can be noted.

Children between 1 and 1½ years of age use only a few sounds correctly in words. The first consonants to appear with any degree of accuracy consist of a few stops—/p, b, d/, the nasal /m/, and the fricative /h/. It is puzzling why children do not draw upon the vast repertoire of sounds acquired during babbling.

The explanation for this discrepancy can be understood in looking closely at what the child is learning. Up to about age 1, sounds are produced as phones or noncommunicative sounds. There is no systematic and consistent use of sound planning having anything to do with using sounds as referents for things or events in the environment. The child has little experience using sounds as phonemes. If speakers used isolated sounds rather than sound combinations as meaningful units, then perhaps the transition from using phones to phonemes might be much easier. But the child must learn to master specific sound combinations and use them consistently in word productions. The child must possess a highly developed system of precise articulatory movement patterns and be able to execute them automatically. This skill is difficult to master, especially when certain sound combinations require complex tongue movement patterns from place to place inside the mouth. For example, the word *grandma* requires the tongue to begin with a backward contact position for /gr/, a slightly forward movement for the /æ/ vowel, then the nasal /n/ is made in the front of the mouth, and finally lip closure when the /m/ is produced and releasing the /ɔ/ vowel. The pronunciation of *grandma* requires a complex set of muscular movements, all of which must be accomplished within a second. It is much easier motorically for the child to say *nanaw*, which requires only two contrastive movements. It is not that the child cannot articulate /g, r, m/ sounds, it is too difficult to make all the contrastive movements necessary to produce the word.

Ease of production may explain why the child reduces many words into simple repetitions such as *mama, dada, bye-bye, nini,* and so on. Ask the 1-year-old to hiss like a snake and this may be accomplished with ease. But ask the same child to say *snake* and it's 100 to 1 that the word will be pronounced *na* or *nat*. The /s/ will be omitted. Certain sound combinations are difficult to say and it is hard for the young child to remember the order of the sounds and the movements required to produce them. That is why a child will say *nana* for *banana, goggie* for *doggie, nini* for *goodnight,* and so on. The child has not yet mastered the voluntary control necessary to make these complex movements.

It may be that the sounds that appear first when children begin saying words are the ones that are easiest to pronounce. Or, the first sounds used in words may reflect those that children have practiced most. Another factor could be the ease with which the child detects the sounds. The ability to discriminate between certain sound classes such as /m, n, w/ and /b, d, p/ occurs at an earlier age than do distinctions between classes within the family of such fricatives as /s, z, f, v, θ / or between the liquids /r/ and /l/ (Shvachkin, 1973). It is not surprising to find that the consonants that appear in the first 50 words of children's speech are /m, n, p, b, d, f, h/ (Ferguson & Farwell, 1975).

By the time the child is 3 years old, all of the vowels that occur in words are used correctly. Vowels do not usually present the problem that consonants do unless the child has a hearing loss. It will be another three to four years before most children master all of the consonants.

Near the age of 4, it has been shown that 75 percent of the children use the following sounds correctly in words (Templin, 1957):

Nasals: /m, n, ŋ /
Front Plosives: /p, b, d/
Back Plosives: /k, g/
Fricatives: /h, f/
Glides: /w, j/

Table 1-2 Comparison of Ages at Which 75 Percent[1] of Children Master English Consonants

Sound	SICD	Templin	Wellman	Poole	Sound	SICD	Templin	Wellman	Poole
m	2	3	3	3–6	g	3	4	4	4–6
n	2	3	3	4–6	s	3§	4–6	5	7–6†
h	2	3	3	3–6	r	3–4§	4	5	7–6
p	2	3	4	3–6	l	3–4§	6	4	6–6
ŋ	2	3	*	4–6	ʃ	3–8	4–6	‡	6–6
f	2–4	3	3	5–6	tʃ	3–8	4–6	5	‡
j	2–4	3–6	4	4–6	ð	4	7	‡	6–6
k	2–4	4	4	4–6	ʒ	4	7	6	6–6
d	2–4	4	5	4–6	dʒ	4+*	7	6	‡
w	2–8	3	3	3–6	θ	4+*	6	*	7–6
b	2–8	4	3	3–6	v	4+*	6	5	6–6
t	2–8	6	5	4–6	z	4+*	7	5	7–6†
					hw	4+*	*	*	7–6

1. The Poole study used 100 percent of the children rather than 75 percent.

*Sound tested but not produced correctly by 75% of subjects at oldest age tested. Wellman: hw reached at 5 years but not 6. Medial ŋ at 3 years.

†Poole: s and z appear at age 5–6, but disappear later and return at age 7–6.

‡Sound not tested or reported.

§Reversal: Reported at earliest age level if only one reversal occurred and percentage at all older age levels exceeded 75%. See text.

Source: Reprinted from "Articulation Development in Children Aged Two to Four Years," by E. Prather et al., by permission of *Journal of Speech and Hearing Disorders* 40, no. 2, pp. 179–191. © 1975.

It can be concluded that in general, nasals and stops are mastered early, followed by the continuants (with the exception of /f, h/, which also are learned early), then voicing distinctions between certain pairs of sounds such as /f, v/, /d, t/, then glides, and finally affricatives.

Table 1-2 shows the results of four studies that investigated the age at which a certain percentage of children produced various sounds correctly in words. The study by Poole (1934) used a criterion of 100% in determining when a sound was mastered. Consequently, ages of children in her study are somewhat higher than those reported in others. The other three studies by Wellman, Case, Mengert, and Bradbury (1931), Templin (1957), and Prather, Hedrick, and Kern (1975) (the SICD) listed age of sound mastery when 75% of the children of that age level produced the sound correctly. Prather et al. (1975) tested children beginning at the 2-year-age level while in the others by Wellman, et al. (1931), Templin (1957), and Poole (1934) testing was initiated with children at the 3-year-old level.

It is interesting to note that the sounds that occur latest in the developmental sequence also are those that children have most difficulty using correctly in words even long after they should have been mastered. The most frequently misarticulated sounds are /s, θ , r, l, tʃ , dʒ / (Winitz, 1969, p. 69). These sounds may reflect problems with discrimination or they may be difficult to produce motorically. It is not sure which is true.

So far, the general order of sound development has been discussed, plus some guidelines concerning the ages at which children begin using these sounds correctly in words. Next, consideration turns to the simplification processes children use to reduce complex adult articulation patterns to a level with which they can cope. There are three general simplification processes young children commonly use between the ages of 1 and 4 according to Ingram (1976). They are (1) changes in syllable structure, (2) assimilation, and (3) substitution.

Changes in Syllable Structure

Young children take a number of actions to simplify words that change the structure of the syllable. They tend to reduce syllables to a simple consonant-vowel (CV) combination. Thus, most final consonants are omitted so that *cat* becomes *ca,* *book* is *boo,* and *make* is *ma.* This tendency continues in some kindergarten and first grade children who have severe articulation problems. Frequently the glottal stop is substituted for final consonants: *book* becomes [bʊ ʔ], *coat* is [ko ʔ], and *top* is [ta ʔ].

Unstressed syllables often are omitted entirely. In fact, most young children speak only monosyllables when they begin using words or they repeat syllables such as *dada, mama, bye-bye, gogo,* and the like. The initial unstressed syllable is omitted so *away* becomes *way, tomato* is *mado,* and *goodbye* is simply *bye.*

Consonant clusters such as /sl, dr, bl, gr, st, pl/, and the like are difficult for young children to produce. As a consequence, they frequently omit one of the consonants or, in some cases, both. *Play* becomes *pay, stop* is *top, try* is *ty,* and *blue* is *bue.* It is not uncommon for the sounds in a cluster to be changed entirely, as in the case of *truck* becoming *fwuck.* They may substitute a different sound for one member of a cluster. Usually, a liquid /r/ or /l/ sound is replaced with /w/ as in the case of *pway* for *play, bwue* for *blue,* or *cwy* for *cry.* Many of the complex consonant clusters are not mastered until the child enters kindergarten even though the sounds involved are used correctly when spoken singly in words.

Assimilation

As noted earlier, neighboring sounds affect the pronunciation of many words. This process of assimilation, in which one sound tends to be pronounced like another, is common in the speech of young children. *Doggie* becomes *goggie* because of this process since the final /g/ affects the initial /d/ sound. The tendency is for both sounds to be made in the same place in the mouth. For this reason, *yellow* becomes *lello, skate* becomes *tate,* and *cheeze* becomes *teeze.*

It is interesting to see how some sounds are omitted because of the influence of surrounding ones. The /mp/ blend in *pumpkin* is omitted because of the influence of the back /k/ sound. The /mp/ blend is produced in the front of the mouth and, since the /k/ is made in the back, the movement required to combine the /mp/ and the /k/ is difficult. Consequently, the nasal sound / ŋ / is substituted for the /mp/ because its position is closer to /k/. Thus, *pumpkin* is pronounced as /p ʌ ŋ k ə n/. Since most adults pronounce this word using the / ŋ / for the /mp/, it is not considered an error, but if the child says *pukin* or *pumpsun,* this would be considered wrong.

Grandma changes to *nanaw* because of the difficulty of the /gr/ cluster. The /n/ takes the place of this cluster and the syllable is repeated. The front sounds /d, m/ are omitted. Sound changes like these occur frequently as young children attempt to simplify complex articulatory movements.

Substitution

The process of *substitution* as a simplification process continues to occur in the speech of many children who enter kindergarten and may be present throughout their first three to four years in elementary school. Lisping, an /s/ substitution, can be observed in the speech of numerous children and adults. As with the other processes, the explanation for substitutions appears to be that it is easier for the child to use the substituted sound than the intended one. Inadequate sound discrimination skills also may explain in part why some substitutions occur.

One of the most common substitutions is *stopping,* in which the stop sounds /p, b, t, d/ replace fricative or affricative sounds. This happens most often in the initial position. It is common to hear young children say *dis* and *dat* for *this* and *that.* Other common substitutions are *tun* for *sun, pinder* for *finger, due* for *chew,* and *ping* for *sing.* But the process does not operate for the stops that occur in the final position, when a fricative may be substituted. *Soap* becomes *soas* or *soaf, cat* may be *cas,* or *pack* might be *pass.*

Another common substitution process is *fronting.* This process has been known to occur in languages other than English. It involves using sounds produced in the front of the mouth for those that should be produced in the mid or back parts. Fronting occurs when a /t/ or /d/ sound is used for /k/ or /g/ as in the case of *tat* for *cat, dirl* for *girl,* or *dun* for *gun.* Several instances also could be classified as assimilation. Even the palatal sounds / ʃ , tʃ , dʒ , ʒ / often are substituted by the front sounds /d, t, s, ts/ as in the case of *sip* for *ship,* talk for *chalk,* and *sues* for *shoes.* The back nasal sound / ŋ / is moved forward to an /n/ when *win* is used for the word *ring.*

Strangely, some children do just the opposite, substituting velar sounds /k, g/ for the front sounds. This is called *velar preference.* It is not a common practice. In such cases, the child says *goggie* for *doggie, kiggie* for *piggie,* and *kink* for *sink.* Here again, assimilation involving a strong influence of the /k/ or /g/ may help explain why this occurs.

Liquid replacement with a glide is a common substitution even through the early elementary grades, although most children master liquids by the time they reach kindergarten. The substitutions consist of /w/ or /y/ for the /r/ and /l/ liquid sounds as illustrated by *wun* for *run, wook* for *look,* or *yook* for *look.* One way to find out how well a child can say the /r/ sound is to ask for a repetition of this sentence: "The rabbit ran around the railroad track." If there is trouble with /r/, it will be apparent immediately. Rather than using a substitution for the semivowel / ɚ / or / ɝ /, most children simply prolong the vowel immediately before / ɚ / or / ɝ /. This prolongation is represented with a colon immediately following the prolonged vowel. *Car* becomes *cah* [ka:], *hurt* is *haught* [h ə :t], and *flower* is *fawa* [fa:wa].

This section has summarized several types of simplification processes young children use during their first attempts to produce adult words. It is during this time that the phonological system develops. This system does not occur with the random addition of sounds but reflects an orderly progressive process regardless of what language they are learning. Of course, children vary as to the type of simplification process they use and how long they employ it, but for the most part, orderly trends in phonological development can be observed as they mature.

If for some reason the child becomes locked into a certain simplification process that continues to be used long after it should have disappeared, the individual is said to have an articulation problem. Consequently, articulation patterns considered normal at the age of 2 are viewed as a problem if continued until the child is 6 or older. The same could be said of many motor development skills. Children of 6 should not be drooling, crawling, or toddling as they may have done at the age of 1.

Completion of Phonemic Inventory

During the ages of 4 through 7 or 8, the simplification processes previously used extensively and especially when the child was 1 or 2 begin to disappear in a series of stages. The child acquires adults' phonological system and learns how to use certain sounds as grammatical markers. These include the use of the /s/ sound to signify plural, the *ed* or /t/, /d/ sound ending for past tense, the *ing* ending for present tense, and irregular verb forms.

Before the child is 4, the following sounds have been mastered (Templin, 1957):

1. Voiced and voiceless stops: /p, b, d, t, g, k/
2. Nasals: /m, n, ŋ /   The / ŋ / is used correctly only in the initial and medial positions of words.
3. Glides: /w, h, j/
4. Fricatives: /f/
5. Liquids: /l/

Sounds usually mastered after the age of 4 are as follows (Winitz, 1969, p. 59):

1. Fricatives: /s, z, v, ʃ , ʒ , θ , ð /
2. Affricatives: / dʒ , tʃ /
3. Liquids: /r/
4. Nasals: / ŋ / in the final position

If the acquisition of sounds is analyzed in terms of distinctive feature development, it is possible to gain insights into why they emerge in a particular order. Figure 1-2 shows that one of the first features to develop is voicing. Although the voiced stops appear later than voiceless ones, this voice-voiceless discrimination appears as one of the first features in the

Figure 1-2 Development of Distinctive Features

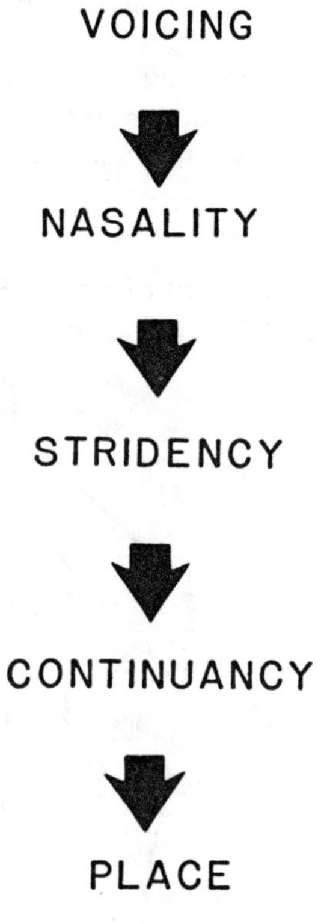

VOICING
⬇
NASALITY
⬇
STRIDENCY
⬇
CONTINUANCY
⬇
PLACE

---

*The place feature includes anterior, coronal, and lateral.

child's contrasts. This is followed by nasality, stridency, continuancy, and place features.

The features acquired last are those in which school-aged children most frequently err. One explanation for this is that such early developing features as voicing and nasality constitute *absolute* contrasts. A sound is either nasal or nonnasal, voiced or unvoiced. But the three other features—stridency, continuancy, and place—are considered *relative* contrasts. There can be various degrees of stridency, continuancy, and place. This absolute-vs.-relative quality of features may be a key to helping understand why some sounds are in error more frequently than others.

28 CLINICAL MANAGEMENT OF SPEECH DISORDERS

Another explanation may be the relative ease of articulation of the features. The movements necessary for producing nasal and voicing features may be easier to accomplish than the others. Finer muscle control may be required to produce contrasts involving stridency, continuancy, and place features.

A model showing the development of features and the sounds associated with them has been designed by Crocker (1969). The development of two sound families, the vowels/semivowels and the consonants, is shown in Figure 1-3.

Figure 1-3 Model on Development of Vowel/Semivowel and Consonant Sounds, by Feature

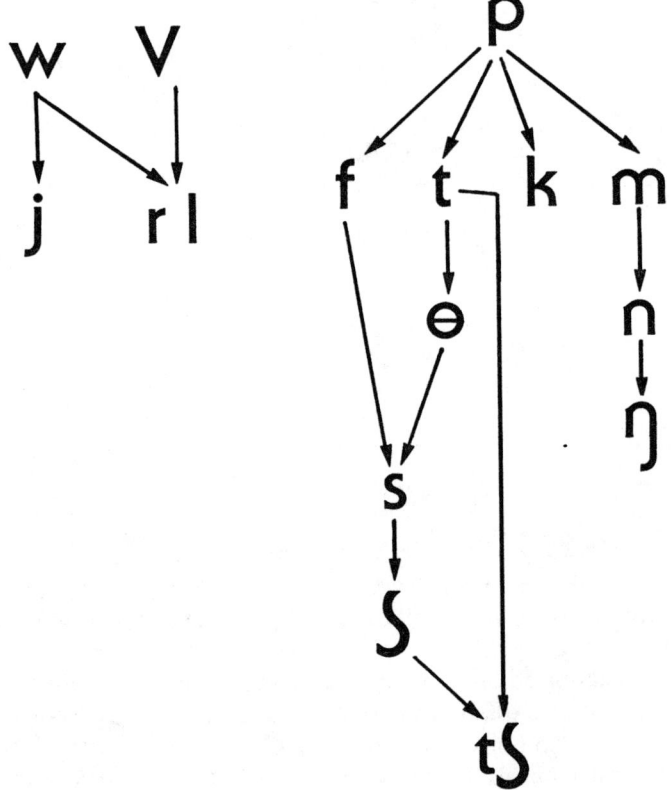

Source: Adapted from "A Phonological Model of Children's Articulation Competence," by J. Crocker by permission of *Journal of Speech and Hearing Disorders* 34, no. 3, pp. 203–213, © 1969.

According to this theoretical model, children possess a group of features called the *prime set* at the time they begin to develop a phonological system. In the case of consonants, this prime set is represented by the features that make up the /p/ sound. By altering a feature, the prime set of features is changed to what Crocker calls the *base set*. This set includes each of four sounds, /f, t, k, m/. Altering a feature in one of the base sets yields other sounds. This progression is illustrated in the diagram. Crocker's model closely parallels what is known from observation about the developmental order of sounds. It also accounts for the fact that certain sounds are substituted for others. Crocker's model provides an important guide for deciding which sounds should be corrected first as well as the order in which they should be taught.

REFERENCES

Brown, Roger. *Words and things.* New York: The Free Press, 1958.

Byrne, Margaret C., & Shervanian, Chris C. *Introduction to communicative disorders.* New York: Harper & Row Publishers, Inc., 1977.

Chomsky, N., & Halle, M. *The sound pattern of English.* New York: Harper & Row Publishers, Inc., 1968.

Crocker, J. A phonological model of children's articulation competence. *Journal of Speech and Hearing Disorders,* 1969, *34*(3), 203–213.

Darley, F., & Winitz, H. Age of first word: Review of research. *Journal of Speech and Hearing Disorders,* 1961, *26,* 272–290.

Delack, J. B., & Fowlow, P. F. The autogenesis of differential vocalization: Development of prosodic contrastivity during the first year of life. In N. Waterson & C. Snow (Eds.), *The development of communication.* New York: John Wiley & Sons, Inc., 1978.

Eimas, P. D., Siqueland, E. R., Jusczyk, R., & Vigorito, J. Speech perception in infants. *Science,* 1971, *171,* 303–306.

Ferguson, C. A., & Farwell, C. B. Words and sounds in early language acquisition: English initial consonants in the first 50 words. *Language,* 1975, *5,* 419–439.

Fourcin, A. J. Acoustic patterns and speech acquisition. In N. Waterson & C. Snow (Eds.), *The development of communication.* New York: John Wiley & Sons, Inc., 1978.

Goldstein, Max A. Speech without a tongue. *Journal of Speech Disorders,* 1940, *5,* 65–69.

Ingram, D. *Phonological disability in children,* New York: Esevier North Holland, Inc., 1976.

Irwin, O. C. Infant speech: Consonantal sounds according to place of articulation. *Journal of Speech Disorders,* 1947, *12*(4), 397–401.

Irwin, O. C. Infant speech: Development of vowel sounds. *Journal of Speech and Hearing Disorders,* 1948, *13*(1), 31–34.

Irwin, O. C., & Chen, H. P. Infant speech: Vowel and consonant frequency. *Journal of Speech Disorders,* 1946, *11*(1), 123–125.

Lieberman, P. Primate vocalizations and human linguistic ability. *Journal of the Acoustical Society of America,* 1968, *44,* 1574–1584.

McNeill, D. *The acquisition of language: The study of developmental psycholinguistics.* New York: Harper & Row Publishers, Inc., 1970.

McReynolds, L., & Huston, K. A distinctive feature analysis of children's misarticulation training. *Journal of Speech and Hearing Disorders,* 1971, *36*(2), 155–168.

Menyuk, P., & Bernholtz, N. Prosodic features and children's language production. *Quarterly Progress Report on the Research Laboratory of Electronics,* Massachusetts Institute of Technology, 1969, *93*, 216–219.

Mowrer, O. H. *Learning theory and personality dynamics: Selected papers.* New York: Ronald Press, 1950.

Murai, J. I. Speech development of a child suffering from a central language disorder. *Studia Phonologica,* 1961, *3*, 58–61.

Myklebust, H. M. Babbling and echolalia in language theory. *Journal of Speech and Hearing Disorders,* 1957, *22*(3), 356–360.

Oller, D. K., Weiman, L. A., Doyle, W. J., & Ross, C. Infant babbling and speech. *Journal of Child Language,* 1976, *3*, 1–11.

Perkins, W. *Speech pathology: An applied behavioral science* (2nd ed.). St. Louis: The C. V. Mosby Company, 1977.

Poole, E. Genetic development of articulation of consonant sounds in speech. *Elementary English Review,* 1934, *11*, 159–161.

Prather, E. M., Hedrick, D. L., & Kern, C. A. Articulation development in children aged two to four years. *Journal of Speech and Hearing Disorders,* 1975, *40*(2), 179–191.

Shvachkin, N. The development of phonemic speech perception in early childhood. In C. Ferguson & D. Slobin (Eds.), *Studies of child language development.* New York: Holt Rinehart & Winston, Inc., 1973.

Templin, M. Certain language skills in children: Their development and interrelationships. *Institute of Child Welfare Monograph 26.* Minneapolis: University of Minnesota Press, 1957.

Wellman, B. L., Case, I. M., Mengert, I. G. & Bradbury, D. E. Speech sounds of young children. University of Iowa Studies in Child Welfare, 1931, *5* (2).

Winitz, H. *Articulatory acquisition and behavior.* New York: Appleton-Century-Crofts, Inc., 1969.

Chapter 2

Assessing Articulation Skills

Usually, a mother's immediate reaction upon hearing her child mispronounce a word is to correct the error. This she does by repeating the word correctly and asking her child to say the word again. This procedure is beneficial for children who have occasional problems with some sounds in certain words but it seldom helps those who have a persistent difficulty learning to articulate specific sounds.

The immediate problem is to determine (1) the nature of the articulation problem and (2) how extensive it is. Once the extent of the problem is known, recommendations can be made as to what could or should be done about it. The decision can be either that the problem is minor and probably will be resolved by parental correction or that more extensive and systematic remedial procedures are appropriate.

Consequently, a systematic procedure is needed to determine exactly what sounds are in error. To this end, a number of assessment measures have been developed to assist the speech/language pathologist (SLP) in making a detailed description and evaluation of a child's articulation ability. These devices differ considerably, depending upon what information is sought.

TYPES OF ARTICULATION TESTS

Articulation tests are given to gather specific information about an individual's performance under standardized conditions. The objective may only be to determine whether or not a problem exists; on the other hand, it may be to describe the articulation errors in great detail. Tests may be administered in an effort to help determine the cause of the problem. Other tests can provide predictive information in helping decide which children are likely to outgrow their speech problems and which will not. Still other tests provide information about how successful the therapy methods are. Articulation assessments can be classified under four categories: (1) screening tests, (2) diagnostic tests, (3) prediction tests, and (4) therapy progress tests.

Screening Tests

One of the first tasks of the speech/language pathologist in the public schools is to survey all or part of the pupil population to identify individuals who have speech problems. Since many students usually are interviewed during this testing period, it is important that the time for examining each individual be kept to a minimum. It is probable that 80 percent to 90 percent of the pupils will have no speech problem, so it would be foolish to administer lengthy articulation tests to them. Screening tests are designed solely to separate those who have speech problems from those who do not. Usually they are of the pass-fail type. They are not designed to help the SLP describe the speech problem or how severe it may be. They simply provide an answer to the question, "Is there a problem or isn't there one?"

Diagnostic Tests

Time is not such a critical factor when using diagnostic type tests. These are designed to provide a thorough description of the articulation patterns and are administered to those who fail the screening tests.

According to Emerick and Hatten (1974), in diagnostic testing, four areas are investigated—those that:

1. describe the error sounds in terms of type of mistake (omissions, distortions, or substitutions), place of error (initial, medial, or final position), and frequency of error (single words or connected speech)
2. describe the speech production mechanism in terms of the function and structure of the oral and respiratory mechanism
3. determine the effect of environmental conditions upon the consistency of the error (effect of auditory-visual models presented, context of utterance, imitative ability, and speaking situation)
4. determine, insofar as possible, the cause of the articulation problem (poor auditory discrimination, low intelligence, inadequate muscular control, organic involvement, functional, etc.)

Such a diagnostic articulation test may be part of a more comprehensive case study inventory that includes medical, social, developmental, and educational histories. No attempt is made to describe such comprehensive tests here since this information can be found elsewhere (see Dickson, 1974; Johnson, Darley, & Spriestersbach, 1963).

Prediction Tests

The primary purpose of predictive tests is to assist the speech/language pathologist in determining which children who misarticulate sounds are likely to persist in their errors during the succeeding years and which will not. The obvious advantage of such test information is that the SLP can identify the children who do not require speech therapy and thus eliminate them as treatment candidates. More time then can be spent serving the children who really need therapy.

The predictive tests currently available are not as sensitive as might be desired. There is always the risk of error in that the test may pass an individual who should have failed. Thus, a child who needs therapy may be denied services. Nevertheless, predictive indicators do provide useful guidelines for selecting children who are more likely to need therapy.

Therapy Progress Tests

One of the most useful articulation tests is the type that provides information about the success of therapy procedures. In one sense, these serve as diagnostic tests since the results can be used as a diagnostic tool in prescribing changes in therapy methods. These tests often are used as a research tool as an indicator of the success or failure of a particular therapy procedure.

These tests usually consist of a spot check of only a few sounds or features that the clinician has been teaching rather than a complete inventory of the child's phonological system. They are designed to be used as comparative tests. By itself, a test may not be informative. It may have value only when its results are compared with other similar tests administered previously to the baseline individual.

When a test is given before therapy begins it is called the baseline—the status of the behavior before remedial measures are taken. The same tests are given again at predetermined times and compared with the baseline results. If desired changes in behavior are evidenced by changes in the scores of succeeding tests, then it is assumed therapy is beneficial. These tests are not standardized; they are tailored to meet the specific needs of each individual. Consequently, a different test usually is administered to each individual.

FEATURES OF ARTICULATION TESTS

Most of the numerous commercial tests of articulation share certain features. For example, pictures are used almost exclusively to evoke speech samples from young children. Older children read from printed textual material. To obtain samples of continuous speech, the tester reads aloud simple stories that are illustrated with appropriate pictures. The individual then is asked to repeat the story while looking at the picture cues.

Most tests examine the person's ability to produce the sound in each of three positions: in the initial position (the /s/ in *soap*), the medial position (the /s/ in *bicycle*), and the final position (the /s/ in *bus*). Sound blends in words such as *slow, stop, sweep, bust,* and *crisp* are tested in both initial and final word positions.

Johnson et al. (1963) argue that a sentence contains only one initial and one final sound and all others are considered medial. Stetson (1951) feels it is more meaningful to describe consonants in terms of whether they initiate or release syllables (*so, fi, ka, te*) or whether they terminate or arrest syllables (*up, it, uk, et*). Thus, a word such as ability has three initiating consonants (*bi, li, ty*) and no arresting consonants. Sound position in terms of initial, medial, and final plays no role in syllable analysis. Only a few tests have been designed to test consonants as they function in arresting or releasing capacities.

Another feature some tests evaluate is the consistency of the error. In a good articulation test, a particular sound will be used several times to determine how consistently the individual misarticulates it. It is not enough simply to test a sound three times, once in each position, and conclude that it will be misarticulated in all contexts. A test designed by McDonald (1964) is designed specifically to test each phoneme in a wide variety of phonetic contexts. Unfortunately, most tests sample each phoneme only a few times so little information about consistency of error is provided.

Stimulability refers to the ease with which an individual can correct a misarticulated sound once it is modeled. A person who then can produce the sound properly is said to be stimulable and, it is anticipated, will progress rapidly if provided with speech therapy. Or perhaps the speech/language pathologist decides therapy may not be required at all if the individual is highly stimulable. Assessing a person's ability to produce sounds correctly when so instructed is an important aspect of articulation testing.

Another important factor is the situation in which the testing is done. In one type of situation, the individual's responses are prescribed by the test items and only specific replies are evoked. The test items usually consist of one-word responses or sentences read by the individual.

The testing usually is done in an examination room. However, different information about articulation ability can be obtained if the test is given in a more naturalistic setting, especially if there is no attempt to place constraints upon the individual's responses. This testing can be accomplished best in a play type situation, preferably in an environmental setting that is familiar to the individual. The disadvantage of this is that the person may not utter some of the responses the pathologist would like to evaluate. This type of instrument also requires a great deal of time, not only during the testing period but also during the evaluation of the tape recorded results later. For these reasons, most pathologists prefer to use tests that restrict responses to a limited number of items.

A good articulation test should contain normative data to enable the examiner to compare one individual's score with those of others of the same age. The severity of the articulation problem must be evaluated in terms of the individual, the number of sounds misarticulated, the frequency with which the sound occurs in the language, and the type of misarticulation. By using a scale or point system, the pathologist can determine how severe the problem is and whether or not therapy is indicated. The normative data used to standardize the test scores should be large enough to make them applicable to a variety of populations.

In the last few decades, there have been attempts to design articulation tests for special populations. For example, bilingual speakers whose first language is Spanish score differently on articulation tests than do native English speakers on whom the test is standardized. The same is true for users of black dialect. Some tests take this into account and are designed and normed for specific populations.

There are a number of related tests designed to accompany articulation testing because their findings can provide important information about possible causes of the problem. These tests, listed by Dickson (1974, p. 31) and Darley (1979, pp. 121–188) include such areas as intelligence, auditory discrimination, auditory memory span, motor proficiency, and laterality. As can be seen, articulation testing is not just a simple matter of asking an individual to repeat a few sounds or words. An accurate appraisal of articulatory ability may require a battery of tests. This is especially true of special disability groups where more careful appraisal is needed. A simple picture type articulation test in itself is inadequate to evaluate the speech of individuals with associated motor problems, neurological involvements, auditory deficits, and so on. It is not enough simply to describe the articulation patterns of these populations in terms of sounds in three positions; it is necessary to know the functional limitations of the oral and respiratory systems as well.

Finally, it is important that an articulation test be both reliable and valid. Reliability refers to the fact that a test provides the same information when given repeatedly. If a person is tested on one day and again one week later on the same questions, and produces vastly different scores, it could be concluded that the instrument is not reliable. Also, different examiners should obtain essentially the same results from a reliable test.

A test is valid if it measures what it is designed to measure. If it does not produce an accurate account of the individual's articulation skills, then it is not valid. This is one of the strongest criticisms of the simple picture type articulation test that examines each sound in only three positions. If the individual happens to misarticulate the sounds in the three test words, it could be assumed (wrongly) that the individual erred on them in all words in all speaking situations. That may not be the case. The individual may produce the sound correctly in a number of different environments.

Winitz (1969, pp. 237-269) lists numerous cautions and criticisms of articulation testing. In addition to test construction, he points out that subject and tester variability can play important roles in determining the validity of results.

DESCRIPTION OF SPECIFIC ARTICULATION TESTS

A wide variety of articulation tests is available. Just which one is selected depends upon what the examiner wants to learn, the time constraints, and the ability of the tester. Some of the different basic types of articulation tests are described briefly next. For a more thorough discussion, see Darley (1979, pp. 89-119) in which he evaluates 13 articulation tests as well as 25 other related instruments dealing with auditory discrimination, auditory memory, digit span, and the like (pp. 121-188).

Screening Tests

Pathologists, clinicians, or special education teachers can devise their own screening test by selecting 10 to 20 words. This self-made test may consist of simply asking the child to count to ten and name seven basic colors (black, brown, red, orange, green, yellow, white). The sounds tested in this manner are the ones that frequently are misarticulated, namely /s/, /r/, /f/, /θ/, /l/, and /v/. Any child who has a moderate to severe articulation problem is sure to have difficulty with several of these sounds and, therefore, will fail the test. Although it is a crude device, the test has the advantages of being easy to administer and/or requiring little time.

For older subjects, reading passages are provided. Since these contain all the sounds in the English language, any substitution or distortion can be detected easily as the examiner listens to the reading. Two frequently used passages are "Arthur the Young Rat," in Johnson, et al. (1963) and "My Grandfather," in Van Riper (1964, p. 484).

Several standardized screening tests also are available. *The Denver Articulation Screening Examination* (Drumwright, 1971) is one. Designed to test children from ages 2½ to 6 years, it can be administered by lay personnel following only minimal instruction. The tester simply asks the child to repeat what the examiner says. Each of the sounds tested (30 in all) is circled if repeated correctly. The number of circles is totaled as a raw score and compared with a column denoting the child's age. The corresponding value is shown as a percentile rank. If the raw score computes to a rank below the 15th percentile, the child fails the test and the articulation is considered abnormal. This test requires about 5 minutes to administer.

A somewhat longer screening instrument containing 66 pictures for testing consonants in all three positions is *The Screening Speech Articulation Test* (Mecham, Jex, & Jones, 1970). The sounds are given in developmental sequence but there is no way of scoring the results. The examiner must decide what criterion is to be used in determining whether the child passes or fails. Test sentences that the child can read are included. Consonants, vowels, and blends are tested. About 13 minutes are required to give the entire test, which is quite long for a screening test. Consonants alone can be tested in 5 to 8 minutes.

The *Triota Ten Word Test* (J. Irwin, 1972) requires only one minute to administer. Pictures of the following words are presented: chair, scissors, Santa Claus, forks, toothbrush, matches, stove, ring, screwdriver, and turtle. The child is asked to name each picture while the examiner evaluates the production of each sound in the word. A total of 54 sounds can be tested in the ten words. A composite error score is obtained based upon the child's age and type of error, from which a pass-fail criterion can be determined.

The remaining three screening instruments are included as part of longer diagnostic tests. The first is the *Templin-Darley Screening Test of Articulation* (Templin & Darley, 1969) composed of the first 50 items of the longer diagnostic test. A total of 22 single consonants, 22 two-consonant clusters, and 4 three-consonant clusters are used. A cutoff score can be obtained for children aged 3 to 8. Those with scores below the cutoff fail and require further testing. The norms used are the children's age, sex, and socioeconomic levels.

The second screening test, which is part of a more complete diagnostic examination, is the *Fisher-Logemann Test of Articulation Competence* (Fisher & Logemann, 1971). The 11 sounds tested are /θ/, /ð/, /ʃ/, /s/,

/z/, /l/, /ʒ/, /tʃ/, /dʒ/, /j/, and /r/. Unfortunately, normative information is not presented.

Finally, McDonald (1964) includes *A Screening Deep Test of Articulation* as a separate section of his diagnostic test. Thirty-one two-word combinations testing ten productions of the following nine sounds are evoked: / ʃ /, /l/, /r/, /t/, / θ /, /s/, /k/, /f/, and /t/. As a screening test, this instrument is quite long and could be considered better as a short form of the longer diagnostic instrument. The information produced concerns the proportion of phonetic contexts in which children of different age levels correctly articulate the tested consonants. No cutoff score is suggested for determining passing or failing.

Thus, a wide assortment of screening tests is available, requiring anywhere from 1 to 15 minutes of administration time. Most practicing pathologists usually rely upon their own self-made tests in screening children.

Diagnostic Tests

The majority of standardized tests involve diagnosis and the evaluation of articulatory proficiency. The first seven tests to be discussed are more thorough diagnostic types, the last four are articulation proficiency types.

Before discussing the available commercial tests, it should be pointed out that pathologists can design tests to suit their own particular needs if they wish. In so doing, they should take into account the many features that good tests usually incorporate. The major disadvantages of a self-made test are its lack of normative information, its validity, and its reliability. It therefore is advisable to administer tests that have been validated and normed, especially if the results are to be used as part of a research project.

One of the most widely used is the *Templin-Darley Tests of Articulation* (Templin & Darley, 1969). It contains 141 items to test single consonants, consonant clusters, vowels, and diphthongs. Pictures are used to evoke responses. Sounds are tested numerous times to check for consistency of error. Sentences are provided for those who can read. Articulation production (stimulability) of the misarticulated sounds is tested in isolation, syllable, and word environments. Finally, conversational speech is evaluated for intelligibility. Norms for several age groups from 3 to 8 years are provided according to sex and upper-lower socioeconomic levels. Several studies of this test have established its validity and reliability.

The *Goldman-Fristoe Test of Articulation* (Goldman & Fristoe, 1969) contains three subtests to help the examiner locate and record articulation errors as an aid in defining problems and providing a guide for selecting effective remedial procedures. The first, Sounds-in-Words Subtest, involves showing the subject 36 pictures. In some pictures several sounds are tested in order to reduce administration time. The second is the Sound-in-Sentence Subtest designed to evaluate articulation skills in connected speech. Two stories illustrated by pictures are told to the child, who is asked to retell them while looking at the picture cues. The third, the Stimulability Subtest, is designed to help the examiner determine the relative ease with which a child's defective articulation might be corrected. The child is asked to repeat specific syllables, words, and sentences that contain the misarticulated sounds. Norm-referencing data for the first and third subtests are provided in percentile tables for children 6 years old or above; no norms are available before age 6. The tests require about 45 minutes to administer and score. Their major strength is that articulation errors can be classified according to type and severity.

Another fairly common instrument is the *Fisher-Logemann Test of Articulation Competence* (Fisher & Logemann, 1971). The Picture Test, designed for younger children, consists of 109 picture stimuli to test 25 consonants, 21 consonant blends, 12 vowels, and 4 diphthongs. The unique feature is that rather than classifying sounds on a developmental basis (that is, when they should appear according to age), it evaluates them according to place of production (10 places), manner of articulation (6 manners), and voicing (2, voice and voiceless). Vowels are classified on a four-feature system, namely, place, height of tongue, tension, and lip rounding. Narrow phonetic transcription is advised, with attention to allophonic variations. Thus, this test offers a distinctive feature approach to the analysis of articulation errors that assists the pathologist in selecting sounds to be taught during therapy.

The Sentence Articulation Test, a second section of this instrument, is designed for use with older subjects. It consists of 15 sentences, 11 testing all the consonants and 4 the vowels. The two versions are not presented as equivalent tests. Rather than appraising sounds in the traditional initial-medial-final position, the Fisher-Logemann tests them in various syllable positions. This holds an advantage over the traditional procedure. Unfortunately, norms by age, sociolinguistic background, or handicapping condition are not available. Interpretation must be made individually by the pathologist. There also is no quantitative expression of the reliability of either version. In spite of these limitations, this instrument has high face validity and adds many new dimensions to articulatory testing. It can be of great aid in planning therapy strategies.

Another innovative test designed to probe factors other than obvious sound misarticulations is McDonald's (1964) *A Deep Test of Articulation*. McDonald feels that the articulation of sounds is a dynamic, ever-changing process consistently affected by adjacent sounds. While a sound may be misarticulated in one context, it may be produced correctly in another. Thus, the purpose of testing should be to investigate all possible contexts in which each sound can be attempted. This procedure obviously leads to a lengthy test.

A Picture Form Test to be used with those whose reading level is below third grade consists of two pictures to be named successively as one word. For example, if the examiner wants to know how /s/ is produced when followed by /t/, a picture of a *bus* is presented with a picture of a *tub* beside it. The child says "bustub." Then a *vase* is presented beside the *bus*, resulting in "busvace" to note the effect of the /v/ on the /s/. Each sound is tested in 30 different two-word contexts as a releasing consonant and in 30 contexts as an arresting consonant. If the child produces the sound correctly in one context, this can serve as a starting point for therapy. Norms for this test are not provided. It is not designed for comparing children with each other. Scoring is based simply upon percent of correct articulations for the sound being tested. This test often is used as a measure of progress before and after treatment.

The *Bzoch Error Pattern Diagnostic Articulation Test* (Bzoch, 1974) is not well known. It is unique in the fact that errors are classified into categories—indistinct, simple substitution, gross substitution, and omission. Each category is presented on a least-to-most-severe continuum. A formula determines the severity of errors in each category. For example, an indistinct production is divided by 1/2, a simple substitution counts as 1, gross substitution is multiplied by 1½, and omissions are doubled. The higher the score, the more severe the problem. Single-word responses are evoked by the use of pictorial stimuli.

An effort has been made to discover the underlying rules that govern articulatory production through phonological analysis. The rationale is that once rules are discovered, the pathologist can direct treatment toward changing the rule system, not simply correcting sounds according to a developmental system (Compton, 1975). To identify the rules operating in a child's phonological system, Compton and Hutton (1978) devised the *Compton-Hutton Phonological Assessment Test*. As in most tests, responses are evoked using pictures representing a phonetically balanced sampling of each initial and final consonant plus consonant blends. Most consonants are sampled twice. All vowels are represented. A narrow transcription is used to record incorrect responses. Once an analysis of sound errors has been made, these data are converted to rules composed of those found to be most common in the speech of young children. A total of 47 rules are listed under place and manner classifications. For example, three rules under the liquid (manner) classification are:

1. l
    [r] → [w]
2. [l] → ϕ   (omitted)
3. [l] → [j]

Once the analysis is completed, the pathologist selects key patterns and key sounds as treatment targets. For example, a key sound that can break down several patterns should be selected first. This test includes no norms, reliability, or validity data. It is not designed to compare children with each other.

A test developed by Weiner (1979), the *Phonological Process Analysis*, focuses on an analysis of the child's phonological processes. Based upon a description of the normal stages of phonological development that children pass through as they master articulation skills, Weiner classifies errors as to (1) syllable structure processes, (2) harmony processes (assimilation), and (3) feature contrast processes. He feels this test is best suited for the unintelligible child between the ages of 2 and 5. He suggests that different treatment strategies be used depending upon the category of sound error and recommends a particular order to be followed in the treatment of specific processes within each major category. Responses are evoked from picture stimuli both as single-word utterances and in phrase contexts. The test requires 45 minutes to administer with a cooperative subject. No norms, validity, or reliability data are presented.

The remaining four tests are concerned chiefly with measures of phonetic proficiency rather than thorough diagnostic measures. They are easy to administer and score and require little time. Of course, the data obtained are not as meaningful as in some other diagnostic tests.

One popular proficiency measure is the *Arizona Articulation Proficiency Scale* by Fudala (1974). It requires 20 minutes to administer. The severity of the problem is determined by the relative frequency with which a sound occurs in the language, so each sound is given a numerical value. /n/, for example, occurs frequently in English and is weighted at 2.0 whereas /θ/, which is used infrequently, is weighted at 0.5. Sounds are tested using pictorial stimuli in single words representing initial, medial, and final positions. The error weightings for each sound are totaled and subtracted from 100 to provide a numerical representation of severity. This is a convenient way to compare a child's progress with the score at the beginning of treatment. A sample of connected speech that can be obtained from using two picture cards or a sentence test is included for those who can read aloud. Age norms from 3 to 12 years are presented. Reliability and validity measures of the test are quite high.

One of the easiest and quickest instruments (5 minutes to administer and score) is the *Photo Articulation Test* by Pendergast, Dickey, Selmar, and Soder (1969). Single words representing 23 consonants in initial, medial, and final positions are evoked by use of 72 colored photographs of familiar objects. The more frequent consonantal clusters as well as 18 vowels and several diphthongs are included. Ability to produce misarticulated sounds correctly is noted. A small sample of connected speech is evoked by a three-picture series. Scoring is accomplished by totaling the number of errors made on tongue sounds, lip sounds, and vowel sounds. Age norms for children 3 to 12 are provided, although they are not particularly useful. Both a short form and long form of the test can be used. Reliability and validity coefficients are high. For a quick appraisal of articulation errors, this test is quite suitable.

A somewhat outdated proficiency examination is the *Developmental Articulation Test* by Hejna (1963). It consists of 26 picture cards depicting single words to test the child's use of consonants, and 14 clusters in initial, medial, and final positions. Developmental norms are provided for each sound. For example, by the age of 3, children should have mastered /m/, /n/, /p/, /h/, and /w/, 4-year-olds /b/, /k/, /g/, and /f/, and so on. No validity or reliability information is available. The test's use is only to provide the pathologist with a general idea of articulatory skills.

Finally, another phonetic proficiency evaluator is the *Ohio Tests of Articulation and Perception of Sounds* developed by R. Irwin and Musselman (1962). As with other measures, single-word productions are evoked using pictures as stimuli to test sound production in the three positions. Sixty-one sounds are tested, using 27 pictures. A revision of this test examines sound production in phrases and in nonsense words (R. Irwin, 1974). It also examines the child's imitative ability with sounds in nonsense words and in meaningful words. Consistency of sound production is investigated with eight productions of the same sound. This test has been standardized and normed for age and sex. The revised version now provides more diagnostic information than just a measure of phonetic proficiency.

Special Articulation Tests

Some articulation tests are designed for special populations. Two are for Spanish speaking children, one for those with cerebral palsy, and one is a measure of intraoral pressure for those with insufficient velopharyngeal closure.

Carrow (1974) developed the *Austin Spanish Articulation Test* for evaluating Spanish phonemes, including consonants, vowels, diphthongs, and consonant clusters that occur in Spanish. Fifty-nine pictures are used to evoke words containing the test phonemes. One limitation is that there is no means of assessing connected speech or accounting for regional dialects. Also, the 25 minutes required to administer this test is rather long considering the limited information it provides. It was tested on 20 Mexican-American children 4 to 7 years of age. No norms, reliability, or validity data are available.

The second example, the *Southwestern Spanish Articulation Test* by Toronto (1977), is designed to rapidly assess articulation of Spanish consonants in single words. Sounds are tested in all three positions in response to naming 47 pictures. No attempt is made to account for dialects or to standardize or validate the test. It is meant to be an informal type evaluative measure of articulation.

As a result of a 13-year study of children afflicted with cerebral palsy, O.C. Irwin (1972) developed one of the few diagnostic tests especially designed and standardized for these children. The *Integrated Articulation Test* consists of five parts. There are four consonant tests and one vowel test suitable for individuals from 3 to 16 years of age. The tests are administered over several days because of the short attention span and fatigue factors so common among these children. Seventy-six consonants are listed in each of the three positions, along with 11 different vowel sounds. The child is asked to imitate words spoken by the examiner. A numerical score is obtained from each part of the test as well as a qualitative assessment of the improvement of each sound in a test-retest situation.

This test has been validated in a series of studies and has been standardized on a population of retarded children, but the results with this group are not as valid as with those who have cerebral palsy. The basic value of this test is to diagnose the child's ability to articulate speech sounds with respect to initial, medial, and final positions.

Another specialized measure is the *Iowa Pressure Articulation Test* (Morris, Spriestersbach, and Darley, 1961), which actually is a subtest of the *Templin-Darley Tests of Articulation*. This was designed to assess the adequacy of oral pressure for speech sound production utilizing 43 items. This subtest helps determine whether or not a child has adequate velopharyngeal closure. It is best suited for children who have a cleft palate. The *Iowa Pressure Articulation Test* was studied by Van Demark, Kuehn, and Thorp (1975), who found it to be a reliable predictor of palatopharyngeal competence.

Predictive Tests

Tests designed to predict which individuals from a given population will continue to exhibit articulation problems providing there is no therapeutic intervention would seem to be of vital importance to the speech/language pathologist. Yet only two such measures have been developed.

One of the earliest attempts was made by Carter and Buck (1958). Their test, designed to be given to children in the first grade, includes 113 pictures representing 13 consonants in each of three positions. Each sound is tested three times in each position with the exception of /θ/. A second part of the test requires the child to repeat 9 nonsense syllables for each of the 13 consonants, three syllables for each position. Percentages of correctness on these tasks are used as predictors of future articulation difficulty. The smaller the percentage of correction articulation, the greater the likelihood that articulation will not be improved later.

The other predictive device, developed by Van Riper and Erickson (1973), the *Predictive Screening Test of Articulation,* is designed to identify children in the first grade exhibiting functional articulation problems who would be most likely to continue to manifest these problems when they reach the third grade, providing they undergo no therapy. The test consists of 47 items presented as words, sentences, sound syllables, imitative hand clapping, and a discrimination judgment. Each item is scored as correct or incorrect, resulting in a possible perfect score of 47. The authors recommend that any child receiving a score of 34 or below be scheduled for therapy, although the tester may wish to choose a different cutoff score depending upon the needs and constraints of that person's program. The complete test requires only 7 to 8 minutes to administer and score. Several studies of this test have found that correction prediction ranges from 72 to 92 percent. It has sufficient criterion-related validity to be useful in selecting children in the first grade who should be given speech therapy.

Therapy Progress Tests

There are no standardized tests specifically designed to evaluate the effects of therapy. Many standardized tests are used as pretest and posttest measures to evaluate progress in articulation ability but it is difficult to determine whether changes in scores result from the therapy or from other intervening factors.

J. Irwin and Weston (1972) suggest taking daily 2- to 5-minute conversational speech samples as an indicator of progress in articulation skills. A graph similar to the one in Figure 2-1 is kept, showing the percent of correct sound productions during each test period. When a certain level of proficiency is reached for a particular sound, work on it can be terminated.

A similar check on the progress of target sounds selected for therapy consists of gathering samples of a child's speech production following each

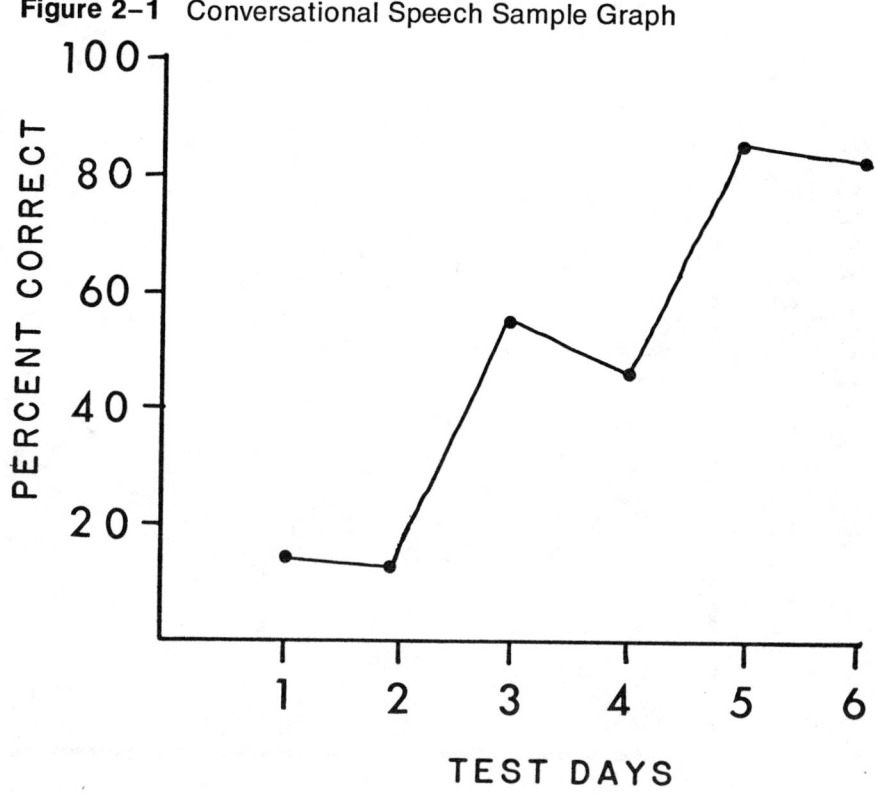

Figure 2-1 Conversational Speech Sample Graph

training session such as used by Wright (1969) shown in Figure 2-2. Two measures are taken: (1) a sound production task (SPT) in which the target is tested in 30 words repeated after the examiner, and (2) an evaluation of 30 target sounds as they appear in the child's connected speech. The data in Figure 2-2 indicate that the child's ability to produce the target sound in isolated words surpasses the ability to produce this sound correctly in conversational speech.

As this rundown has demonstrated, numerous and varied tests are available to assess articulation skills. Each has its specific merits and unique application. Some can be administered by lay persons who have received only minimal training, others should be conducted only by speech/language pathologists. Certainly, anyone who accepts the responsibility of providing speech therapy to individuals with articulation problems should be well acquainted with the assessment devices available. Obviously a number of other measures such as hearing assessment, motor ability, discrimination

Figure 2-2 Progress on Target Sounds Graph

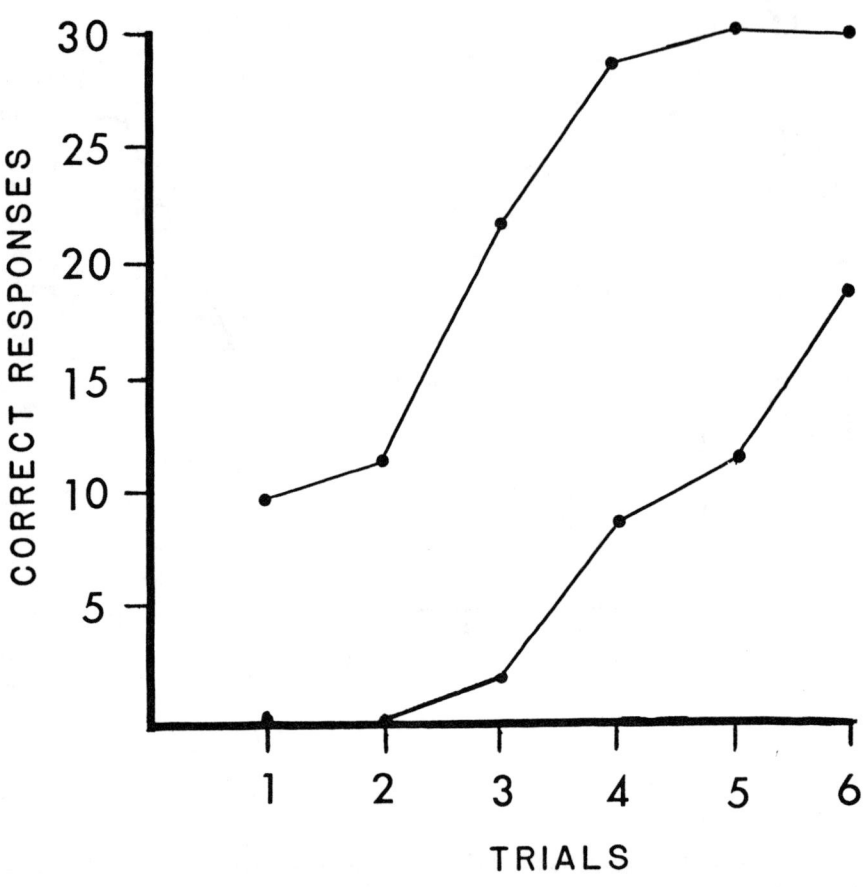

ability, and the like should be given in conjunction with articulatory diagnostic and proficiency tests before a course of treatment can be outlined.

TESTS RELATED TO ARTICULATION ABILITY

Oral Examination

It is important to examine first the structure and function of the oral region. An oral examination consists of looking inside the mouth to note any structural anomaly of the teeth, hard palate, tongue, and velum.

Assessing Articulation Skills   47

The Hard Palate

The roof of the mouth should be examined to determine whether its shape is within normal limits. For example, it should not be arched high so that it appears ʌ-shaped. The shape of the alveolar ridge just behind the upper front teeth also should be noted.

The Tongue

Mobility and flexibility of tongue movement are extremely important. Abnormal width or length of the tongue should be checked. The individual may be asked to move the tongue from left to right as well as up and down. One movement pattern that may predict tongue problems is the act of saying "pu-ti-ku" ([pʌ tik ʌ]) several times in rapid succession. When the tongue is lifted, any restriction that might be caused by a short frenum should be noted, as should the action in producing such words as *thumb, soap, lamb, toy,* and *key*.

The Velum

The velum must be sufficiently long and mobile to provide adequate closure so air does not escape through the nasal cavity except for the nasal sounds. Any tendency for the velum to slope to one side should be noted. The individual should be asked to phonate an "ah" and the clinician should watch for velar movement, which should be clearly evident. The simple task of blowing up a balloon requires good velar closure and is a fair test of how sufficient the closure is. The presence or absence of tonsil and adenoid tissue also should be checked.

The Jaws and Teeth

Normal teeth closure should include the rear molars and a slight overlapping of the upper front teeth over the lower front ones. Any deviancy of this condition should be noted. Occasionally, there will be a case of open bite where there is a wide space between the front teeth. This condition makes it difficult to produce the /s/ and /z/ sounds correctly. Conditions of an undershot or overshot jaw as reflected in deviancies with closure should be observed. Missing or irregular teeth that could affect sound articulation should be noted.

Test of Auditory Memory Span

Sometimes it may be important to determine how many digits or syllables children can remember if they seem to have difficulty producing sounds that occur in multisyllabic words. Generally, children who have problems articulating sounds do not have deficiencies in auditory memory span, so this subject usually is not included as part of the routine test battery. Beebe (1944) found that children aged 4 through 7 should be able to repeat about four syllables in a nonsense word. Nonsense syllables such as *galubi, samuta,* and *labeeta* are suggested. Beebe's article provides detailed information regarding the procedure for testing auditory memory span.

Test of Phonetic Discrimination

It may be necessary to evaluate a child's phonetic discrimination ability, especially if there is a hearing loss. Several tests designed to evaluate phonetic discrimination are available but only two popular ones are discussed here. The first, designed by Templin (1957) contains 50 pairs of nonsense syllables. Two nonsense syllables are presented, one following the other. The child is asked to judge whether the two are alike or different. Examples of syllable pairs are: /ð e-de/, /θe-θe/, /fi-θi/, /en-em/, and /eð-ed/. Each item is scored as a correct or an incorrect discrimination. The total score is compared with age norms to determine whether the child passes or fails the test.

The second test, by Wepman (1958), consists of 40 pairs of words such as *sought-fought, tall-tall, shack-sack,* and the like. These word pairs are read to the child, who decides whether each pair is the same or different. A difference in word meaning as well as sound value is created by using meaningful words rather than nonsense syllables.

Tests of Oral-Motor Coordination

In some instances, it may be necessary to evaluate adequacy of tongue movement. Van Riper (1964, p. 481) suggests five imitative activities that should help in evaluating the adequacy of voluntary tongue control. Each one involves a demonstration by the teacher, who tells the child to:

1. Stick out your tongue like this.
2. Curl up the end of your tongue like this.
3. Move your tongue from side to side like this.
4. Open your mouth and lift your tongue up like this (in position for /l/).
5. Put your finger between your teeth (at the incisors) and click like this (tongue moves from /l/ position downward as air is sucked in to produce a clicking sound about three times per second).

Children as young as age 3 should have no difficulty following these directions if tongue mobility is adequate. If they are unable to accomplish these tasks, they may either have difficulty following directions or their motor coordination may be insufficient to articulate sounds in words.

SUMMARY

As this chapter has shown, a wide variety of tests is available for evaluating articulation skills. They are designed to elicit different kinds of information. Some provide essentially the same inventory of a child's phonetic skills, so the tester's personal preference determines which test to use. Other tests are designed to produce different kinds of information. If pathologists expect to be seeing numerous individuals who misarticulate sounds, they should be familiar with all of these tests, although they may use only a few of them regularly. Once they have determined the nature of the problem, they can proceed to the treatment phase of the program.

REFERENCES

Beebe, H. H. Auditory memory span for meaningless syllables. *Journal of Speech Disorders*, 1944, *9*(3), 273–276.

Bzoch, K. *Bzoch error pattern diagnostic articulation test*. Gainesville, Fla.: University of Florida Press, 1974.

Carrow, E. *Austin Spanish articulation test*. Hingham, Mass.: Teaching Resources Corp., 1974.

Carter, E., & Buck, M. Prognostic testing for functional articulation disorders among children in the first grade. *Journal of Speech and Hearing Disorders*, 1958, *23*(2), 124–33.

Compton, A. J. Generative studies of children's phonological disorders: A strategy of therapy. In S. Singh (Ed.), *Measurement procedures in speech, hearing, and language*. Baltimore: University Park Press, 1975.

Compton, A. J., & Hutton, J. S. *Compton-Hutton phonological assessment test*. Hayward, Calif.: Carousel House, 1978.

Darley, F. L. (Ed.). *Evaluation of appraisal techniques in speech and language pathology*. Reading, Mass.: Addison-Wesley Publishing Co., 1979.

Dickson, S. (Ed.). *Communication disorders: Remedial principles and practices*. Glenview, Ill.: Scott, Foresman and Co., 1974.

Drumwright, A. *The Denver articulation screening examination*. Denver: Ladca Project and Publishing Foundation, 1971.

Emerick, L., & Hatten, J. *Diagnosis and evaluation in speech pathology*. Englewood Cliffs, N.J.: Prentice-Hall, Inc., 1974.

Fisher, H., & Logemann, H. *The Fisher-Logemann test of articulation competence*. Boston: Houghton Mifflin Company, 1971.

Fudala, J. B. *Arizona articulation proficiency scale*. Los Angeles: Western Psychological Services, 1974.

Goldman, R., & Fristoe, M. *Goldman-Fristoe test of articulation.* Circle Pines, Minn.: American Guidance Service, Inc., 1969.

Hejna, R. F. *Developmental articulation test.* Ann Arbor, Mich.: Speech Materials, 1963.

Irwin, J. The Triota: A computerized screening battery. *Acta Symbolica,* 1972, *3,* 26–38.

Irwin, J., & Weston, A. J. Articulation. In A. Weston (Ed.), *Communicative disorders: An appraisal.* Springfield, Ill.: Charles C Thomas, Publisher, 1972.

Irwin, O. C. Integrated articulation test. In O. C. Irwin (Ed.), *Communication variables of cerebral palsied and mentally retarded children.* Springfield, Ill.: Charles C Thomas, Publisher, 1972.

Irwin, R. Evaluating the perception and articulation of phonemes of children ages 5 to 8. *Journal of Communication Disorders,* 1974, *7,* 45–63.

Irwin, R., & Musselman, B. A compact picture articulation test. *Journal of Speech and Hearing Disorders,* 1962, *27*(1), 36–39.

Johnson, W., Darley, F. L., & Spriestersbach, D. C. *Diagnostic methods in speech pathology.* New York: Harper & Row, Inc., 1963.

McDonald, E. *A deep test of articulation.* Pittsburgh: Stanwix House, Inc., 1964.

Mecham, M. J., Jex, J. L., & Jones, J. D. *The screening speech articulation test.* Salt Lake City: Communication Research Associates Inc., 1970.

Morris, H., Spriestersbach, D. C., & Darley, F. An articulation test for assessing competency of velopharyngeal closure. *Journal of Speech and Hearing Research,* 1961, *4*(1) 48–55.

Pendergast, K., Dickey, S. E., Selmar, J. W., & Soder, A. L. *Photo articulation test.* Danville, Ill.: Interstate Printers & Publishers, Inc., 1969.

Stetson, R. *Motor phonetics.* Amsterdam, the Netherlands: North-Holland, 1951.

Templin, M. Certain language skills in children: Their development and interrelationships. *Institute of Child Welfare Monograph 26.* Minneapolis: University of Minnesota Press, 1957.

Templin, M., & Darley, F. *Templin-Darley tests of articulation* (2nd ed.). Iowa City, Iowa: University of Iowa, Bureau of Educational Research and Service, 1969.

Toronto, A. S. *Southwestern Spanish articulation test.* Austin, Texas: Academic Tests, Inc., 1977.

Van Demark, D. R., Kuehn, J., & Thorp, R. F. Prediction of velopharyngeal competence. *Cleft Palate Journal,* 1975, *12,* 5–11.

Van Riper, C. *Speech correction: Principles and methods* (4th ed.). Englewood Cliffs, N.J.: Prentice Hall, Inc., 1964.

Van Riper, C., & Erickson, R. L. *Predictive screening test of articulation* (3rd ed.). Kalamazoo, Mich: Western Michigan University, Continuing Education Office, 1973.

Weiner, F. F. *Phonological process analysis.* Baltimore: University Park Press, 1979.

Wepman, J. M. *Auditory discrimination test.* Chicago: Language Research Associates, 1958.

Winitz, H. *Articulatory acquisition and behavior.* New York: Appleton-Century-Crofts, Inc., 1969.

Wright, V. A. *Comparison of imitative and spontaneous speech samples in the evaluation of articulation change with therapy.* M. A. thesis, University of Kansas, 1969.

Chapter 3

The Treatment of Articulation Disorders

Once having administered the appropriate articulation tests plus any others that seem indicated, the speech/language pathologist (SLP) or special educator should try to eliminate or reduce the effect of factors that may contribute to the problem. For example, if the teeth are positioned in such a way that they interfere with the production of some sounds, referral to a dentist or an orthodontist should be considered. Correction of the dental problem may be possible. If the individual's hearing acuity falls below normal standards, say a loss of 20dB or more of two or more frequencies in one ear, referral to an otologist or audiologist may be necessary. If the individual is unable to make the rapid tongue and jaw movements normal for that age, referral to a physician for further diagnosis of motor ability may be advisable.

After these steps to eliminate any causal factors, the pathologist or special educator should be ready to begin teaching the individual how to articulate sounds correctly. But where to begin? What is the first step?

PRELIMINARY CONSIDERATIONS

Should the Problem Be Explained to the Individual?

Some pathologists feel it is important to explain the nature of the problem to the individual before beginning treatment (Van Riper, 1964). Just how extensively this is done depends upon the age of the individual. If it is a preschool child or one in the early elementary grades, it would be foolish to review for that person why it is important to speak correctly or to discuss at length which sounds are in error. A simple explanation that the child will be helped in learning to say some sounds differently is adequate. With older children, a brief explanation of the importance of effective articulation may be appropriate. Adults and parents of these children may appreciate being told about the test results. The pathologist also could explain the goals set for treatment and what kind of a time schedule is anticipated for seeing the individual and completing goals that are established.

Establishing Rapport

It is difficult to explain how to establish rapport with an individual. So much depends upon the setting and the personality of both the individual who has the problem and the person who will provide the therapy. Many young children associate their first trip to the speech pathologist with a visit to a doctor or dentist that previously may have been a painful experience. The tears may flow freely. If this is the case, it may be necessary to engage the child in play activities for 10 to 20 minutes until cooperation can be established. When working with older individuals it is advisable for pathologists to be as pleasant as possible yet establish themselves as knowledgeable persons who know exactly what to do. It is not advisable to spend a great deal of time getting to know the individual. During the first session, much time can be wasted in irrelevant conversation in the name of establishing rapport. Normally, rapport can be established during the first five minutes.

Auditory Discrimination Training

Some pathologists believe that children misarticulate sounds because they are unable to discriminate between correct and incorrect ones. If not a direct cause of the articulation problem, it has been shown that poor auditory discrimination is at least associated with articulation difficulties. Several textbooks outline detailed procedures for teaching children sound discrimination skills (Van Riper, 1964; Anderson, 1953). These procedures consist of a variety of listening activities that require the child to indicate when two sounds are alike or different and to identify the target sound when produced by the pathologist in isolation and in words. The teaching of sound production usually is delayed until sufficient auditory training has been provided.

In recent years, this initial phase of therapy involving the teaching of auditory discrimination skills has been challenged. For example, McReynolds, Kohn, and Williams (1975) in their study of auditory discrimination skills find few differences in the discrimination scores of children who have articulation problems and those who do not. They feel it is not appropriate or necessary to provide sound discrimination training to these children.

Another study (Williams & McReynolds, 1975) reveals that when auditory discrimination training alone is provided to children with articulation errors, the only change that occurs is that their test scores improve in this area only. Their ability to produce the target sounds they misarticulated did not improve. On the other hand, the study finds that training in the actual production of sounds results in improved scores on both production and discrimination tasks. It concludes that if improvement in sound production is desired, therapy must be aimed toward teaching production, not discrimination.

Weiner (1967), reviewing the literature concerning the importance of auditory discrimination skills as they relate to faulty articulation, concludes that there may be a relationship between poor auditory discrimination skills and poor articulation. This relationship seems most marked among children below the age of 9 who have multiple articulation errors. However, this does not mean that training in discrimination skills will help them learn to produce the misarticulated sounds correctly.

Many pathologists now feel that auditory discrimination training is not as useful as once thought, especially with children who have normal hearing and misarticulate only a few sounds. When administering an instructional program emphasizing production training, Mowrer, Baker, and Schutz (1968), found that 85% of the children scored 90% correct or better on a criterion test administered following termination of three sessions of instruction. No attempt was made to provide auditory discrimination training. Most of the children in this study misarticulated only the /s/ and /z/. It is possible that young children who have multiple sound errors would profit from auditory discrimination training. It may be possible that production training could be facilitated by discrimination training but as yet, we have no evidence to support this belief.

There can be no doubt that children who have a hearing loss would benefit from auditory discrimination activities. In instances where hearing loss plays a key role as a causal factor in faulty articulation, auditory discrimination training plays an important part as a prerequisite to sound production training.

Two levels of discrimination skills have been identified. One is the ability to identify differences in someone else's speech production of a sound (interdiscrimination); the other is the ability to discriminate between one's own correct or incorrect sound production (intradiscrimination). This latter skill, intradiscrimination, seems to be more important in learning correct articulation than the interdiscrimination skill. Weiner (1967) pointed out that little systematic research has been conducted on this topic. Many pathologists frequently ask the children to judge the accuracy of their own responses (intradiscrimination). This practice appears to facilitate the correction process by helping them learn to be their own judges.

Selecting Sounds for Correction

If only one or two sounds are in error, the pathologist may begin by teaching correct vocal production. But many children misarticulate several sounds. Which ones should be taught first? And in what order? Speech/language pathologists use several different criteria to select sounds for treatment.

Developmental Age

One often-used criterion is to choose sounds that children tend to master first. A number of charts that show the maturational levels of various sounds are available (Poole, 1934; Wellman et al., 1931; Templin, 1957; Prather, Hedrick, & Kern, 1975). Some feel that the sounds that are mastered first developmentally are the same ones that should be taught first. The ages at which children are expected to master consonant sounds are shown in Table 3-1.

The first sound selected for correction in the speech of a 7-year-old child who misarticulates /s, r, θ, k/ is /k/, then /r/, /s/, and /θ/ since this is the order in which youngsters acquire them. The theory here is that the sounds that appear first should be those that are easiest to learn. It should be pointed out that this theory has never been proved. There are no data to indicate that developmental norms should be relied on in selecting the order in which sounds should be corrected. Nevertheless, many pathologists do use them. While this procedure may appear to be logical, experts cannot be sure it is the most effective.

Stimulability

One of the best predictors of success in articulation therapy is the degree to which the child is able to imitate a sound produced by someone else. The pathologist simply asks the child to repeat the target sound in isolation, in nonsense syllables, and in words. It is highly probable that the child who correctly imitates these models on the first attempt will be successful in learning to use this sound even without the assistance of an SLP. The clinician who picks the sounds the child can imitate correctly will be assured of success. One of the chief advantages of this procedure is that it increases the likelihood that the child will experience immediate success.

Table 3-1 Summary of Studies Reporting Age of Mastery of English Consonant Sounds

SOUNDS MASTERED NEAR AGE 4	SOUNDS MASTERED NEAR AGE 6	SOUNDS MASTERED NEAR AGE 7
m n ŋ p f h w j k b d g	r s ʃ tʃ t θ v	l ð z ʒ dʒ hw

On the other hand, children may not need help with sounds that are imitated easily. Clinicians who choose sounds that the child cannot master easily without help should select those that are least stimulable. Some pathologists justify their selection of sounds based upon this latter criterion.

Consistency

This refers to how consistently the child misarticulates the sound. Sounds that are in error only infrequently are more likely to be mastered with or without help than are those that are misarticulated consistently. To make sure the child experiences success during treatment the pathologist selects sounds that are in error inconsistently because they should be easier to correct. However, those that are in error consistently are in more need of attention.

Visibility

It might be thought that the more visible the sound is, the easier it would be to teach. /f/ should be easier to teach than /k/ since the lip and teeth structures can be seen easily when /f/ is produced but not when /k/ is spoken. Consequently, a clinician might pick the front sounds such as /f, v, θ, ð p, b, m/ and perhaps /t, d, n, l/ before teaching /tʃ, dʒ, ʒ, r, k, g/ simply because the former are more visible. But there are factors other than visibility that also are important in learning sounds. Children master vowels that are not visible long before they acquire some of the more highly visible consonants. If visibility were the chief factor in learning sounds, then the reverse should be true. Also, / θ / , ð , v/, which are highly visible sounds, are among the last consonants to be mastered. Selecting sounds on the basis of visibility alone does not appear to be a valid procedure.

Frequency

The frequency with which a sound occurs in English may be a helpful criterion in selecting a sound. If a child misarticulates / θ / and /r/, it is best to select /r/ rather than / θ / since /r/ occurs much more frequently. Correction of the /r/ may result in increased intelligibility since it occurs more often. No consideration is given to ease of production. The important factor is how well others will understand the child when a particular sound is corrected, not how easily it will be learned. A list of the consonants and their frequency of occurrence is shown in Table 3-2.

Error Type

Articulation errors are classified into three types: omissions, substitution, and distortions. McDonald (1964) states that children progress through four stages in learning correct sound production: first they omit sounds, then they substitute one sound for another, next they distort the sound by using one that is a close approximation of the target, and finally they pronounce it correctly. According to this progression in the sound learning process, the types of errors in need of most help are omissions, followed by substitutions and distortions. Consequently, sounds that are omitted should be chosen to start treatment. If no sounds are omitted, substituted sounds are the next choice, followed by those that are distorted.

The only problem with McDonald's concept is that it is not known whether children do in fact progress through these three stages. This may be the case for some sounds but not for others. The position of the sound in a word also is a factor to be considered. A sound in the initial position may follow these stages but the same one in the final position may not. Usually, the condition of children who omit sounds is considered more severe than those whose articulation problems are limited to substitutions and distortions.

Table 3-2 Frequency of Occurrence of English Consonant Sounds in Speech

Number	Phoneme	Percentage of occurrence
	Consonant	
1	t	6.60
2	n	6.12
3	s	5.04
4	d	4.68
5	r	4.65
6	l	3.78
7	k	3.09
8	z	2.88
9	w*	2.88
10	m	2.60
11	ð	2.37
12	h	2.34
13	b	1.74
14	v	1.74
15	p	1.68
16	g	1.62
17	f	1.50
18	ŋ	1.25
19	j	1.02
20	ʃ	0.88
21	tʃ	0.77
22	θ	0.66
23	dʒ	0.62
24	ʒ	0.04
	Vowel	
1	ə	6.4
2	ɪ	5.4
3	i	4.0
4	a	3.5
5	æ	3.1
6	ɛ	2.5
7	ɔ	2.5
8	ɝ	2.42
9	ɚ	2.23
10	u	2.0
11	e	1.8
12	ʊ	1.5
13	ʌ	1.4
14	o	0.7
		100

*/hw/ has been combined with /w/.

Source: Reprinted from *Clinical Management of Articulation Disorders* by C. Weiss, H. Lillywhite, and M. Gordon, St. Louis, C.V. Mosby, p. 55, © 1980.

Distinctive Features

In the discussion of distinctive features in Chapter 1, each sound is composed of a bundle of features such as presence or absence of voicing, continuant, consonantal, strident, and so on. What if a child's error pattern reveals that the youngster experiences difficulty with /f, v, s, z/ but not with /θ, ð, r, l/? Both groups of sounds are members of continuants (that is, they are + continuant) but they differ in that the first set has + stridency as the common factor. The second group does not have a + stridency feature. Therefore, the pathologist selects all four sounds, /f, v, s, z/, that have stridency as a common feature and works on all of them together. In this way, the pathologist treats the + stridency feature, not the separate sounds. McReynolds and Huston (1971) recommend that if a child omits a feature, all the sounds sharing that feature should receive attention. The features of stridency and continuancy tend to be in error most frequently.

Crocker (1969) presents a theoretical model based upon the development of distinctive features in the child's speech (Figure 1-3, supra). He feels this model best represents the progressive development of consonant sounds. It seems to be a practical means of selecting sounds that is much more useful than the norms presented in several studies of developmental mastery.

Numerous criteria thus are used in selecting a sound or group of sounds to begin therapy. Unfortunately, they do not all agree. The question remains, which criterion should be chosen? The answer depends partly upon the expert's training. If not trained in the distinctive feature approach, the pathologist or special educator may not feel comfortable using this technique. Most of the procedures have not been validated.

A combination of procedures is considered next. It is important that children experience success when learning new articulation patterns. The highly motivated child usually makes rapid progress whereas the poorly motivated one lags behind. The pathologist also should take into account which features of sounds appear to be contributing to the articulation problem. It is more economical to work with groups of sounds providing they share certain distinctive features that are relatively easy to learn, and are visible, stimulable, and inconsistent, if the highest degree of success is desired. The more difficult sounds, the omissions, the consistent error types, and those that are not easily visible then are added. The use of developmental charts is not too helpful in selecting the first target sounds. Crocker's (1969) model showing the development of features and the resulting acquisition of sounds (Figure 1-3, supra) appears to provide a logical selection sequence. Pathologists who use this model as a developmental guide have found it useful.

Some authors make no distinction in selecting sounds but simply prefer to work on all defective ones simultaneously (McCabe & Bradley, 1975). This position is difficult to defend since it is not based upon a theoretical model. However, from a pragmatic standpoint, it is reported to be effective.

PROCEDURES FOR EVOKING CONSONANT SOUNDS

Evoking the target sound is one of the most important tasks to be performed with an individual who misarticulates. Speech/language pathologists spend many hours learning to use various techniques designed to help children produce sounds correctly. They soon learn special techniques that consistently result in helping the child produce the sound correctly. Some of these techniques that have been found effective are reviewed next. The pathologist will learn other techniques by talking with or observing other professionals, by working with children, or by reading about techniques suggested by other authors. The more techniques the pathologist has available, the better that expert will be prepared to deal with all types of children.

The pragmatic approach seems to be a useful method. Some SLPs have reported what appear to be impractical procedures but often use of these procedures results in correct sound production. Procedures such as telling children that their teeth are a train track and by placing that train (the tongue) on the tracks (teeth) and moving it backward while vocalizing often results in the production of /ɝ/. This seems to be a roundabout way of teaching the /ɝ/ sound but often it works.

The suggestions that follow should help pathologists, therapists, or educators to evoke the consonants that children and adults misarticulate frequently and cannot produce through imitation of a model. These consonants are /s, ʃ, tʃ, f, θ, k/ and their paired voiced cognates plus the liquids /r, l/. Since evoking sounds is a live and ever-changing dynamic process, it is not possible to spell out exactly what the pathologist should say, for it will vary somewhat with every individual. A better understanding of the actual process is derived by listening to recorded sound-evoking sessions or by observing treatment sessions.

Evoking /s/

Anatomical Features

/s/ is an alveolar voiceless, sibilant, fricative, continuous consonant. Its voiced counterpart is /z/.

This sound can be produced using one of three basic tongue-tip positions: up, midline, and down. The up and down positions are used most frequently and are recommended in comparison with the midline one. In all instances the airstream is directed over a small groove in the central portion of the tongue. In the up position, the forward part of the tongue is elevated so the tip is placed in near contact with the upper teeth and gum ridge. A small central groove in the tongue allows rushing air to escape and produce the high frequency /s/ sound, which sometimes results in a whistling /s/.

In the tongue-tip down position—the preferred method to teach to most children—the tip is placed behind and touching the lower front teeth. A hump in the tongue is formed so the blade is elevated against the alveolar gum ridge. A small central groove allows the airstream to escape, producing the /s/. In both cases the turbulent airstream is generated in the small space between the tongue and the alveolar ridge. The lips and teeth are slightly parted.

Methods of Evoking /s/

The method chosen for evoking /s/ depends largely on how it is misarticulated. This requires a procedure for lateral emission of /s/ different from the one used for frontal lisping. If any structural deviations such as open bite are present, procedures must be adapted to accommodate these differences.

Frontal Lisp

Slight protrusion of the tongue between the front teeth constitutes the most common /s/ misarticulation. This type of /s/ substitution is found chiefly among children in kindergarten through second grade.

The pathologist first tells the child to close the teeth and say /i/. The teeth, tongue, and lips now are in a position close to /s/ production. Next, the child is told to keep the teeth closed and say /is/. The result may be either an acceptable or a distorted /s/ but the pathologist should not be concerned with the correct sound at this point; the tongue and teeth positions are the important features.

After practice with /is/, the /i/ is dropped and practice continues with the /s/ in isolation for several trials until the sound improves in acoustic qualities. It should not be necessary to tell the child where to put the tongue tip, but if positioning seems necessary, the pathologist can demonstrate by opening the mouth, placing the tongue behind the bottom teeth, and, by closing the teeth, produce the /s/. The child then is asked to imitate this placement while the pathologist models the action slowly.

One important point is the manner in which the child closes the teeth. The molars, not the front teeth, must be touching. Frequently, children understand, "Close your teeth" to mean jutting the lower jaw so the front teeth close. If this happens, it must be explained that the back teeth, not the front, should close. Of course, some children's back and front teeth close at the same time in a normal bite position and the pathologist should not attempt to alter this pattern.

Lateral Lisp

Children also produce /s/ laterally as an unvoiced /l/. The chief problem here is not teeth position as in the frontal lisp but airstream direction. There are three procedures to try.

The first procedure has been found to be very successful. It begins with a /t/ production and moves into an /s/. The child is told to produce a few /t/ sounds, greatly aspirated. This produces the frontal airstream direction desired for /s/, but with a plosive release instead of a sibilant fricative. To attain this second goal, the child is told to push hard on the /t/ and let it out a little at a time. Thus, the /t/ is changed to a fricative and the resultant sound resembles /s/. The child is directed to smile during the prolongation of /t/ so the /s/ will be more distinct. This results in a tongue up /s/ production. If a tongue-tip down /s/ is desired, it is begun by producing /t/ from a tongue down position. It seldom is necessary to refer to tongue position since the child will adopt whatever one is easiest to manipulate during coarticulation.

If the first procedure is not successful, the second should be tried. The child is asked to produce /ʃ/. If this sound is correct, that is, using the frontal airstream, the sound is changed from an /ʃ/ to /s/ by asking the child first to produce /ʃ/ and then spread the lips slowly into a smile position. This is done in one smooth action. The moment lateral emission is heard during this transition period, the child is asked to stop and the pathologist says, "No, you let the sound slip out the sides." Even if the initial attempts to produce /s/ result in distortion, the child should be rewarded for producing frontal airstream direction. Once this feature has been acquired, the /s/ always can be shaped with tongue placement instructions.

The third technique is simple: the child is asked to say /θ/. This produces frontal airstream direction immediately but the /θ/ will lack the sibilant characteristics of /s/. To achieve this feature, the child is told to retract the tongue slightly. The pathologist provides a model for the child to follow. This position change is practiced several times, then the tongue is retracted a little more. This process is continued until the tongue is far enough behind the teeth so they can be closed. The child is directed to close the teeth and make a distorted / θ / sound imitating the instructor's model. The /s/ is improved by telling the child to move the tongue tip either down or up, whichever produces a better sound. Once a good /s/ is being produced, tongue placement is ignored. Using a mirror may help the child position the tongue.

/s/ Omission

This problem is more common among kindergarten children than at older ages. Since the child produces no /s/, a direct procedure is to evoke it through imitation. The pathologist simply tells the child to do just what the instructor does. The child imitates some other fricative sounds such as / θ , f, ʃ /, then /s/ alone. There should be no problem evoking /s/ in isolation. Combining it with other sounds is more difficult. The procedure here is to model the sound for the child and provide teeth closure or tongue placement cues as needed.

/t/ for /s/ Substitution

Teaching /s/ to a child who has a /t/ for /s/ substitution is similar to the way to teach a child who has an /s/ omission. The pathologist provides a model and asks the child to imitate it. If the youngster has trouble, the pathologist makes sure that the tongue tip is positioned behind the bottom teeth. The teeth are closed slowly so the back molars meet and force the air out to produce /s/. The chief problem comes in trying to join /s/ with a vowel. In most cases the child will produce /s/ followed by /t/ and then the vowel. If /s/ is requested, the response is [t a]. One of the best ways to eliminate the /t/ is to teach the substitution of /h/ for /t/. First /h a / is taught, then /s-h a /. Another procedure is to teach /nei/, then /snei/, then /sneik/. These sound combinations help eliminate the /st/ blend.

/s/ is not a difficult sound to teach, although gaps caused by missing front teeth may hinder learning it. If teeth are missing, it may be advisable to wait until new ones emerge before an attempt is made to teach /s/.

No mention has been made of /z/, the paired cognate of /s/. It usually is not necessary to teach it as a separate sound once /s/ is mastered. Some /z/ words are included in the practice list such as *is, was, his,* etc. The child should experience no difficulty adding voice to the /s/.

Evoking / ʃ /

Anatomical Features

/ ʃ / is a postalveolar, voiceless, sibilant, fricative, continuous consonant sound. Its voiced counterpart is / ʒ /. In producing / ʃ /, the tongue tip is raised but expanded and more blunted than for /s/. The sides of the tongue touch the upper side teeth but not the front ones. The opening is somewhat wider than for / s / and the resulting airstream is more diffuse. The sound still retains a sibilant quality. The teeth are separated slightly and the lips are rounded in a puckered fashion.

Methods of Evoking / ʃ /

The simplest procedure for evoking / ʃ / is to model the sound for the child. The pathologist explains that this is the "quiet sound" and is used when it is desired that people be quiet. The pathologist places a finger vertically in front of the lips and makes the / ʃ / as people usually do to indicate quiet, then asks the child to imitate that production.

It usually is not beneficial to provide instructions concerning tongue placement. It may be appropriate to squeeze the cheeks together so lateralization of air does not occur, using a mirror to help the child imitate the lip position.

If the / ʃ / is produced laterally, the pathologist first teaches frontal airstream direction for /s/ and, when /s/ is produced correctly, presents /ʃ/ by shifting from /s/ to / ʃ /. The instructor proceeds from a smile lip position to a puckered lip while producing the sound shift. If lateral air is heard, the pathologist stops immediately and goes back to correct /s/ production. The chief difference between /s/ and / ʃ / is the lip position and slight retraction of the tongue to provide a larger opening.

As in the case of the paired cognate of /s/, there is no need to teach / ʒ / in isolation. Few words contain / ʒ /, and adding voice should present no problem.

Evoking / tʃ /

Anatomical Features

/tʃ / is a tip postalveolar stop consisting of two consonant sounds blended together. The tongue is raised and the tip contacts the hard palate slightly farther back than in /t/ production. The airstream is blocked completely and allowed to escape suddenly in a plosive manner as the sound of / ʃ / is produced. The lips are slightly rounded and protruded when the sound is initiated. The lower jaw drops as the sound rushes out.

Methods of Evoking / tʃ /

In most cases, a child will distort this sound or will produce it laterally. It is not a sound that is misarticulated frequently. Evoking it could begin with a /t/ if the child says [s ɛ ɚ] (*share*) for *chair*. Once this is established, the pathologist distorts the sound by squeezing the cheeks together to pucker the lips. This should result in a distorted /t ʃ / sound that then can be shaped toward the desired one. Practice in opening the mouth follows after the /t/ is released. Models should be provided during demonstrations. It should be explained that the /t ʃ / explodes like a firecracker. The lips must be puckered. There is no need to teach the paired cognate / dʒ / separately.

If the child says [t ɛ ɚ] *(tear)* for *chair,* the pathologist may have to begin by adding /s/ after the /t/ to get /ts/. A fricative feature should be added following the /t/. The /ts/ then can be modified to a /t ʃ / sound.

Evoking /f/

Anatomical Features

/f/ is a labiodental, voiceless, fricative, continuous consonant. It is produced by moving the lower lip slightly upward and inward against the bottom edges of the upper front teeth. The tongue plays no part in the production of this sound. The airstream passes centrally between the edge of the teeth and the lip.

Methods of Evoking /f/

Evoking /f/ is not difficult. The child is simply asked to bite the bottom lip and blow—but not laterally. If this occurs consistently, one end of an ear swab stick is placed centrally between the lip and teeth. The child is directed to blow over the stick. Or the pathologist strikes a match and asks the child to blow it out while saying the /f/. A few models from the SLP and the instruction to "bite your bottom lip and blow" should be sufficient to evoke this sound. There is no need to teach /v/ alone; the inclusion of /v/ words with practice on /f/ words should suffice.

Evoking / θ /

Anatomical Features

/ θ / is a linguadental, voiceless, fricative, continuous consonant sound. To produce / θ /, the tongue tip is thrust slightly between the central incisors. A small groove is formed on the top of the tongue so the airstream rushes centrally through the groove just under the front teeth. The lips are parted slightly.

Methods of Evoking / θ /

The most effective instruction to evoke this sound is, "Stick your tongue out and blow." The usual response is an extended tongue protrusion with lots of saliva flying in the pathologist's direction. If so, the response should be, "Don't blow so hard." Better /θ/ sounds usually can be evoked with more blowing practice.

If the air comes out laterally, a small stick (not a tongue depressor) is placed on the midline of the tongue and the child is told to blow over the stick. A straw also can be used. The desired feature is central airstream direction.

The second fault may be too much tongue protrusion. This may be ignored at first, but if it continues, the child is simply told the tongue is sticking out too far and that it should be kept back more. A tongue depressor could be put slightly in front of the lips and the child told to just touch it with the tongue and blow over it. /θ/ should be an easy sound to evoke; there is no need to work with /ð/ separately.

Evoking /k/

Anatomical Features

/k/ is a velar, voiceless, stop-plosive consonant sound. It is produced using the back part of the tongue raised high against the front of the soft palate, which is raised. The tongue action causes a blockage of air—the "stop" part of the consonant. The tongue drops quickly, allowing the air to "explode" through the oral cavity. The lips are in a relaxed position, the teeth parted slightly.

Methods for Evoking /k/

This sound may be difficult to evoke primarily because it is not easy to observe the movement. The closest sound position to it is /ŋ/. If the child can learn to produce /ŋ/ and then block off the sound completely (by closing the soft palate), the first element, the stop, will have been acquired. Another procedure is to produce /ŋ/ by blocking the sound with upward and backward movement of the tongue plus soft palate closure. It should be a simple matter to release the air pressure to produce the plosive part of the sound.

The pathologist may prefer to evoke the sound as an entire unit, both stop and plosive, rather than working on one, then the other. This can be done best through modeling the sound a few times and stressing the backward and upward position of the tongue.

The handle of a spoon or a tongue depressor can be used to assist in pushing the tongue back into position. The tongue tip must be held down so the bulk of the tongue is pushed back and upward to fill the rear oral cavity. The probe is removed quickly when the sound is to be released.

The child may wish to use a finger to push the tongue back in position. It also may be desired to touch the rear of the hard palate with a tongue depressor to give the child a sensory target position for placing the tongue for closure.

Sometimes it is helpful to suggest that the child make a cough-like sound. In demonstrating this sound, the pathologist produces an aspirated /k/ somewhat like an /h/. More plosive characteristics are added to the sound gradually. Production of /g/ should be no problem once /k/ is achieved. If the sound is not evoked in 20 or 30 attempts, it is best to discontinue it until the next session.

Evoking /l/

Anatomical Features

/l/ is an alveolar, voiced, lateral, continuous consonant. It has no voiceless cognate. The blade of the tongue rests against the alveolar ridge and is spread out somewhat to leave space for lateral emission of the airstream. Two types of /l/ sounds can be produced: dark or clear. The dark sound is made by dipping the midportion of the tongue while humping the posterior section; the clear sound is produced by keeping the blade of the tongue high toward the hard palate. The clear /l/ resonates more toward the forward portion of the oral cavity, the dark sound more toward the rear.

Methods of Evoking /l/

It is unnecessary to distinguish between clear and dark /l/ sounds. The major problem in evoking /l/ is in airstream direction, which tends to be central instead of lateral. The common substitutions for /l/ are /j/ and /w/, both central airstream sounds. Therefore, it is necessary to concentrate on lateral airstream. There are several ways to do this. One is to ask the child to repeat /a/ and move the tongue tip up to the alveolar ridge while still producing /a/. If the tongue blocks the central airstream, thus forcing it out laterally, an /l/ should be produced. The lips must be kept spread to allow lateral emission. By snapping the tongue down, /la/ should be produced.

Another technique involves distorting a sound that has some of the components of /l/. This may be somewhat more difficult. /n/ and /d/ have approximately the same tongue positions but /d/ releases centrally and /n/ is a continuant. If the child can be instructed to release either of these two sounds laterally, a close /l/ production should result. For example, in the case of /d/, the child is told to keep pressing the front part of the tongue in the /d/ position but, instead of dropping the tongue tip, to hold it up in that position and let the air out over the sides of the tongue. It is important to retain the voiced element of /d/ or something like a lateral lisp will be produced. For /n/, the nostrils are pinched shut while producing /n/ and the child is told to continue pressing the tongue in the /n/ position while allowing the air to escape laterally.

Of course, the most direct approach is to instruct the child to lift the tongue up high against the upper front teeth, push up, and imitate the pathologist's /l/ sound. It is recommended that the pathologist try this procedure first; it is helpful to practice in front of a mirror.

Evoking /r/, /ɝ/, and /ɚ/

Anatomical Features

/r/ is a postalveolar, voiced, fricative, continuous consonant sound. /ɝ/ and /ɚ/ are postalveolar voiced vowels. The unstressed /ɝ/ is written as /ɚ/. Both sounds can be produced in a variety of ways using one of several possible tongue positions to shape the oral cavity. Typically, the tongue tip is elevated behind but not touching the alveolar ridge. The sides of the tongue are spread, forming contact with the sides of the upper gums along the region of the molar teeth. This tongue shaping allows the airstream to be emitted centrally.

Methods for Evoking /r/, /ɝ/, and /ɚ/

These sounds often are difficult to evoke. The reason is that the correct tongue-cupping position is not visible and the individual must acquire correct sound production by auditory means alone. Outlined next in specific terms are five programs designed to evoke /ɝ/; once /ɝ/ is acquired, /r/ can be evoked by adding a vowel to /ɝ/ and by progressively shortening /ɝ/.

Five programs (A, B, C, D, E) are presented. Programs A and B represent procedures used by the majority of practicing speech/language pathologists according to a survey conducted of more than 500 such experts in public schools. Programs C and D are used to a lesser degree. While Program E is a procedure unknown to many pathologists, it is highly successful. If after using all five programs the child still is unable to say /ɝ/ correctly, the pathologist should wait a month and readminister them.

Since it is unlikely that a child will produce a correct /ɝ/ during the first attempts, the pathologist should accept close approximations. It is impossible to anticipate the sounds various children will make during their initial attempts. The pathologist must be flexible in adjusting the program to fit the needs of each individual child. For example, if correct /ɝ/'s are produced immediately upon request, these programs can be omitted and the child can advance directly to the next stage of treatment.

68 CLINICAL MANAGEMENT OF SPEECH DISORDERS

PROGRAM A

Objective: To lift the tongue up and back to produce /ɝ/.

1. "Curl your tongue like this." (This action is demonstrated and the child is asked to look at the pathologist's tongue. The pathologist should lift the tip of the tongue up and curl it back so that the tip almost touches the hard palate (Figure 3-1)).
2. "Now curl your tongue back there again and make this sound, [ɝ]." (The sound is prolonged for 2 seconds.)

Figure 3-1 Illustration of the Tongue Curled Upward and Backward in the Oral Cavity

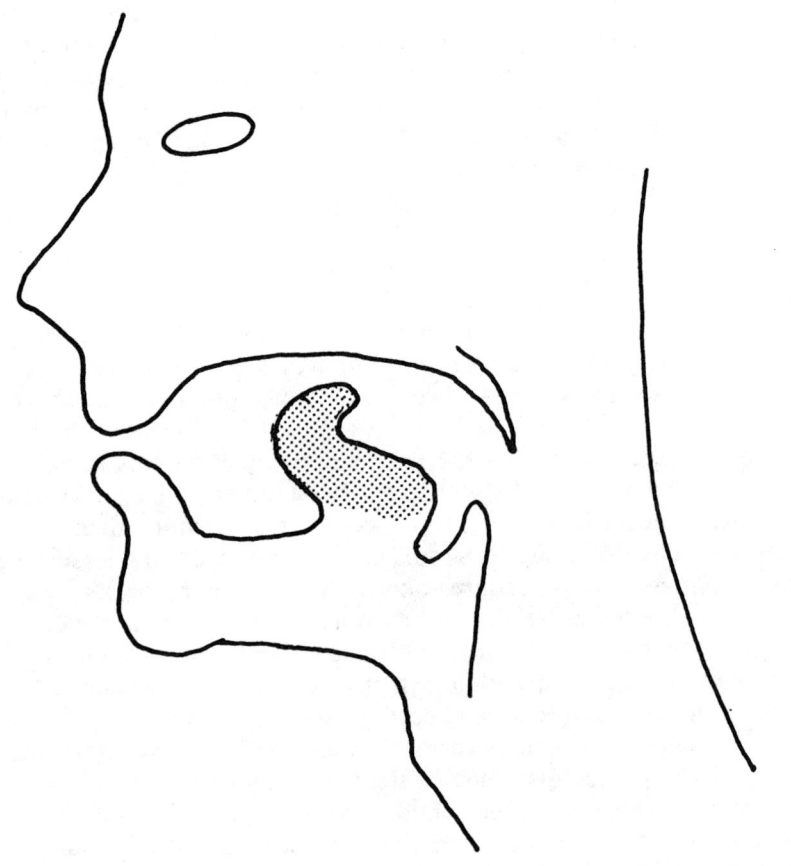

3. "Keep your tongue back there and say it each time I raise my finger." (The pathologist raises five fingers, one at a time. It is important to tell children how well they are progressing. Each time a child makes a sound, the pathologist should evaluate it and say what is appropriate, such as "That's pretty good," "Better," "Yes," "Almost," "No," "That's worse," "Fine," etc. The pathologist should look directly in the child's mouth to see whether the tongue is up and back. There is no need to worry much about the sound at this point. Correct tongue position is more important.)
4. "Watch my tongue again." (The child must look in the mouth of the pathologist who makes three /ɝ/ sounds.) "Now you try it some more." (It is helpful to provide the child with a mirror to check tongue position. The youngster should be encouraged to make about five more /ɝ/ sounds. The pathologist should be sure to follow each sound with a brief verbal comment.)
5. If the child is making good /ɝ/ sounds, the pathologist should ask that this be continued, with pauses of 2 or 3 seconds between each attempt. This will provide time to say "Good, "Better," "No," or whatever. If good /ɝ/ sounds are not being produced, the child should be directed to put the tongue back farther, lift it up higher, or curl the tip back more. The pathologist should ask the child to say five /ɝ/ sounds between each cue. It is important to announce whether the child is getting closer to or farther away from the /ɝ/ sound on each attempt. The pathologist may wish to use a hand to demonstrate how the tongue should move. (See Figure 3-2.)
6. "Keep making the [ɝ] sound until you can say ten of them in a row all correct." (The pathologist still may need to continue giving cues about lifting the tongue back farther if the child has some trouble saying /ɝ/ correctly. When satisfied the youngster can say ten correct /ɝ/ sounds in a row, the pathologist proceeds to the next stage of treatment.)

PROGRAM B

Objective: To lift the tongue, placing its sides against the upper rear molar teeth to produce /ɝ/.

1. "I'm going to lift my tongue up and put the sides of my tongue against my back teeth and say a sound." (The pathologist demonstrates and says /ɝ/ as the child looks inside the mouth.) "Now let's see if you can touch your teeth with the sides of your tongue. First, pull your tongue way back and feel your teeth with your tongue." (Tongue

Figure 3-2 Illustration of Hand Moving from the Prone Position Resembling /a/ Production to the Approximation of the Tongue Position for /ɝ/ Production

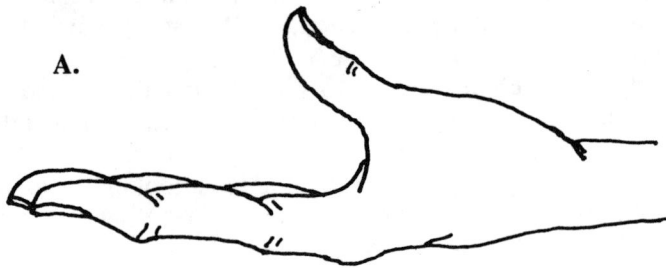

A.

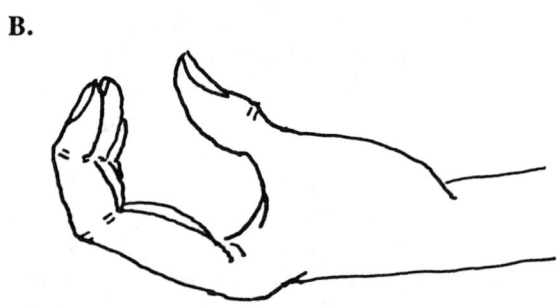

B.

---

position should be checked; the tip should not be up but should just flatten into the midportion.)
2. "Now keep your tongue up there against your teeth and make this sound, [ɝ]." (The child is asked to continue trying to say /ɝ/ five times. If the sound is close to /ɝ/, the child is told "Good," "That's better," or "Fine." If the resulting sound is a very poor approximation of /ɝ/, the child is directed to pull the tongue back farther or lift it up higher. The pathologist should look in the youngster's mouth to check tongue position.)
3. "Now say the sound after me, [ɝ]." (The pathologist says the sound ten times. The child attempts to imitate this. If the imitations are close to the pathologist's, the child should be told "Good," "Better," or "Close." If the child still is unable to approximate /ɝ/, the pathol-

ogist should say, "Move your tongue back a little farther," "up higher," or "touch the back teeth.")
4. "Keep trying to make the [ɝ] sound. We want ten good [ɝ]'s in a row so we can go on to the next part of our lesson." (The /ɝ/ attempts, good and bad, should be noted. Cues should be used as the pathologist feels they are needed to direct the child toward producing better /ɝ/ sounds. When ten correct /ɝ/ sounds are produced in a row, the case proceeds to the next phase of the treatment. If the child still experiences considerable difficulty saying /ɝ/ correctly, another program should be selected.)

PROGRAM C

Objective: To produce /i/ and, by moving the tongue back through three positions, produce /ɝ/.

1. "Say [i]" as in *eat*.
2. "Feel your tongue up there on the top of your mouth? Say [i] again. Look in the mirror. See your tongue up there when you say [i]. Say it again."
3. "Pretend your tongue is a train and your teeth are the tracks like this picture (Figure 3-3). Keep your tongue on the tracks and move your tongue back a little so you make this sound [ɪ]." (This should not sound exactly like /ɪ/ but will contain a sound more like /i/.)
4. "Say it again and keep your tongue up."
5. "Now the train is leaving the station so make it go back farther and make this sound [ɝ]ᴅ." (The ᴅ stands for a distorted /ɝ/ sound. There is no sound like this in English. It is a mixture of /ɪ/ and /ɝ/.)
6. "That was a funny sound wasn't it? Let's make it a couple more times. Remember, keep the train up there on the tracks." (Or the pathologist can say, "Keep your tongue up there on your teeth," if it gives the child a better idea of what to do. The child should be asked to say the sound four times.)
7. "Now, make your tongue go back a little farther and say this sound [ɝ]. Keep it on the tracks. Try it." (The child should produce a sound fairly close to a good /ɝ/ and should be told to continue saying it. The pathologist should praise the youngster after every sound that resembles /ɝ/. If the sound begins to drift away from /ɝ/ or if it is desired to help the child make a sound closer to /ɝ/, the pathologist should go on to instruction 8. It also may be advisable to go through all four steps, /i/, /ɪ/, /ɝ/ᴅ, /ɝ/, during each attempt.)
8. "Keep your tongue up there like before only pull it back some more. Make the sound after me: [ɝ]____ [ɝ]____ [ɝ]____ [ɝ]____

Figure 3-3 Illustration Demonstrating Analogy of a Train Positioned on the Upper Teeth

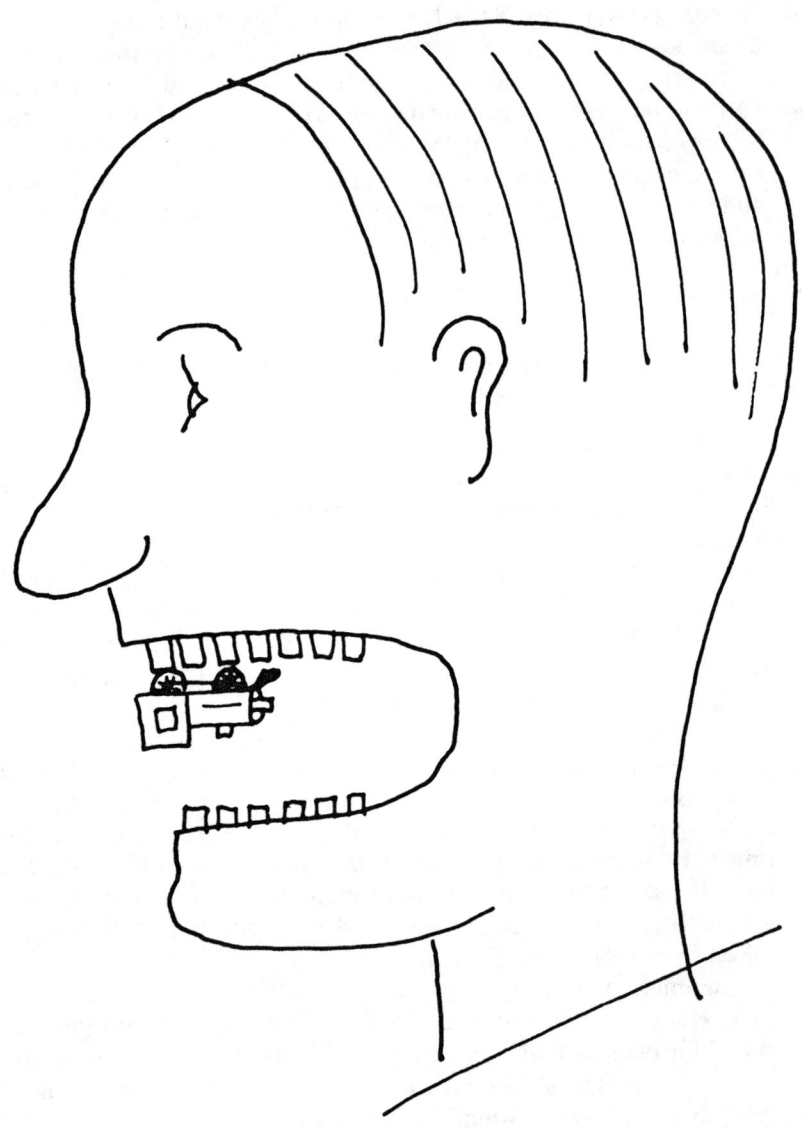

[ɝ]___." (The key instructions are to keep the tongue up against the teeth and pull it back. If the tongue is positioned correctly so a sound close to /ɝ/ is produced, it often is possible to get a better /ɝ/ simply by the pathologist announcing when the child is getting closer to or farther away from the sound. When ten good /ɝ/s have been produced, the case moves on to the next phase of treatment.)

PROGRAM D

Objective: To produce /l/ and, by moving the tongue tip back against the hard palate, produce /ɝ/.

1. "Put your tongue tip up and say [l] like this: [l]." (The pathologist demonstrates by producing /l/ and maintaining the sound 3 seconds.)
2. "Now we're going to drag the tongue tip along the roof of our mouth back like this." (The pathologist demonstrates but does not produce sound, just shows the tongue movement. The child is asked to do this several times. Use of a mirror is helpful.)
3. "Now, let's drag our tongue back and make a sound like this [l-ɝ]." (The pathologist demonstrates by slowly moving the tongue from the /l/ position to the /ɝ/ position while vocalizing. This will produce several different sounds while moving from /l/ to /ɝ/. The /ɝ/ sound is prolonged longer than the others. The child practices moving from the /l/ to the /ɝ/ ten times. When a close approximation to /ɝ/ is produced, the case goes on to the next item.)
4. "Let's see if you can make that last sound all by itself. Put your tongue way back there and say [ɝ] like this: [ɝ]." (The pathologist demonstrates, then asks the child to say it ten times. During these trials the pathologist should praise sounds that are closer to /ɝ/. When the sounds are not like /ɝ/, the child is told to put the tongue back farther or up higher and try some more.)

PROGRAM E

Objective: To lift the tongue tip up and, by moving it in a circular direction around the surface of the hard palate, produce close approximations to the /ɝ/ sound.

1. "Lift your tongue up and move it all around the top of your mouth like this." (The pathologist demonstrates, producing the constantly changing sound continuously for five seconds, moving toward and away from the /ɝ/ sound.) "I'll tell you when you're getting close to

the right sound. OK, you try it." (The child will produce a variety of sounds, some closer to /ɝ/ than others. When a sound resembles /ɝ/, the pathologist immediately says, "Good," "That's it," or "Fine." When the sound drifts away from the /ɝ/, nothing is said. If the sound does not even come close to /ɝ/, the child is told to move the tongue around more or back farther and to draw a circle on the top of the mouth with the tongue tip. When the child has produced 15 or 20 close /ɝ/ sounds, the case moves to Item 2.)

2. "Now, just say that [ɝ] sound that you've been saying so well. Make it sound just like you did before. Try it." (If the child is unable to replicate the /ɝ/ sound, it may be advisable to return to Item 1. When /ɝ/ is produced, the youngster is told to hold on to that sound and keep saying just that one. Item 2 then is repeated.)

3. "Now, say [ɝ] 10 times in a row. If you can do that, we'll go to the next lesson. Try it." (When the child can produce ten consecutive correct /ɝ/ sounds, the case goes to the next treatment step.)

These suggestions should help evoke the target sound quickly. It should not require more than seven to ten minutes to evoke the sound and stabilize it so the child is able to say it correctly at least five consecutive times within five seconds. Once this goal is reached, the case proceeds to the next treatment step, which is to incorporate this sound within contexts of vowels and consonants.

INCORPORATING THE TARGET SOUND IN WORDS AND PHRASES

Syllable Production for Consonants Frequently in Error

Once the target sound can be produced correctly in isolation with no hesitation, it is taught in combination with some vowels. The child will experience more success using the sound with single vowels rather than with words. The reason is that familiar words tend to trigger old responses. This is especially true with preschool children. A child may be taught to say /θ/ correctly in isolation but when words such as *thumb, think,* and *both* are introduced, the child may revert to the habitual sound substitution. These patterns are not strong when using nonsense syllables like *thu, thi,* and *oth.* Since the consonant-vowel nonsense syllable has no meaning to the child, it is more likely to be spoken correctly, thus building a repertoire of new articulation patterns.

The SLP begins by blending the five long vowels—a, e, i, o, and u—with the target sound. Except for the voiced consonants /l/ and /r/, which have no voiceless counterparts, only the voiceless sounds are discussed here. It usually is a simple task to evoke the voiced cognate once the voiceless sound is produced.

If /s/ is being taught, the child is asked to say *see*, with the instruction, "Keep your teeth closed and say see." Then *so, si, su,* and *sa* are introduced. When saying the syllable *sa*, the pathologist encourages the child to open the mouth during production of the /a/ vowel. The same procedure is used for all other consonants except /r/ and /ɝ/, which are discussed separately following this section.

If it is difficult to move from production in isolation to these vowel nonsense syllables, the consonant-vowel transition should be practiced more slowly. The consonant should be prolonged if it is a continuant such as /s, f, ʃ, θ, l/, blending it into the vowel gradually.

These consonant-vowel combinations need be practiced only until they can be pronounced rapidly without hesitation and without error. Usually, 10 to 30 productions are sufficient, after which words can be attempted.

Once the target sound is established in syllable context, the child may already be saying some words without realizing they are meaningful. In that case, it may be appropriate to move directly into phrase contexts. For example, the consonant-vowel combination /si/ can be placed in the context of *I see, you see, we see,* and *the sea.* /so/ can be extended to *I sew, so can he,* and *sew the coat.* /ʃi/ becomes *she can, she did,* and *she will.* Adding a consonant to the final position produces words for other consonant-vowel combinations. Some examples are: *feet, fight, shine, sheet, fuss, lick, lease, thumb,* for continuants; and *take, team, peek, paint, chase, chime, jip,* and *jeep* for stops and affricatives.

The simple addition of another word to the beginning or to the end of these key words produces phrases incorporating the target sound. At first, the words can be spoken more slowly than normal if necessary. As the child becomes accustomed to using the new sound, speech rate can be increased to a normal speed.

Up to this point, the child has been asked to repeat words. It is advisable to introduce pictures as evoking stimuli, thus reducing the child's dependence on the use of auditory models. At first, the child simply names the picture. Then short phrases such as *blue ball, red car, shiny car, big fox, red cherry,* etc., may be required. When the child can use the target sound correctly in response to 30 to 50 pictures or words, longer phrase and sentence structures are introduced. But before that stage is considered, a close look at techniques for establishing /r/ and /ɝ/ is appropriate.

Special Instructions for Teaching /r/ and /ɝ/

The consonants /r/ and /ɝ/ present special problems. It is not advisable to begin teaching /r/ in the initial position of a syllable. It is much easier to begin with the /ɝ/ as it occurs in the final position. The use of /ɝ/ in the initial position can be taught using one of the programs in the sound-evoking section. Only a few words such as *earth, early,* and *earn* begin with /ɝ/. Instructions for teaching /r/ are not included in the sound-evoking section. Teaching /r/ in the initial position is easier once the child learns to produce the /ɝ/ with several vowels.

The simplest way to introduce words once /ɝ/ can be produced correctly is to begin with the breathy /h/ sound followed by /ɝ/ to produce *her*. From that point, instruction can move immediately into phrases such as *her coat, her hat, her boot,* etc. It is equally simple to insert other consonants in the initial position to produce words such as *fur, burr,* and *sir*. The ending *ger* can be added to make two-syllable words—*hunger* and *finger; er* can be added, resulting in *mother, father,* and *brother*. Consequently, sounds added to the beginning of /ɝ/ can generate a large number of one- and two-syllable words.

When the vowel sound preceding /ɝ/ is changed, it often is more difficult for the child to retain the correct /ɝ/. If asked to say *door,* the child probably will produce something like *dowah.* Seven vowel combinations influence the /ɝ/: /aɝ/ as in *car,* /ɛɝ/ as in *air,* /oɝ/ as in *door,* /uɝ/ as in *endure,* /aiɝ/ as in *fire,* /iɝ/ as in *ear,* and /auɝ/ as in *hour.* These combinations usually are not produced with equal ease. /oɝ/ seems to be the most difficult, /aɝ/ the easiest. It usually is advisable to begin teaching the /aɝ/ combination once /ɝ/ has been mastered.

In teaching /aɝ/, the child is asked to open the mouth, say /a/, and slowly lift the tongue tip up and at the same time pull it back toward the position to produce /ɝ/. This tongue position is taught in Program A in evoking /ɝ/ in the previous section. The child should glide from /a/ to /ɝ/ while producing one continuous sound as the tongue moves up and backward. Once this sound is practiced several times, initial consonants may be added, resulting in such words as *car, far, bar, scar, tar,* etc. Numerous words can be used as drill material for this sound if the child can produce just /ɝ/ and /aɝ/.

Once these two sounds are produced easily, the next sound to be introduced is /ɛɝ/. When it can be used correctly in 10 to 15 words, /aiɝ/, /iɝ/, /auɝ/, /uɝ/, and finally /oɝ/ are introduced. It may not be necessary to follow this order exactly but for many children, these last five sounds usually are more difficult than /ɛɝ/ or /aɝ/.

In most cases, the /w/ is substituted for the /r/ as illustrated by /wop/ for /rop/, /kwai/ for /krai/, /əwound/ for /əround/, and so on. Once the /ɝ/ can be produced correctly, it is not difficult to structure situations to evoke /r/ by using contexts that require /ɝ/ to be blended into /r/. The two-word combination *car ran* is one. A slow blending of the final /ɝ/ sound in *car* into the initial /r/ of *ran* can evoke the /r/ in a word environment. There may be a tendency to say *car wan* rather than *car ran*. The SLP must be careful that /w/ is not inserted. Once *carran* is produced as one word, *tar ran, car rode, mother read, teacher rode,* and similar combinations are practiced. The child then is asked to whisper the first word and say the second one aloud. This should result in correct /r/ sounds in the initial position. Next, the pathologist simply eliminates the first word and has the child practice saying words that begin with /r/.

Once this task is mastered using 15 to 20 words, the /r/ blends such as *cry, try, street, friend,* and *gray* are introduced. Some 30 to 40 are practiced until the child has no difficulty including /r/ in the blend position.

When the consonantal /r/ and postvocalic /ɝ/ sounds are produced correctly in one- and two-word combinations, picture cues are introduced to evoke responses, as mentioned earlier. The child is now ready for the extended phrase and sentence stage once 30 to 50 pictures can be named correctly. There is no need to teach the unstressed /ɚ/ separately.

USING THE TARGET SOUND IN CONNECTED SPEECH

The transfer from phrase to sentence context should be easy since by this time the target sound has been used repeatedly in phrases. By using pictorial stimuli, sounds can be evoked easily in sentence contexts. Action pictures depicting the key word(s) as the predominant factor are useful stimuli. The pathologist should assemble a group of magazine or newspaper pictures that depict key words. Several publishing firms make picture card stimuli available to speech/language pathologists.[1]

Children in upper grade levels may be asked to read sentences rather than use the picture stimuli. It is not wise to spend more than a few sessions reading sentences or naming pictures. The important task is to use the sound habitually in automatic speech. Practicing words and sentences allows the child an opportunity to establish correct sound production at the conscious level. Once this task is mastered, the child should advance to the automatic speech level.

USING THE TARGET SOUND AT THE AUTOMATIC SPEECH LEVEL

During this stage, the pathologist should engage the child in conversations about various topics in an attempt to establish the new sound in automatic speech patterns. Some stimuli are necessary as a reminder to use the sound correctly. The presence of the SLP serves as one reminder, as do certain picture cues used in prior sessions. It is important to use supportive cues at the beginning of this stage. By gradually changing these cues through providing new pictorial stimuli, new topics, other audiences, and other environmental conditions, the pathologist paves the way for the child to begin using the target sound at the automatic speech level.

Picture sequences that depict a story are selected first. Examples are cartoons used in newspapers or comic books. The pathologist tells the story, illustrated by the picture sequence, emphasizing key words incorporating the target sound. The child repeats the words singly, making sure the target sound is pronounced correctly. The child then is asked to retell the story as the pathologist points to the pictures in the sequence.

To illustrate this procedure, the SLP selects /r/ as the target sound. The child can produce the sound in isolation and can combine it with nonsense syllables, words (including blends such as /br/, /kr/, /tr/, etc.), phrases, and some sentences. The pathologist now is ready to present stories that the child will retell. The following key words are selected from a picture story about a bear's walk into the forest: *brown, bear, rabbit, forest, scared, tree, ran,* as shown in Figure 3-4.

The child repeats these words after the pathologist, who makes sure the /r/ is correct. When the child can repeat them correctly, this short story is told:

> One day, a big brown bear went walking in the forest. A rabbit jumped out from behind a tree and scared the big brown bear. The big brown bear ran away.

After the story is read aloud, the child is asked to fill in the correct words as it is retold, as follows:

> One day a _____ was walking in the _____. A _____ jumped out from behind a _____ and scared the _____. The big _____ _____ ran away.

Next, questions about the story such as the following are asked:

a. Who was walking in the forest? _____
b. Where was he walking? _____
c. What jumped from behind a tree? _____
d. What did the brown bear do? _____

By this time, the child has had ample opportunity to practice the target sounds in the key words and is familiar with the story. While looking at

Figure 3-4 Sequence Illustrating Story of Bear in Forest

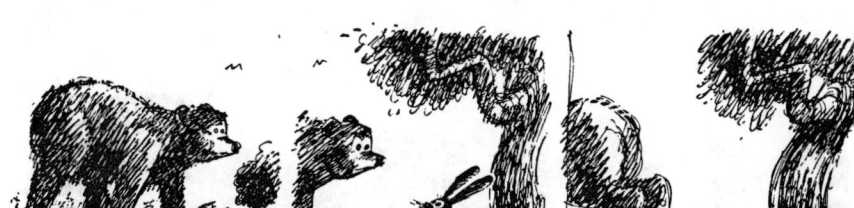

the pictures, children should be able to retell the story in their own words. This activity resembles conversational speech, yet the key words are well controlled. If children do not produce the target sound correctly in any of the key words or others they use in the story that contain /r/ sounds, they should practice saying these words separately. The child then retells the story at a slower rate. Upon hearing an error the second time, the pathologist should interrupt and have the child practice the word several times in several sentence contexts. The child then continues retelling the story.

Another example is a story activity taken from S-PACK, an instructional program by Mowrer, Baker, and Schutz (1974) (Figure 3-5) designed to correct frontal lisping. The key words in the picture are *Chester, bus, stop, street,* and *saw.* Others contain /s/ or /z/ such as *was, his, see,* and *last,* but these are not considered key words. If the /s/ is used correctly in these words, then it is obvious the child is generalizing the correct sound to other words at the automatic level. Generalization is important. It is impossible to teach the child every word containing /s/ in it. Generalization accounts for the fact that words other than the practice ones can be produced correctly. The story is told:

> This is a story about Chester and his bus ride. I'll tell it to you first:
>
> Chester was waiting at the bus stop for a bus. He looked up and down the street for the bus. At last, he saw the bus coming so he put up his hand for the bus to stop. The bus stopped and Chester got in. Then the bus drove off from the bus stop with Chester inside.

After the story is told, the child is asked to say all the key words correctly. If this is done, the child fills in the missing words as the story is retold. Then the child is asked to answer the following questions:

Figure 3-5 Sequence Illustrating Story of Boy at Bus Stop

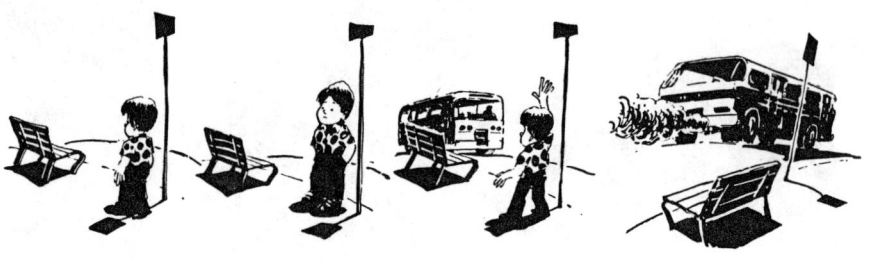

1. What was the boy's name? (Chester)
2. Where did Chester look for the bus? (up and down the street)
3. What did Chester do when he saw the bus? (put up his hand to stop the bus)
4. What did the bus do? (stopped)
5. Who got in the bus? (Chester)

Finally, the child retells the story while looking at the pictures.

The pathologist, or special educator, should collect 15 to 20 story sequences about each sound that is being taught. These stories should give the child ample practice saying the sound in connected speech. The pictures can be collected from magazines or newspapers, photographs taken by the instructor, or sketches the pathologist asks talented high school students to draw. The art teacher often can help obtain pictures. Picture card sequences are available commercially from publishers.[1]

Once these stories have been told to the child several times, spontaneous speaking situations can be planned. This can be done by asking the child to make up a different ending to the story or to continue it by adding another sequence of events. In the sequence about Chester, the child can describe where Chester was going after he got off the bus. The pathologist can suggest that Chester was going to the zoo, or to a store to buy his mother a birthday present, or to school. The child should be encouraged to explain what might have happened. The story can be related to the child's own experience of riding a bus or going somewhere by car, train, or plane. This can initiate dialogues that will allow the pathologist to evaluate how well the child is using the target sound in conversational speech situations. When mistakes are heard, the pathologist makes a note of the words and has the child practice them, first in isolation and then in sentences. For example, if the child says /θpun/ for /spun/, the practice consists of saying *spoon* several times. Practice words also can include those similar to *spoon*, such as *spook*, *spoke*, *spool*, *spell*, *span*, and *spin*. These words then are included in sentences such as the following:

I have a spoon.
The spoon is in the cup.
Where is the big spoon?
His spoon is dirty.
Can you spell?
A spook scared him.
He couldn't spell spoon.

Tongue twisters should not be used as they are difficult even for accomplished speakers and rarely have relevance in ordinary speaking situations.
It is important at this stage that children practice words they used in their conversational speech, not words the SLP might choose from a book.
Older children may find the picture-naming activity too juvenile. In this case, they can be asked to read textual material, starting with sentences in which key words are underlined, then paragraphs with similar underlining, and finally, material from their classroom textbooks. The pathologist may underline a few of the words that include the target sound, eventually eliminating the underlining, then ask questions about the material and discuss it. The pathologist monitors their pronunciation of words that contain the target sound, picks out those not voiced correctly, and has the children practice them in sentences until they can say them correctly.
The final stage of treatment involves discussing topics with the child in a conversational setting, monitoring the accuracy of articulation as the chat progresses. It also is important to include other people in the conversation. The child may invite one or two friends to attend the session. This provides the child with an opportunity to practice using the sound correctly in the presence of persons other than the pathologist. It also is important to arrange for speaking situations outside the therapy room. The pathologist can accompany the child to the playground, cafeteria, principal's office, school secretary, classroom teacher, or school nurse. The pathologist tells them the child is practicing the newly learned sounds in a variety of speaking situations and their help is needed. The child also can be sent on errands to talk to people. Afterwards, the pathologist can check with these individuals to find out how well the child articulated.
Involving the parents to assist in the therapy process is an important part of the program. Most parents are interested in helping their child learn correct speech habits, although there always are a few who will not cooperate. For those who wish to help, speech assignments are sent home with the child. However, the pathologist should confer with the parents first to

explain what sounds are being studied and how they can help. The homework assignments should be as specific and detailed as possible. Parents should not be asked to look for and cut out pictures or construct materials. They should be provided with the necessary instructions and practice materials for ten-minute speech lessons in the home. If three to five of these lessons are completed each week, it will speed up the remediation process. The child must not be reprimanded if homework is not completed. Forcing practice by causing the child to feel guilty seldom results in positive motivation. If the necessary cooperation cannot be obtained from parents and the child, the pathologist should try to get this assistance from school personnel. Many staff members are happy to assist, providing this does not infringe on their time.

Once the target sound is produced correctly in words used in conversation, the pathologist need only make sure the new articulation skills are maintained in the child's daily speech. This can be done best by conversing with the child occasionally, perhaps once a week or biweekly for a month or two. The teacher and parents can be asked how well the child is articulating at school or at home. If a reversion to old speech habits is apparent, the pathologist should begin seeing the child more frequently in a variety of situations. Additional practice should be assigned to make sure the target sound is pronounced correctly. Most children will not require follow-up training once they begin using the sound correctly in conversational speech.

The procedure described here has been used successfully by many speech/language pathologists. Van Riper (1964) outlines this basic approach by beginning with the sound in isolation, then building longer speech sequences until conversation situations are established. The procedures presented here are not new. If they are followed, correction of articulation problems can be accomplished quickly and effectively.

MOTIVATION

Aside from the technical aspects of teaching correct sound production and use of the sound words, pathologists must consider the importance of motivating the child. It is important from a motivational standpoint to keep the pupil well informed regarding the success of the various efforts. The proverb, "Nothing succeeds like success" certainly applies when working with a child who has a speech problem. The pathologist should be sure to reward the child immediately when a correct response occurs, and do this frequently.

When the child is first learning a new task, there should be a reward almost every time the response is correct. After the new response has been practiced so well that the pupil rarely makes a mistake, a good rule is to reward about every fourth response. What is meant by reward? A reward may consist of verbal praise in statements such as: "That's good," "Fine," "Swell," or "Great." It also may be worthwhile to use a point system by keeping a tally of all correct and incorrect responses during a session. The percent correct can be determined and plotted on a graph. Special bonus points can be earned for each session in which correct response is above 80 percent. Points also can be assigned to each correct answer or to groups of correct ones. A fair ratio might be one point for every ten correct responses.

The child should be encouraged to save points later to be redeemed for prizes, privileges, or whatever the pathologist observes will be rewarding. Many teachers offer a menu of items to choose from, each item having an assigned point value. For example, a plastic soldier could be worth 10 points, a ring 25 points, a whistle 50 points, a toy car or bracelet 100 points, and so on. This token economy system works very much like the merchandising stamp system many grocery and department stores used rather extensively during the 50s and 60s in which books of stamps could be exchanged for gift items listed in a catalog.

Use of Game Activities

The speech activity chosen to assist in the acquisition of correct articulation should be enjoyable for the child. This will help ensure that the child is motivated to practice the speech activities the pathologist selects. Many pathologists incorporate a game activity as a device to encourage the child to speak. These games generally consist of interest-provoking activities that serve well both in motivating children to respond and in keeping their interest. The games can be used advantageously to help generate a good deal of speech practice.

However, some game type activities are of little use even though they are enjoyable and provide high levels of motivation. For example, horse race games, speech bingo, or others may require the child to repeat stereotyped phrases or sentences such as, "Please can I spin," or "The name of the picture is ____." These types of contrived speech activities bear little resemblance to children's common conversational patterns. They also do not generate sufficient speech responses and do not provide the variety of word practice needed. Consequently, little generalization can be expected from speech patterns used in stereotyped responses. Speech activities should be made as relevant and as meaningful to the child as possible. In selecting practice words, the words found in the pupil's daily speech vocabulary or reading books should be used. Relevancy is much more important than just having a good time in speech class and winning games.

The second important factor aside from relevance of words chosen in speech activities is rate of response. It is useless to design a speech activity that generates only a few responses from a child. The proverb "Practice makes perfect" is especially applicable to changing articulation. This proverb also applies to behaviors that require motor learning—skiing, typing, and speaking. Little is accomplished when the teacher monopolizes speaking time with long explanations of how to play a game or by chatting with the child about topics unrelated to speech. For example, when the simple statement "Good" would suffice following a correct response, one also could say, "Oh boy, Johnny, that was a good sound. You did just what I told you to. I think you're really getting the hang of it. We'll have to be sure and keep it up now that you've learned how to say your sound correctly." By the time the teacher stops talking, the child may forget how the sound was said. Mowrer (1977) reports a study in which some pathologists outtalked children in speech class at a rate of 10 to 1. It should be remembered that the child, not the teacher, is the person who needs practice speaking.

Some game activities require that participants spend considerable time moving objects around a game board. These nonspeech activities conflict with opportunities to produce the target sounds. If it is true that practice makes perfect, then when the child is not practicing the target sounds, little progress in learning new articulation skills can be expected. Van Riper (1964) cautions the speech/language pathologist against letting the game activity take precedence over speech practice.

It is important to remember that the focus of therapy should always be upon correct sound production, not upon winning in competitive games or simply having fun while playing. A good game activity is one that allows the child to have maximum opportunity to produce target sounds correctly while maintaining high motivation.

BEHAVIORAL OBJECTIVES

Much has been written about the use and value of behavioral objectives in education (Mowrer, 1977). There can be no doubt that writing objectives helps the teacher pinpoint the behavior to be learned, organize learning activities, and accomplish goals.

Mager (1962) outlines a simple procedure for writing behavioral objectives based on these factors: (1) a *do* statement, (2) a statement about the *conditions* of the learning tasks and (3) a statement about the *criterion* the child is expected to meet.

The *do* statement reflects what the learner is to do. It is the verb component of the behavioral objective. Some examples are: to *write*, to *say*, to *identify*, to *point* to, etc. Verbs used in the do statements must be measurable and observable. Since it is not possible to observe a person understanding, knowing, or appreciating, these verbs cannot be used in the statement of objectives. It is possible to infer that a person knows something only by observing some other measurable behavior such as pointing, listing, identifying, or saying. For example, if a person is tested on the ability to discriminate between two sounds, one method is to observe as the individual points to one of two pictures after one is named aloud. Pointing is not the objective the person is intended to accomplish. Pointing behavior is used only as an indicator of being able to discriminate between sounds.

The *conditions* consist of all relevant variables in the learning environment that may affect performance. If the pathologist is presenting picture cards and modeling them to the child in the therapy room, these three conditions (the pathologist, picture cards, modeling) should be listed in the objective. But the color of the walls, the temperature and shape of the room, and the pathologist's hair style are not relevant conditions, so they are not included. Relevant conditions include the cues, how they are provided, where, and by whom. These are conditions that always should be listed.

Finally, the *criterion* statement should include what the pathologist expects in terms of accuracy of performance. This usually is stated as a number, such as 9 out of 10 times, 85 percent of the time, with 80 percent accuracy. Time constraints can also be included in the accuracy statement. Within 5 seconds, during a 20-minute session, or immediately are statements that refer to how fast the person should respond. Time and accuracy of response are the two important statements in the criterion statement.

Objectives can be written for each behavior or task taught during the entire sound-learning process. Terminal objectives may be written as the final behavior desired that the person exhibit. The following examples may clarify how behavioral objectives are written:

The child is required:

a. to say /s/ in isolation correctly five consecutive times immediately following one model presented by the pathologist
b. to read aloud, in the presence of the pathologist, five words containing /l/ in the initial position that have not been included in the treatment material, with 100 percent accuracy

c. to say /b/ in all positions of words in all speaking situations with 100 percent accuracy

So far many topics that relate directly to changing articulation behaviors of children have been discussed. By presenting a treatment program designed for a young child who displays multiple articulation errors and by following this individual's progress, all of this information can be tied together in a way that should be meaningful.

EXAMPLE OF CHILD WITH MULTIPLE ARTICULATION ERRORS

Clifford, a 5-year-old boy, attended kindergarten in a small rural community. His articulation skills lagged far behind those of his peers. His parents, concerned about his slow development, arranged to have an examination at a university speech and hearing clinic.

Testing Procedure

The *Goldman-Fristoe Test of Articulation* (1969) was selected to aid in assessing Clifford's articulation skills. His responses to the Sounds-in-Words Subtest are shown in Table 3-3. At first glance, it is difficult to see any sound substitution or omission patterns that could help in devising a plan for treatment. One way to help clarify Clifford's phonological system is to superimpose it over the adult rule system. As discussed in the classification of sounds (Table 1-1, supra), sounds can be classified in terms of the place where they are articulated in the mouth as well as the manner in which they are articulated. First, only the stop, fricative, and affricative sounds are considered.

Analysis of Sound Substitutions and Omissions in Terms of Place and Manner Features

Analysis of Stop, Fricative, and Affricative Sounds

The 16-stop, fricative, and affricative sounds are shown in Figure 3-6. Manner of articulation is shown across the horizontal plane and place of articulation on the vertical.

A comparison of each of Clifford's articulation attempts on the sounds in the *Goldman-Fristoe Test* with those that should be present (the adult phonological system) shows how the two systems differ. Using a circle containing cross marks to indicate the omission of a sound and arrows to designate a sound substitution, pathologists and special educators can get a better understanding of Clifford's phonological system (Figure 3-7).

Table 3-3 Clifford's Responses to Test Words of "Sounds-in-Words Subtest" of the Goldman-Fristoe Test of Articulation

Test Word	Clifford's Response	Test Word	Clifford's Response
house	[aʊ]	this	[dɪ]
telephone	['tɛləfon]	carrot	['tɛw't]
cup	['tʌp]	orange	[ɔn]
gun	[dʌn]	bathtub	[bæf'tθb]
knife	[naɪf]	bath	[bæ]
window	[fɪndo]	thumb	[dʌm]
wagon	[fædən]	finger	[fində]
chicken	['tɪʔn̩]	ring	[fiŋ]
zipper	[ipə]	jumping	[dʌmpɪn]
scissors	[idə]	pajamas	[pədæmə]
duck	[duʔ]	plane	[pen]
yellow	[io]	blue	[bu]
vacuum	[bæʔum]	brush	[bʌ]
matches	[mæʔə]	drum	[dʌm]
lamp	[l̩æmp]	flag	[fæg]
shovel	[fʌbə]	Santa Claus	[æntə 'tɔ]
car	['taː]	Christmas tree	['timʔ 'ti]
rabbit	[fæbɪt]	squirrel	['tɛə]
fishing	[fɪʔn̩]	sleeping	[ipən]
church	['təʔ]	bed	[bɛd]
feather	[fɛʊ]	stove	['to]
pencils	[pẽnɔ]		

* ['] unaspirated
** [ˌ] syllabic consonant

Figure 3-6 Arrangement of Stop, Affricative and Fricative Consonants by Manner, Place, and Voicing Features

	Frication		Affrication		Plosive	
	vl	v	vl	v	vl	v
Front	θ f s ʃ	ð v z ʒ	tʃ	dʒ	p t	b d
Back					k	g

Figure 3-7 Clifford's Phonological Errors Overlaid on Classification System Shown in Figure 3-6

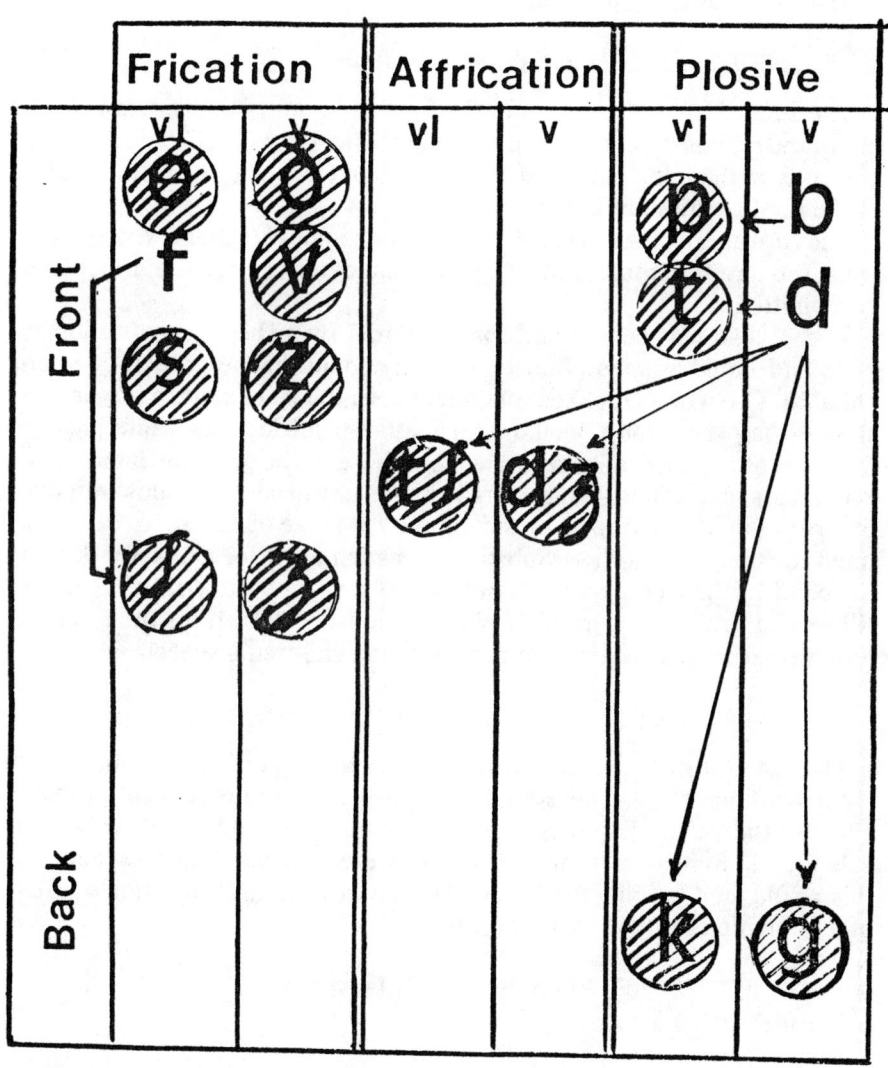

By comparing the representation of the two sound systems in Table 3-5 it can be seen how /b/ and /d/ are used as substitutions for /k, g, p, t, tʃ, dʒ /. Actually, /t/ and /p/ are unaspirated, making them sound like /b/ and /p/ substitutions. In the area of frication, only the /f/ is present. It sometimes is used as a substitution for / ʃ /.

Analysis of Liquids and Glides

The second area of concern in Clifford's phonological system is in the use of the liquids /r/ and /l/ and the /j/ glide. The /l/ appeared to be produced correctly in the initial and medial positions but not when near the /j/ glide, in the final position, or in clusters.

The /f/ was substituted for the initial consonantal /r/ but a vowel or /w/ was used as a substitution for the postvocalic / ɝ / or / ɚ /. The /r/ in blends was omitted.

The /f/ also was substituted for the initial /w/. The /f/ substitution for glide and liquid sounds is not commonly found in the speech of young children. Crocker's (1969) developmental sequence of sounds (Figure 1-2) shows that the group including fricatives, affricatives, and plosives develops along lines quite separate from those in the group including vowels, liquids, and glides. While sounds in one group could be substituted for others within that group, it is uncommon for those of one set to be substituted for those in another. Substitutions such as /f/ for /s/, /t/ for /k/, and /s/ for / ʃ / might be expected, but not /t/ for /r/, /f/ for /r/, or /k/ for /l/. While Clifford's /f/ for /r/ and /w/ is difficult to explain, his other substitutions and omissions are common in young children's speech.

Analysis of Nasals

The last group of sounds, the nasals, present no particular problem with the exception of / ŋ /. This sound was not present in his speech, probably because the velars /k/ and /g/ were not present, /d/ and /'t/ being used as substitutes. Since the front consonants were utilized almost exclusively, this would tend to bring the / ŋ / toward the front to an /n/ position because of assimilation, as in the case of [fɪndɚ].

Analysis of Clifford's Phonological Rules According to Simplification Processes

The previous discussion covered the three sound simplification processes children pass through during early stages of learning during the ages of 1 through 4. It is worthwhile comparing Clifford's rule system with each of these processes.

Syllable Structure

1. Omission of final consonants: This feature does not characterize Clifford's articulation pattern. The final sounds of *cup, gun, knife, lamp,* and *rabbit* are clearly present.
2. Reduplication: Clifford does not reduplicate syllables.
3. Cluster reduction: A definite problem exists here. Clifford usually omits the second consonant, which usually is a liquid or glide, and the first one if it is a fricative. He appears to be in the second stage of cluster production, the first stage being omission of both clusters and the third the substitution of one sound in the cluster for another.
4. Omission of unstressed syllable: There was no evidence of this characteristic.

Thus, syllable structure appears to present no problem in Clifford's phonological system with the exception of his difficulty with clusters.

Assimilation

1. Vowel assimilation: There appeared to be no strong evidence of vowel assimilation.
2. Vowels affecting voicing: While it is possible that the voiced component in vowels influenced the tendency to voice /t/ and /p/, it seems likely that lack of frication was more responsible for unaspirated /t/ and /p/ productions than was vowel influence.
3. Consonant assimilation: There was little evidence of consonant assimilation.

Substitution

Clifford's problem was most evident in substitution. Each of the six areas in this group are discussed next.

1. Stopping: The use of stops for fricatives and affricatives was present to a large degree, but not always. He simply omitted many of the sounds rather than using stop substitutions. In other instances, the /f/ was present regardless of its position in a word. If stopping was predominant, stops would be used in place of /f/.
2. Fronting: Fronting was present on most occasions because /b/ and /d/ were used in place of the velars. But the glottal stop / ʔ / was used on occasion as in [tʌʔi] for *turkey*. Consistent fronting would have necessitated [tʌti] for *turkey*. Fronting of the /r/ was evidenced by the substitution of /f/ for /r/.

3. Use of alveolar nasal /n/ for velar nasal / ŋ /: This, too, was a common error possibly because of the assimilation effects of the predominant front consonants /b, d, f/ as in the case of [f ɪ ʔ ŋ] for *fishing* and [find ə] for *finger*. One exception was [fi ŋ] for *ring*.
4. Liquid replacement: The liquid /l/ was correct most of the time but the consonantal /r/ was replaced with /f/. Therefore, the liquids as a group were not defective—only one element was. This is not uncommon even for children in the first and second grades.
5. Syllabic /ɝ/ replacement: The postvocalic /ɝ/ and /ɚ/ sounds were replaced with either /w/ or /ə/. This was consistent and, again, is typical of speech in first and second grades.
6. Omission: Omission of sounds probably best characterizes Clifford's articulation pattern. Those omitted were the alveolar, dental, palatal, and glottal fricatives /s, z, θ, ð, ʒ, ʃ, h / and often the palatal affricatives / tʃ, dʒ /. /f/ for / ʃ / was an inconsistent substitution.

Summary of Clifford's Phonological System

As a result of this analysis, Clifford's articulation errors can be summarized in terms of five categories dealing chiefly with the addition of sounds:

1. Frication needs to be added to his system. This will allow for the production of eight consonants, namely, /s, z, θ, ð, v, ʃ, ʒ, h / which are missing from his repertoire.
2. Affricatives need to be added to obtain /tʃ, dʒ /. This should follow the addition of the fricative feature.
3. Velars /k/ and /g/ are needed. This probably will result in more consistent use of the / ŋ / because of assimilation.
4. Consonantal /r/ and liquid /ɝ/ need to be added. These are two distinctly different sounds and require slightly different teaching strategies, although mastery of one should facilitate learning of the other.
5. One member of consonant clusters needs to be added to complete cluster development.

These five goals provide the direction needed to help Clifford reorganize his phonological system to conform more to that of adults. The addition of the fricative sounds should contribute greatly to intelligibility. They also are relatively easy to master. Consequently, treatment should begin with the addition of these sounds.

EXECUTION OF THERAPY PROCEDURES

One feature that complicated the organization of the therapy program was the fact that Clifford lived in a remote area far from those served by speech/language pathologists. The solution was to install a telephone amplifier in Clifford's house so instructions could be delivered from the office of the speech/language pathologist some 1200 miles away. Although this constrained traditional treatment procedures, it had the advantage of necessarily involving Clifford's mother in treatment as well as providing treatment in the home setting in which the child felt secure. The distance factor in no way influenced the selection and execution of treatment goals. Cost was not a factor since a telephone WATS line was used. Calls were placed at least three times per week even through the holiday seasons.

Motivation

Since the pathologist could not be present during treatment, some means of motivating Clifford to respond were required. This was accomplished by establishing a token economy system. Clifford's mother was instructed to give him a token for each correct response. The definition of a correct response for each objective was spelled out clearly to the mother, whose job was to monitor the child's replies. Clifford could exchange the tokens for small toys. Thus, the contract was that he could exchange tokens earned by responding correctly for toys of his choice. The more correct responses he made, the more toys he could earn.

Establishing Frication

The first goal was to teach Clifford the production of several sounds that contained frication. Using Crocker's (1969) model as a guide (Figure 1-2 supra), it was decided to begin teaching /s/ and /θ/ first. Since an /s/ correction program, S-PACK (Mowrer, Baker, & Schutz, 1974), was available, teaching /s/ was the first target.

This program consists of a step-by-step hierarchy of tasks beginning with /s/ in isolation production followed by /s/ in nonsense syllables, words containing /s/, phrases containing /s/, and finally /s/ used in words simulating conversational speech situations. Cues are faded gradually and the reinforcement schedule changes from continuous to intermittent.

The pathologist mailed a copy of the /s/ correction program to Clifford's mother so she could follow the instructions and evaluate the boy's responses. It was difficult for the pathologist to evaluate correct /s/ production using the phone. Any attempt to produce frication during /s/

production was rewarded. His mother was able to monitor correct usage more closely.

Once the first three parts of S-PACK were concluded, Clifford's mother was instructed to administer the program on a daily basis for three consecutive weeks. A program similar to the S-PACK designed to correct the /ð/ and /θ/ was mailed to the parent and administered by the pathologist by phone as soon as the three-part S-PACK was completed (five 15-minute sessions). This program also began by teaching /θ/ in isolation and progressed through a series of nonsense syllables, words, and sentences containing /θ/ and /ð/ sounds.

Introduction of Velars

Next the /k/ was introduced when it was noted Clifford spoke the word *think* using the /k/ correctly. Admittedly, this was a fortunate occurrence. The /k/ was imbedded into carrier phrases as a final sound in the word *make*, releasing a variety of other sounds that followed it. Here are some examples:

Make a book.
Make a man.
Make a boy.
Make a goat.
Make a sun.
Make some food.
Make some money.
Make the bell.

As is evident, these were close to nonsense phrases but were selected for practice in coarticulation sequencing. They were spoken rapidly with no pause between words. *Make a boy* was modeled as /ˈmækəˈbɔɪ/ in rhythmical fashion, one phrase quickly followed by another. Other phrases were introduced to practice rapid articulation sequences of /s, z, θ, ð/. Fricatives were introduced between and after vowels:

It's a boy.
It's a girl.
It's a cake.
He's a son.
He's a cook.
There's a man.
There's a girl.

Both are big.
Both are soap.
Take a bath.

This phase of therapy is best typified as a drill and practice routine. Following 3 to 5 minutes of this drill, the pathologist conversed with Clifford for a few minutes about school activities, his rabbit, the weather, and home duties. His articulation errors were noted as they occurred in certain phrases. These were recorded and used as variations of practice phrases. For example, Clifford once said [aiædəæmbəgə] (I had a hamburger). A series of phrases featuring the use of /h/ was generated and used for practice during the next session:

I had a hamburger.
I had a coat.
I had a comb.
I had a soup.
I had a goat.
I had a thumb.

These phrases were used as the fricative /h/ was introduced.

The voiced cognates were introduced in phrase contexts rather than taught as separate units. Taking advantage of assimilation of voicing components in the phrase, the pathologist could establish the voiced feature easily. Examples involve surrounding the target sound by vowels: "He's a man," where the /s/ becomes /z/ when surrounded by two vowels; "Even you," where /v/ is surrounded by vowels; and "He goes," where /g/ also is surrounded by vowels. In this way the voiced features of the vowels influence the voicing in the consonant.

Phrases also were constructed to maximize contrast in place and manner features. Place features were contrasted by the use of phrases that required rapid successive movements from front to back as in the following examples:*

It's a bug body.
$\quad\quad\;\;\overline{b}\,\overline{f}$
There's a tugboat.
$\quad\quad\quad\quad\;\overline{bf}$
It's a flag pole.
$\quad\quad\;\;\overline{b}\,\overline{f}$
He makes buildings.
$\;\;\overline{f}\;\overline{b}\quad\;\;\overline{f}\;\overline{b}$
Grandpa comes home.
$\quad\;\overline{f}\;\;\overline{b}$

Manner changes are illustrated by these phrases:*

Like some tar.
$\overline{\text{s}}\ \overline{\text{f}}$
Cook for me.
$\overline{\text{s}}\ \overline{\text{f}}$
Dig some dirt.
$\overline{\text{s}}\ \overline{\text{f}}$
Give him pepper.
$\overline{\text{s}}\ \overline{\text{f}}$
There's papa.
$\overline{\text{f}\ \text{s}}$

*f = front; b = back
s = stop; f = fricative

Following a month of this practice, it was clearly evident that Clifford's use of frication during conversational speech had increased greatly. The /s, z, θ, ə, v, ʃ, h/ fricatives were included in his daily conversations with his mother and his speech for the most part was intelligible. Previously, only about 10 percent of his speech had been understandable.

Introduction of /ɝ/ and /r/

After the fricatives and velars were well established, it was decided to introduce /ɝ/. There was doubt that this could be taught by telephone since evoking /ɝ/ usually requires shaping fine sound distinctions. After directions were provided regarding tongue placement (up and back), Clifford was able to produce an acceptable /ɝ/ following presentation of the pathologist's model. His mother also provided models that the child could imitate.

Once the /ɝ/ was produced in isolation several times, the word *her* was introduced and was imitated easily. From that point, phrases were used as follows:

her coat
her comb
her gun
her gas
her cold

Velars were used following /ɝ/ to minimize place contrasts. Later, two-syllable words were added: *mother, father, sister, heater, bumper, feather,* etc. The addition of some vowel changes expanded the number of /ɝ/

Treatment of Articulation Disorders

words that could be used. / a ɝ / vowel combinations added words such as *car, far, tar, bar, arm, barn,* etc. These words were incorporated immediately into phrase drills as follows:

See her arm.
The bar is big.
His car is nice.
Far away.

Other vowel changes practiced were such words as *hurt, early, air, fire, ear, tear, fear, four, door,* etc. These words also were used as parts of phrases. The fricatives and velars were included to provide additional practice on those elements.

The consonantal /r/ was introduced in phrase context by paring a postvocalic / ɝ / with the consonantal /r/ in phrases illustrated by:

car over
car ran over
the car rolled
mother read
father ran
fire rope

Introduction of Affricatives

The affricative / tʃ / was introduced last, although Clifford had been producing close approximations of this sound while practicing the fricatives. Words were selected containing / tʃ / in the final position: *match, catch, batch, latch,* etc. Sentence-phrases were as follows:

Catch a man.
Catch a boy.
Catch a girl.
Match a book.
Latch a door.
Pitch a ball.

Introduction of Consonant Clusters

The final phase of treatment involved selecting consonant clusters that would provide practice first with /s/ clusters /sm, sn, sk, st, sp, sl/ followed by the liquid and velar clusters /kl, bl, gr, kr, pl, gl/. Clifford already was beginning to use some of these clusters correctly even though they were not taught. They simply were incorporated into daily practice phrases.

Treatment sessions included engaging the child in increasing amounts of conversational topics as a check on the use of correct articulation of the sounds practiced during the drill sessions. It was noticed that correct use of the target sounds during treatment sessions always was more frequent than their inclusion in conversational speech.

EVALUATION OF PROGRESS

Clifford was tested three times over a four-month period to provide a more detailed account of articulation change. While the first two tests did not reveal great changes, significant advances were noted during the third test. Fricatives and velars almost always were correct. /ɜ/ and /r/ were correct about 50 percent of the time and the affricatives were present but somewhat distorted. A few of the clusters were being used correctly five months after treatment was initiated.

It was decided therapy could be terminated at this time. Another articulation test administered two months later showed continued improvement. His speech was entirely intelligible although he continued to make occasional errors.

Following summer vacation, Clifford attended first grade. An itinerate speech pathologist who was unaware that Clifford had received treatment tested his articulation. Her recommendation was that his few errors were so minor that speech remediation was not warranted. By the time Clifford completed first grade, his articulation skills matched those of his peers.

It is important to point out that several favorable factors helped achieve rapid success in learning articulation skills:

1. Clifford seemed to have no neurological or motor problems that could have impeded progress.
2. Clifford's hearing appeared to be quite acute; the presence of a moderate or even slight hearing loss could have affected progress adversely.
3. Clifford was highly motivated to follow instructions and engage in the drill activities.
4. Clifford's mother cooperated in following instructions and created a favorable learning environment.

Obviously, there is much more involved in the execution of effective articulation remediation than simply a well-structured plan. Motivational factors, good relationship with the pathologist, and interest level all are important factors.

This chapter has provided a strategy that should help in designing an effective plan to modify articulation skills. If it is possible to create suitable motivation, obtain client cooperation, and eliminate or reduce causal factors, the pathologist should be successful in changing articulation patterns. In summarizing, the important points to remember are: (1) make an adequate diagnosis of the problem, (2) develop and execute the treatment program, and (3) control motivational factors.

REFERENCES

Anderson, V. *Improving the child's speech*. New York: Oxford, 1953.

Crocker, J. A phonological model of children's articulation competence. *Journal of Speech and Hearing Disorders*, 1969, *34*, 203–213.

Goldman, R., & Fristoe, M. *Goldman-Fristoe test of articulation*. Circle Pines, Minn.: American Guidance Services, 1969.

Mager, R. *Preparing instructional objectives*. Palo Alto: Fearon Publishers, 1962.

McCabe, R., & Bradley, D. Systematic multiple phonemic approach to articulation therapy. *Acta Symbolica*, 1975, *6*, 1–18.

McDonald E. *Articulation testing and treatment: A sensory-motor motor approach*. Pittsburgh: Stanwix House, Inc., 1964.

McReynolds, L., & Huston, K. A distinctive feature analysis of children's misarticulation training. *Journal of Speech and Hearing Disorders*, 1971, *36*, 155–168.

McReynolds, L., Kohn, J., & Williams, G. Articulatory-defective children's discrimination of their production errors. *Journal of Speech and Hearing Disorders*, 1975, *40*, 327–338.

Mowrer, D. *Methods of modifying speech behaviors*. Columbus, Ohio: Charles E. Merrill Publishing Co., 1977.

Mowrer, D., Baker, R., & Schutz, R. Operant procedures in the control of speech articulation. In H. Sloane and B. MacAaulay (eds.), *Operant procedures in remedial speech and language training*. New York: Houghton Mifflin Co., 1968.

Mowrer, D., Baker, R., & Schutz, R. *S programed articulation control kit*. Tempe, Arizona: IDEAS, 1974.

Poole, E. Genetic development of articulation of consonant sounds in speech. *Elementary English Review*, 1934, *11*, 159–161.

Prather, E. M., Hedrick, D. L., & Kern, C. A. Articulation development in children aged two to four years. *Journal of Speech and Hearing Disorders*, 1975, *40*, 179–191.

Templin, M. Certain language skills in children: Their development and interrelationships. *Institute of Child Welfare Monograph 26*. Minneapolis: University of Minnesota Press, 1957.

Van Riper, C. *Speech correction: Principles and methods* (4th ed.). Englewood Cliffs, New Jersey: Prentice Hall Inc., 1964.

Weiner, P. Auditory discrimination and articulation. *Journal of Speech and Hearing Disorders,* 1967, *32,* 19–29.

Wellman, B. L., Case, I. M., Mengert, I. G., & Bradbury, D. E. Speech sounds of young children. *University of Iowa Studies in Child Welfare,* 1931, *5* (2).

Williams, G., and McReynolds, L. The relationship between discrimination and articulation training in children with misarticulations. *Journal of Speech and Hearing Disorders,* 1975, *18,* 401–412.

NOTE

1. Picture card stimuli publishers include the following:

   IDEAS
   Box 741
   Tempe, Ariz. 85281

   Word Making Productions
   Box 15038
   Salt Lake City, Utah 84115

   Communication Skill Builders
   Box 42050-S
   Tucson, Ariz. 85733

   Teaching Resources
   50 Pond Park Road
   Hingham, Mass. 02043

Section II
Voice Disorders

Chapter 4

Voice Therapy in the School System

Among the many disorders of communication found in primary, intermediate, or secondary schools, those of voice traditionally comprise the lowest percentage of a speech/language pathologist's (SLP's) caseload. Gillespie and Cooper (1973) report a low 1.2 percent incidence of voice disorder among school children, Silverman and Zimmer (1975) a much higher incidence of 23.4 percent. Senturia and Wilson (1968) report a moderate incidence of 6 percent among more than 32,000 children. Regardless of whether the actual incidence in a given school population approaches any of those figures, the SLP's typical voice therapy caseload does not seem to reflect the expected incidence of such children. There could be several reasons for this: poor identification procedures, priority judgments of the SLP that place other forms of communication disorder higher than voice cases, or a feeling of incompetency about how to proceed to identify and remediate these students.

The intent of this chapter is to provide practical suggestions to the SLP who may need help in identifying, evaluating, and treating students with voice disorders. The identification and treatment concepts are practical and workable without requiring the SLP to abandon principles of voice science. While most SLPs have the background and experience to be competent with voice disordered students, others do not. Many are not comfortable with such factors as pitch identification, pitch modification, vocal range, voice quality analysis, and a multitude of additional details involved in voice therapy.

One case illustrates the frustration many SLPs experience in working with voice clients. R.D., a 15-year-old male high school student, was referred by a local otolaryngologist because of persistent dyplophonia (double-pitched voice) and extremely high pitch. Another physician had treated him for contact ulcers on the vocal processes of the arytenoids by placing him on two months of voice rest. At the end of that period, the contact ulcer had improved but voice quality and pitch had not. R.D. also had been receiving voice therapy for a year at school by a recently graduated SLP with a master's degree.

In the first session, it was apparent immediately that R.D.'s voice disorder was not based on contact ulcers or any organic condition but resulted from his inability to let his voice change after puberty, a voice disorder known as puberphonia. The specific treatment involved in this case is explained later in this chapter, but suffice it to say that 30 minutes after beginning therapy, R.D. had a new masculine voice that included normal quality and pitch parameters. A few days later, the school SLP who had been working with R.D. called to express frustration about working so long and unsuccessfully with a student, only to have someone else correct the problem in 30 minutes. Perhaps the most significant aspect of this case was that the SLP had not been trained to work with puberphonia. The individual had been exposed to it academically but not in practice—and both were needed.

This chapter cannot replace a well-taught graduate course in voice disorders with associated practicum experiences. However, it does provide the SLP who has a background in voice disorder with the information necessary to work with the cases usually found in school systems. This includes general information about professional relationships with physicians and support personnel in the schools, about voice parameters of a normal nature, and about evaluation and treatment steps for specific problems. No attempt is made to cover voice disorders not typically found in the school.

MEDICAL EVALUATION AND REFERRAL PROCESSES

One of the most troublesome concerns school SLPs experience when working with voice cases is knowing when to refer for medical consultation. Many SLPs have been trained never to work with a voice case until there has been a medical inspection of the larynx and the physician has cleared the student for therapy. This becomes frustrating because medical referral requires parental support and usually a significant amount of money. Often a student is identified as having a voice disorder and the referral process is begun, only to be stopped by a parent who is not willing to take the child to a physician who can view the larynx and report on its condition. Or the SLP refers a child with a voice disorder to a physician who reports "nothing is wrong." Then parents ask, "Why the referral? Why the expense?"

Although there are no easy solutions to these problems, some recommendations are presented next. Medical referral is an important part of voice management. When deliberate and well-thought-out processes are followed, a significantly greater number of referrals will be well handled. But this cannot be done casually. It requires hard work in developing professional relations with local medical communities.

Communication with medical personnel must occur. Some otolaryngologists (ear, nose and throat physicians) are happy to work closely with SLPs but others are not so cooperative. This is a reality of the professional relationships between these disciplines. SLPs seeking good relationships should obtain an appointment with an otolaryngologist to whom a referral is likely. SLPs then should explain that they realize referral to the medical community is important in the management of voice clients and ask to discuss how this best can occur. They should ask questions such as:

- How do you feel about referring all persistently hoarse children for a laryngoscopic examination?
- Who should not be referred?
- What happens when you examine a student who is hoarse and your evaluation does not identify any vocal fold pathology?
- How do you feel children with vocal nodules should be handled? With surgery? Vocal therapy? Both?

Each SLP should have specific attitudes about these questions but this dialogue with the physician might influence both professionals. At any rate, this communication process allows the SLP to establish good rapport and help decide which physicians are receptive to voice referrals. Open communication is essential for this rapport.

Parental support of the referral process is most important. Many problems must be overcome to gain parental support, but once again, communication is essential. A note home usually produces results in only a few cases. A telephone call is better. A personal appointment is best and much needed for successful referral follow-up. The SLP should call the parents and set up the appointment and must be prepared to convince them that a voice disorder exists. It is hard to do this with words only so the SLP must communicate with pictures, models, and tape recordings. These are commercially available.

Wilson and Rice (1977) have published a voice disorder kit that constitutes an excellent method to help convince parents to be concerned about these problems. The kit contains slides of normal and abnormal vocal folds plus taped samples of children and adults with various voice disorders. These can be used to explain in either a simple or complex manner why there should be a medical referral. The student also should be present during this explanation. At the end of the presentation, the parents and student should understand what comprises a voice disorder, its long-term and short-term consequences, possible causes, why the medical referral is necessary to determine the specific reason, and whether medical treatment is necessary before or during therapy. This communication process greatly increases the probability of a successful referral.

SCREENING AND IDENTIFICATION PROCESSES

Students with voice disorder usually are identified by means of screening by an SLP during the early weeks of the school year or by teacher referral. To identify these students accurately, both the SLP and the teacher must have a working knowledge of what normal voice is and is not. It is appropriate for the SLP to hold a short workshop early in the school year to teach the faculty basic listening skills to help the identification process. Once again, the Wilson and Rice (1977) kit is helpful by providing slides and taped examples of specific disorders.

Many teachers have little understanding of the voice and the bases of voice disorder. A voice disorder workshop should be directed at general listening skills necessary to help identify the two most common areas of voice disorder found in schools: hoarseness and excessive nasality. Many other voice concerns could be taught, but it is wise to keep the instructional process simple and manageable. The lecture should cover one disorder that causes hoarseness, e.g., vocal nodules, and one that produces excessive nasality, e.g., cleft palate. It is a good idea to show slides that illustrate the laryngeal and pharyngeal bases of these disorders, play taped samples of voice and speech characteristics, and provide practice in listening and judging recorded samples. The one or two hours needed for such a presentation should open considerable dialogue between the teaching staff and the SLP and improve voice management.

Problems in Voice Screening

When screening children, it is necessary to keep in mind that voice patterns and conditions are highly changeable and capricious. Many severe voice disorders are a result of temporary conditions. A child may have a severe cold or allergic reaction that causes changes in the laryngeal structures that produce hoarseness. It is inappropriate to enroll such a child in voice therapy until more is known about the persistency of the vocal pattern. Since the same voice characteristics can be caused by temporary as well as by more persistent etiologies, it is necessary to follow up on screening to ensure the child has a condition that requires remediation. Questions should be asked of the child at the screening, such as: "Does your voice always sound as it does today? Do you have a cold? How long has your voice sounded like this?" The reliability of the information the child provides may be questionable but the answers can provide some insight as to whether the voice disorder is temporary or persistent. These same questions should be asked of the classroom teacher about a child identified as having hoarseness.

Regardless of the information gained from such questions to the child and teacher, the pupil should be screened again two weeks later. To compare vocal patterns two weeks apart, it is necessary to have a taped sample of the child's voice. At the initial screening, a recording should be made of any child whose voice is abnormal. The pupil should state date, name, and school, and count from 1 to 20. That is the only sample needed to compare the child's voice upon rescreening. When the question of persistency of voice disorder has been determined and vocal pattern judged abnormal, the next question is whether medical referral is necessary.

When to Refer to a Physician

To be on the safe side of this question, the SLP can refer every child with any kind of voice disorder for medical clearance before initiating therapy. However, such a conservative approach is unnecessary. The primary concern is that a child might have a serious medical condition in the laryngeal structures requiring surgery or medicine rather than therapy. Such conditions do exist and the concern is legitimate. A question often is raised as to whether the SLP should be concerned about laryngeal cancer in children. That is so rare in children that the SLP need not refer them just to make sure they do not have cancer. But there are nonrare medical conditions that can be progressive and interfere with breathing, and the SLP should be aware of these possibilities.

Juvenile papillomatosis is a condition resembling wart-like growths in the body. The growths can occur in the larynx and obstruct the airway. The vocal symptoms are not easily distinguished from those produced by a less threatening condition such as vocal nodules, but the treatment is radically different and entirely medical. Other conditions such as laryngeal web, polyps, laryngeal paralysis, and laryngeal trauma all can produce similar voice symptoms. Medical investigation of the larynx thus is necessary to determine the exact cause of the vocal symptoms.

Therefore, a safe but not necessarily conservative position is that any child with a voice disorder stemming from abnormal functioning of the vocal folds that produces abnormal voice quality, or in any way makes breathing difficult, should be evaluated medically before management by SLP. The abnormalities that constitute this criterion include breathiness, tension, hoarseness, dyplophonia, or any combination of these. They are discussed in detail later. The SLP also may refer pitch problems without these characteristics of voice quality, or resonance problems not involving velopharyngeal closure, or loudness, but such disorder will not likely be found to have an organic basis. Experience with these youths can help shape the philosophy of each SLP as to when referrals should be made. Before sufficient experience has been obtained to shape the philosophy, it is well to be more liberal in selecting those who need medical referral. It is better to err on the side of overreferral.

PARAMETERS OF VOICE

The parameters of voice production discussed next are critical to understanding the clinical aspects of human phonation. Each of these must be evaluated in the screening and management of students suspected of voice disorder.

Pitch

The pitch of a human voice is a psychological or perceptual correlate of the physical dimension of frequency of vocal fold vibration. When exhaled air from the lungs reaches the closed vocal folds, pressure builds until it is sufficient to blow the vocal folds apart setting them into vibration. The frequency of vibration establishes the pitch. Stated more simply, a person's voice is high, low, average, appropriate, or inappropriate for a given age and sex, depending on how many times per second the vocal folds vibrate when activated by exhaled air. There are complex anatomical, physiological, and acoustical bases in this process and the reader should investigate references that detail them (Daniloff, Schuckers, & Feth, 1980; Minifie, Hixon, & Williams, 1973).

Frequency of vocal fold vibration is determined by the critical variables of (1) vocal fold length, (2) vocal fold mass, (3) vocal fold tension, and (4) airflow and subglottic air pressure factors. These variables interact in a complex fashion to determine the pitch of a person's voice. Age and sex differences are apparent and reflected in pitch.

The SLP evaluating the student is not capable of determining the status of the vocal folds with regard to length, mass, and tension except by listening to and determining the pitch of the voice. Then only subjective judgments about the actual sizes of the vocal folds can be made. It therefore is the student's pitch that is critical to evaluate, seldom the length, mass, and tension. Is the pitch appropriate for the age and sex of the student being evaluated? Is it too low? Too high? Monopitched?

Essentials of Pitch Evaluation

In pitch evaluation, the SLP's task is to determine the student's habitual pitch level and determine how that relates to the level that would be optimal. The *habitual pitch* is the modal or average level heard in a continuing vocal stream. It is the level around which normal pitch inflections up and down occur. It is the one heard most commonly as a person talks—the central tendency of pitch. The *optimal pitch* is the one best suited for the length, mass, and tension of the student's larynx. Under the best of conditions, the habitual pitch level used (the most common) should be the same as the optimal (the best suited). This often is not the case. It is necessary to evaluate both the habitual and optimal levels to determine whether they are the same or different and, if different, how clinically significant the variance is.

Pitch can be evaluated by means of complex and elaborate equipment, or with a simple pitch pipe that can be purchased for a few dollars at any music store. The SLP can use the pitch pipe to determine the essential pitch characteristics of students when a few basic procedures and concepts are followed and understood. The pitch pipe is a miniature harmonica-type instrument that produces 13 specific tones in an octave. The tones include sharps and flats, which are half-tone steps either up (sharp) or down (flat) from the reference tone. Many SLPs become uncomfortable when asked to deal with musical language such as octaves, tones, sharps, flats, etc. To evaluate pitch in a student, some basic concepts in musical language are needed. Here are the basic ones:

- The range of musical tones in the human voice can be compared to the notes on a piano or on a pitch pipe.
- The piano tones range from 27 Hz to 4186 Hz.
- These tones can be divided into octaves.
- An octave represents a doubling of the numbers of vibration, so a tone of 100 Hz doubled to 200 Hz would constitute an octave jump.
- A numerical indication is given from the lowest octave (1) to the next octave (2), to the next (3), etc.
- Each octave is divided into eight whole tones, with each tone represented by a letter of the alphabet (ABCDEFGA)
- From A to B is one whole tone step. A sharp (A#) represents half a tone step up. A half tone stepped up from A is either A# or Bb (A sharp or B flat).

- Each tone on the musical scale is indicated by its alphabetic note (ABCDEFGA) in the octave it represents such as (A_4), or by its actual numerical frequency (Hz), such as 220 Hz. Thus, A in the fourth octave (A_4) also is 220 Hz. A in the fifth octave (A_5) is 440 Hz.

The human voice is capable of producing tones that can be closely matched to notes or tones on the musical scale, whether a pitch pipe or piano is used as the source. Some SLPs have difficulty matching the pitch of a person's voice to a note on a piano or pitch pipe. However, there are many voice disorders in which the habitual and optimal pitch levels must be determined to manage the disorder properly. Therefore, how an SLP can sample a person's voice to obtain pitch information is outlined step by step. The age and sex of the person being evaluated must be known since pitch appropriateness is based on these factors. In the following steps to help identify the habitual or most commonly used pitch level, the SLP will:

- Have the student count from 1 to 10. This lets the SLP hear the pitch level used in typical speech.
- Have the student repeat counting the first three numbers, i.e., 1, 2, 3 ... 1, 2, 3 ... 1, 2, 3 ... and so on.
- Ask the student, after that counting, to hold onto the vowel sound in "thr*ee*." It appears like this: "One, two, three ... one, two, threeeeeeeee."
- Blow notes on the pitch pipe until one that matches the student's voice on the "eeeee" is heard. When the matching tone is found, the habitual pitch level probably has been found.
- Verify that the pitch level found is the habitual one used by having the student talk or read as the tone is played on the pitch pipe. The SLP checks as to whether the student's pitch matches the tone being played. If so, the habitual pitch has been found.
- Mark on a piece of paper the tone found on the pitch pipe that represents the students habitual pitch level, e.g., $A\#_4$, which would mean A sharp in the fourth octave.

Finding the habitual pitch level is only the first step in determining the appropriateness of the one the student is using. The SLP then must determine the optimal pitch, the one best suited for the student's voice structure. The typical person has a pitch range of about two octaves from lowest tone to highest, and the optimal pitch level usually is found about three or four whole tones from the bottom of the range. Therefore, here are steps to follow in locating the optimal pitch level of a student. The SLP will:

- Have the student hum the tone that was established as the habitual pitch level, e.g., $A\#_4$.
- Start at the habitual pitch and have the student hum down the scale in whole tones until the lowest tone possible has been produced. This is the basal tone.
- Have the student hum up the musical scale in whole tones until about four above the basal. This should produce a tone that is close if not the optimal pitch.
- Determine when the optimal pitch has been reached because the student's voice suddenly becomes a little louder and the tone easier to produce.
- Verify the optimal pitch by having the student start at the lowest pitch again and hum up in whole tones until reaching the fourth tone above the basal. Each tone upward from the basal should be easier to produce and its loudness will increase without greater effort. If repeated attempts at this procedure produce the same tone that suddenly increases in loudness without effort, the optimal probably has been found.

The SLP must keep in mind that the optimal pitch level is a subjective one at which voice production seems easiest for the student. It usually is found about four tones above the basal. This is not to say that the tone four whole steps from the basal is the only optimal pitch, but merely the lowest that should function as the best habitual pitch for the student. The pupil should be able to speak comfortably in a narrow range of pitches beginning no lower than the optimal and ending a few tones above. The student using the optimal pitch level habitually takes much less effort to produce voice with the normal pitch inflections and loudness changes necessary to provide dynamic characteristics.

As noted, the typical human voice has a pitch range of about two octaves. An octave contains eight whole tones, so most people have a speaking range of about sixteen tones. Since the optimal pitch usually is about four tones above the basal of that 16-tone range, this means that a person typically has much more potential for pitch inflection upward than downward when speaking at the optimal pitch. This is exactly what voice scientists and SLPs have found in their work with pitch for children and adults, males and females.

Significance of Pitch in School Children

Although accurate evaluation of pitch in school children requires skill knowledge, it may be of some comfort to know that pitch is seldom such a critical factor in voice disorder among children in the primary grades that it needs to be changed. Pitch becomes more critical in some of the disorders in teenagers, which is analyzed later. However, when the need to evaluate pitch in a student's voice is necessary, it constitutes a great challenge to even the experienced SLP. The steps outlined in this chapter are intended to simplify somewhat the process of pitch evaluation.

When pitch is a factor in a given voice case, the SLP should (1) find the habitual pitch, (2) identify the optimal pitch, (3) determine whether they are the same, and (4) bring them into conformity if they are different. If the habitual pitch level is too low for the age and sex of the student, e.g., one or two tones from the basal, it probably will need to be raised to the optimal level to produce a voice that is used more efficiently. Speaking at too low a pitch level can abuse the vocal folds and produce tissue damage. This is discussed in more detail later in this chapter. On the other hand, if the habitual pitch level is too high, it usually is a concern only if it causes sex confusion (male student with a high voice mistaken for female on the telephone). Rarely will a too-high pitch be a cause of vocal abuse unless it is so high it approaches the upper extreme of the pitch range. This rarely is the case.

Voice Quality

In addition to pitch, another important voice parameter is overall quality of production. This is a confusing dimension for most SLPs since the terms used to describe human voice quality have little scientific basis or semantic uniformity. Such abstract terms as *mellow, rich, harsh, raspy, piercing, twangy,* and *throaty* are difficult to imagine, let alone to describe. Unfortunately, there are few if any terms that can describe voice quality in a uniform way without using the strict language of voice science, which working SLPs usually do not understand clearly. Some terms used to describe voice quality seem to have more clinical relevance and semantic uniformity than others, and are used in this chapter.

Voice quality in humans is determined either at the vibrating vocal fold level or by the shaping and resonating of sound produced by the vocal folds in the chambers of the pharynx, oral, and nasal cavities. When quality is negatively affected at the vocal fold level, it is because the folds are not vibrating properly as a result of some organic or functional condition in the larynx. The resonance processes cannot mask the negative effect produced by the vocal folds when they are vibrating abnormally. Normal voice quality requires a sound source at the vocal fold level that involves uniform vibration of the two folds, a process described as vocal fold periodicity. To have normal periodicity of vocal fold vibration, the mass, length, and tension factors of each must be uniform so a constant and sufficient airflow from the lungs will have the same effect on each fold. This sets them into uniform or periodic vibration and the tone produced (glottal tone) will be normal.

Hypofunctional and Hyperfunctional

Several conditions in the larynx might affect this process. The vocal folds might vibrate with too little approximation, allowing excessive air escape through the glottis (the space between the vocal folds). The voice will sound breathy. On the other hand, too much approximation can result in a voice quality marked by excessive tension. These conditions are described as being hypofunctional (too little approximation) or hyperfunctional (too much approximation) voice quality.

Extremes of hypofunctional and hyperfunctional voice quality occur often. An extreme of hypofunctional approximation is no voice at all (aphonia). An extreme of hyperfunctional approximation produces a voice quality that is so tense that airflow from the lungs cannot overcome the resistance of the taut vocal folds, producing a quality that is called a spastic voice. Between these extremes are the gradients of voice quality that reflect a continuum from hypofunction to hyperfunction. The voice qualities reflected in this continuum of function are described next in what it is hoped is sufficient detail to allow the SLP to be comfortable with each one. Exhibit 4-1 illustrates this continuum of function at the vocal fold level.

When voices are described as having one or more of these six factors, the term is used merely in a general sense to define the vocal characteristics that can be heard. The following is a description of each of the voice characteristics indicated on the continuum:

Aphonia

This quality is not likely to be heard in a student because it is rare in any population. A person who is a true aphonic has no voice at all. It would be comparable to someone who had lost the larynx surgically (laryngectomy). Other than the person who has been laryngectomized, the aphonic individual is someone who for psychological reasons makes no attempt to produce voice or who is so weak from illness or neurological disease that voice production is not possible. Stated simply, when listening to an aphonic person, nothing is heard.

Whisper

This quality is easy to understand and identify because everyone has had an occasion to use it deliberately in such instances as in the library or

Exhibit 4-1 Continuum of Voice Quality

Hypofunction	Normal Function	Hyperfunction
Aphonia...Whisper...Breathiness...	Normal Tension...	Excessive Tension...Spasticity

church, or behind someone's back. The person who can *only* whisper, however, has a serious voice disorder. It could be caused by organic disease or psychological difficulty. The quality of whisper voice is emitted by vocal folds that are so far apart during speaking attempts that only articulated airstream is heard. This articulation of sounds without voice support is the distinguishing characteristic between the whisper quality and aphonia. In other words, the consonant sounds articulated by the tongue, teeth, or lips are heard in the whisper quality, but no voice supports them.

Breathiness

This is a mixture of voice with an excessive escape of air during speaking attempts. On the low end of the continuum, it is almost like a whisper except that a slight amount of voice is heard. There are degrees of breathiness ranging from the near whisper just described to nearly normal voice. The significance of these subtle degrees of breathiness is important to recognize in the clinical management of many voice disorders.

Normal Voice Quality

This is difficult to describe because of the numerous differences between individuals' voices. However, there are characteristics that must be present to produce normal vocal fold vibration. The vocal folds must be completely but not excessively approximated at midline when air from the exhaled lungs hits them. This complete approximation must be along the entire length of the folds. If the tissue length and mass are equal on each vocal fold and if the vibrating edge of each is uniform, air pressure below the closed folds will cause them to vibrate passively.

This vibration is the sound source of the human voice. This sound is then resonated in the chambers of the vocal tract (pharynx, oral cavity, and nasal cavity) and shaped by the articulators (tongue, teeth, velum, lips) into speech. The symmetry of the two vocal folds constitutes the primary basis for normal voice quality. Key factors such as tissue symmetry, complete approximation along the entire vibrating edge, an adequate air supply to drive the vibration, and proper resonance to shape and modify the tone all are needed. Otherwise, the voice quality will be abnormal. The SLP usually can tell whether these factors are present by listening and critically analyzing the quality of the voice.

Excessive Tension

A significant factor in many voice quality disorders is excessive tension. This is heard when there is too much approximation of the vocal folds at midline during voice production. Tension can exist on a continuum from slight (beyond normal) to a degree that stops the passive vibration process. It is a factor of excessive glottal resistance to airflow and subglottal air pressure. The more tension present, the greater the factors of airflow and subglottal pressure needed to cause vibration.

Spasticity

When vocal tension from too much approximation of the vocal folds is so great that even increased effort is not sufficient to overcome the resistance, voice is stopped and vocal spasticity has occurred. In most cases, vocal spasticity is an intermittent phenomenon during voice production rather than a complete stoppage at all times. Typically, the person with a voice quality described as spastic manifests periods of excessive tension with periodic moments of spasticity.

In addition to the voice quality parameters just described, which represent variances along the continuum from hypofunction to hyperfunction, several voice characteristics are comprised of combinations of factors. The most common of these is hoarseness.

Hoarseness

Many different organic conditions affecting the vocal folds can produce the quality described as hoarseness. When a person has a cold and accompanying laryngitis, the voice quality heard is called hoarseness. Hoarseness is caused by upper respiratory infections, allergies in the larynx, growths on the vocal folds (including cancer), and numerous other conditions, many of which are described in detail later in this chapter. Because the etiologies of hoarseness are so varied, the patterns of voice quality falling within its characteristics similarly are varied.

Most varieties of hoarseness result when the condition of the vocal folds prevents normal approximation and symmetrical vibration. For example, folds swollen from an infection usually are not affected uniformly. The mass characteristics of each fold therefore are different. In addition, the vibrating edge of each fold may be rough and uneven, resulting in incomplete approximation while speaking. This incomplete approximation produces a breathy quality.

Tension is introduced when the person attempts to overcome breathiness. These factors of breathiness and tension, coupled with vocal folds that vibrate aperiodically because of mass differences, form the bases of hoarseness. Some forms of hoarseness involve a wet quality when excessive mucous secretions are present on the tissue of the folds. Other forms sound excessively dry when there is insufficient lubrication of those tissues. For example, when vocal folds have been exposed to extreme amounts of radiation, as in one treatment of cancer, they are affected in many ways, including excessive dryness for a period of time (see Chapter 7). Hoarseness in all its many forms can range from slight to severe.

Resonance

Many voice disorders have nothing to do with how the vocal folds vibrate but what happens to the tone they generate in the resonation chambers of the oral and nasal cavities. This process adds richness and fullness to the voice but only when normal resonance factors occur. Many children and adults have poor vocal resonance, which affects the quality of the voice. The most common resonance disorders of children occur when the nasal cavity is not used properly as a resonator. When inadequate or excessive nasal resonance occurs, the disorder is known as hyponasality or hypernasality, respectively.

Hyponasality

Under normal conditions, the nasal cavity is used as a resonator when the following sounds are produced: /m/, /n/, and / ŋ /. Whether the nasal cavity is used properly in producing these sounds is determined by its overall condition and that of the structure that opens and closes access to it from the oral cavity, the palatopharyngeal or velopharyngeal mechanism, hereafter called velopharyngeal mechanism. When the nasal cavity is normal and the velopharyngeal mechanism is working properly, sound is introduced into the cavity during speech attempts to produce the nasal consonants /m/, /n/, or / ŋ /. However, when a condition exists in the cavity that decreases the space available for nasal resonance, such as during a cold or severe nasal allergy, proper production of these sounds cannot occur. The overall quality is perceived as a lack of nasal resonance on sounds that ordinarily require it. The /m/ sound is heard essentially as a /b/, the /n/ as a /d/, and the / ŋ / as a /g/. Evaluation and treatment considerations of hyponasal voice quality are discussed later in this chapter.

Hypernasality

When the velopharyngeal mechanism is working properly during speech, the oral and nasal cavities are separated completely except during the production of the nasal consonants /m/, /n/, and / ŋ /. Several conditions in the speech mechanism can affect negatively the ability of the velopharyngeal mechanism to close and separate the oral and nasal cavities. The result is a voice quality that sounds excessively nasal. All vowel sounds are nasalized and, when the condition is severe, many consonants are affected by leakage of air pressure out the nose. The specific conditions that cause hypernasality are explained later in this chapter along with evaluation and treatment considerations.

SPECIFIC DISORDERS OF VOICE

A number of voice disorders are described next in sufficient detail to allow the SLP to evaluate and remediate each one. The descriptions include case examples of persons seen by the author of this chapter. Only disorders commonly seen in the school system are discussed.

Mutational Falsetto (Puberphonia)

During puberty, the typical male experiences major body changes as a result of growth and hormone development. The larynx changes rapidly in concert with general body growth. Voice quality and pitch change significantly. The pitch of a young man's voice manifests the most significant and noticeable vocal change. As a result of rather sudden increases in vocal fold length and mass, the typical male's pitch will drop about one octave, or eight whole tones. The voice also becomes more resonant and acquires a richer and fuller quality. Essentially, in a few short months, the boy's voice has become a man's.

In some instances the transition from boy to man is not easy. Not only is it difficult to handle increased responsibility in life, but the rapid body changes often are confusing and difficult to accept and understand. When a boy experiences difficulty in making these adjustments to the voice, a disorder can develop that is termed mutational falsetto, or puberphonia (Aronson, 1980). It is a functional voice disorder that results when a boy is not able to make the vocal transition to manhood. The main symptom is maintained or raised pitch when growth of laryngeal tissue normally would dictate a significant lowering of the pitch. The result is a boy's voice in a man's body.

The actual development of this disorder is not understood clearly other than from the perspective of clinical experience. Several cases seen by the author of this chapter provide the following profile.

The male who develops puberphonia usually is one who is shy and somewhat insecure in personal relationships. Case history data from parents and clients verify this point. It is the authors' opinion that most males experience some embarrassment about the rapidly changing voice during puberty but this is a momentary concern. During this changing period, pitch breaks and other voice adjustment problems occur. These pitch breaks can produce momentary concern and embarrassment even to the well-adjusted male. However, when they occur in one who has a poor self-image, or who has experienced inadequate social relationships, the effect can be prolonged embarrassment and concern.

For example, should a pitch break occur around a friend or group of peers, teasing may result. Nobody enjoys being teased, but the boy who has a poor self-concept and is not secure in peer relationships can be psychologically devastated by it. When the source of the teasing is a pitch break or squeaky voice, the concern is directed at the voice. The boy is likely to become concerned about a repeat occurrence. It is almost as though he becomes so worried about a pitch break that it is on his mind each time he begins to talk, especially if he is in a socially difficult situation such as with a girl. The boy may think such thoughts as, "I wonder if my voice will squeak or break if I talk to her. I hope it doesn't happen here."

This concern about pitch stability before speaking sets the stage for the development of puberphonia. To secure pitch patterns and ensure that breaks will not occur, the boy may attempt to keep his pitch at the familiar level he has always used, i.e., his prepuberty level. He has experienced the physical changes of puberty, including those in his larynx, but has not allowed his voice to change into the lower pitch. He has functionally kept his pitch from lowering when structurally it should have. It is not long before his old pitch becomes stabilized in his new structure and the puberphonic voice disorder has been established.

The following are typical voice characteristics of the male who has developed mutational falsetto or puberphonia.

Pitch Factors

The typical pitch level in puberphonia is more closely matched to a female who has completed puberty. It is close to the tone of G in the 3rd octave (G_3). This is the lowest habitual pitch level the typical puberphonic male will use, although instances of extremely high (falsetto) samples are not uncommon. By contrast, a postpuberty 17-year-old male has a normal pitch of $C\#_3$, with an acceptable range of G_2 to $D\#_3$ (Wilson, 1979). The pitch frequently breaks upward or downward. The youth may even experience moments of "low voice" that occur when he is relaxed and not threatened by the speaking situation. Except for the breaks, the habitual pitch level of the typical puberphonic male is a monotone, devoid of natural inflections. Diplophonia (double pitch) is common. However, it is the unnaturally high voice that is the striking characteristic of this disorder.

Quality Factors

The voice of the puberphonic speaker usually is of normal quality in terms of laryngeal vibration and resonance. Hoarseness is rare. A slight amount of tension is heard at times but is a minor concern and probably results from the speaker's using a pitch level that is not optimal, with increased effort necessary to maintain voice continuity.

Loudness Factors

The boy with puberphonic voice has essentially normal loudness ability in conversation, but sometimes complains of not being able to yell. This is related to using a pitch level that is not compatible for the voice under optimal conditions, thus limiting its projection potential.

Evaluation Procedures in Puberphonia

Developing a Case History

Developing a case history is fairly straightforward. The SLP asks questions about the onset of the pitch disorder, the onset of puberty, what was happening socially during the puberty change, whether there were instances of speaking avoidance because of embarrassment about pitch breaks, and whether any conscious attempt was made to keep pitch at a high level.

Generally, it is necessary to gain perspective only about the relationship between puberty and the current state of the voice. Aronson (1980) suggests exploring such additional factors of etiology as delayed maturation of the laryngeal structures because of endocrine imbalance, severe hearing loss that makes pitch monitoring difficult, neurological disease during adolescence change, and general debilitating illness during puberty. All of these possibilities need exploration in a thorough case history. From this information it can be determined whether medical referral is necessary. If any question exists after such a case history as to the possibility of a physical basis for the pitch disorder, it is important to obtain current medical information on the student by appropriate referral.

Voice Evaluation

The voice characteristics of the puberphonic student are rated first on the parameters of pitch, quality, and loudness. This is important in obtaining a measurement of the habitual pitch level using procedures previously outlined. The SLP then tape-records a five-minute conversation during which the student reads a short paragraph. Any instances of low-pitched voice should be noted.

In most cases, after a case history and voice evaluation have been completed, it should be apparent that puberphonia is the basis for the disorder. It is particularly helpful to have medical information on the student either before or shortly after the evaluation indicating that the laryngeal structures are normal for voice production.

Stimulation Techniques

Once puberphonia is established as the basis for the pitch disorder, the SLP should explain to the student the likely relationship between the onset of puberty and the pitch problem. The SLP then states that techniques will be used in an attempt to find the boy's true pitch. One of the following two techniques should help facilitate normal pitch function:

- Cough: A human cough creates a sound that is a result of air vibrating the closed vocal folds. It is a rough form of phonation using the same mechanisms of normal voice production. Coughing, as compared to normal phonation, is a biological act and is not subject to the emotions associated with phonation in human communication. Therefore, the student coughs and the sound usually reflects the condition of the vocal folds in a natural state. The pitch of the cough roughly approximates the optimal pitch of the voice. A cough can facilitate the use of the optimal pitch.
- Digital Manipulation: Gentle pushing on the thyroid cartilage of the larynx during phonation suddenly relaxes the vocal folds and the pitch drops approximately one whole tone. The technique is to have the student relax and say "ah" as the SLP pushes gently on the thyroid cartilage. The pitch goes down and, when the dropped tone is heard, the youth is instructed to hold onto it as the pressure on the thyroid cartilage is released. The process is repeated as the student lowers his pitch in whole tone steps. When the pupil has a pitch that is optimal for his age, the SLP stabilizes and shapes it into conversation using techniques explained next.

A Case Example of Puberphonia

This example illustrates how the evaluation and treatment procedures for puberphonia can be handled. R.D., the 15-year-old male referred to at the beginning of this chapter, was referred to the author of this chapter by an otolaryngologist because of persistent dyplophonia (double-pitched voice) and an inappropriately high-pitched tone. He also had been treated by another physician who had diagnosed R.D. as having contact ulcers on his vocal folds. His case history revealed nothing of significance in relation to his pitch disorder other than the fact that his "voice did not change when it was supposed to." It seemed apparent that since recent examinations by otolaryngologists indicated normal laryngeal structures and the case history was devoid of significance other than the delayed voice change at puberty, R.D. was a true puberphonic. The following explanation to the youth as recorded by an SLP is an example of how voice management of this disorder could occur.

> Let me explain what has happened to your voice. During the years of puberty change, as your body was growing and changing, you probably experienced some frustration handling the pitch of your voice. This frustration led you to keep the pitch of your voice with which you were most familiar rather than let it change. We are going to try some techniques to help you find your best pitch. It may be easy, it may be hard, let's find out.
>
> First, I want you to cough like this. (SLP demonstrates cough.) Did you notice the sound of your cough was low . . . much lower than your speaking voice. That is because your vocal folds were vibrating at a pitch which was natural for them.
>
> Now, try it again. (R.D. coughs at $D\#_3$.) Good, try it again . . . and again. Now cough and prolong the cough into an "ah" sound like this. (SLP demonstrates.) (R.D. coughs, followed by an "ah" at the same pitch level.) Good. Notice your pitch stayed low with both the cough and the "ah." Do it again . . . and again.
>
> Now I want you to "think" of a cough without actually coughing and say "ah" at that pitch. (R.D. does it.) Good. Do it again. Now say "ah" like you have been, then go into an "o" sound like this. (SLP demonstrates.) (R.D. does it.) Good. Now you can say any sound at that pitch level. Say the following sounds after me. (R.D. repeats ten different vowel sounds after model.) Now count to 20 at the low pitch level. (R.D. does it with two slight breaks into a higher pitch.)
>
> Now say the ABCs at that pitch. (R.D. does it.) Now tell me your address and phone number. Good. Now I want you to read

this list of sentences using your new pitch level. If you get confused at where your pitch should be, just cough gently or think of a cough and speak at the cough level.

In a few minutes, using a biological state of the larynx to facilitate normal phonation at an optimal pitch level, R.D. learned to control his pitch and left the therapy session with a new voice. As he became comfortable with his new pitch, he relaxed and his voice lowered to an optimal and habitual pitch of A_3 (approximate Hz of 110). During the first session, he was able to read orally, converse with the SLP about school, and then chat for 20 minutes with his sister who had accompanied him. This conversation was monitored by the SLP to determine that the youth maintained his new pitch level.

As he left the clinic, R.D. was instructed to use his new pitch in any situation in which he felt comfortable. Called a few hours later by the SLP, the youth reported he had no difficulty using his new pitch in all speaking situations, including those with close friends. He mentioned that several persons had commented on his new voice, but he dismissed these by saying he had a cold. Four days later R.D. returned to the clinic and was recorded in conversation. All aspects of his voice were judged normal, including pitch, quality, and loudness. He was using his voice in all speaking situations and felt comfortable with it.

Special Considerations in Puberphonia

Although puberphonia is a functional voice disorder and easy to remediate when done properly, a few cautions need to be stated. As the SLP begins to change the student's voice, care should be taken not to indicate that if one specific technique is used the proper pitch level will occur, i.e., cough and the proper pitch will emerge. Rather, the SLP should indicate that several methods will be attempted to help the student find his new pitch and one of them should work. Then, if failure occurs on the first technique, the youth will not become discouraged easily. All the eggs have not been placed in one basket, so a new technique can be attempted easily.

Often when a youth hears his new low-pitched voice he will comment that he does not like it. This is understandable since he has never heard himself speaking low. Since he does not like it because he is not used to it, he may be somewhat reluctant to use it with others, assuming that they will not like it either. The SLP should tell him he soon will be used to it and that others will like it immediately. He should test his new voice with strangers, such as store clerks, and he will notice no negative reaction to his pitch. As he experiences such instances, he will develop confidence in the normal nature of his new pitch.

Care also should be taken not to lower the student's voice too much. Rather, the SLP should seek an optimal pitch level about three or four tones from his basal pitch. This new level will allow all downward inflections in his voice without approaching the basal, which would produce tension. Even when the pitch still seems somewhat high after lowering it, it should be kept in mind that as the student matures into adulthood his voice will become deeper in pitch and richer in resonance.

When the student expresses concern about using his new pitch around persons other than the SLP, it may be necessary to carefully control the process of generalization from the clinic or school therapy to other situations. This can be done through ranking in task difficulty all speaking situations, called hierarchy analysis of typical speaking situations (Boone, 1977) and by assigning the student to speak with his new voice first in situations low on the task hierarchy before moving onto the more stressful levels.

It is important that the change of pitch from the puberphonic level to the normal level occur quickly as compared to typical school communication disorder therapy durations of weeks and months. Within two or three days, the change should be complete. Even in settings such as the school where youths may be seen only a few minutes a week, it is important to change the schedule to accommodate intense therapy. The SLP must be assertive in expecting the student to use the new pitch in situations that may be rather uncomfortable for him at first. The youth should be told that the discomfort he experiences will be momentary and people soon will not even notice the change.

Working with youths who have puberphonia can be most satisfying to the SLP, who is used to seeing only slight change in communication performance even under prolonged therapy. To see a boy significantly change, in a few hours or days, a voice pattern that has caused so much concern and embarrassment can compensate for more frustrating therapy efforts.

Vocal Abuse in School Children (Vocal Nodules)

Perhaps the most common organic change in the laryngeal structures of children is the development of vocal nodules. Senturia and Wilson (1968) screened 32,500 school children for voice disorder and found 6 percent with abnormal patterns. Of those examined later by indirect laryngoscopy, the largest pathology type noted was vocal nodules and localized hyperplasia (excessive tissue). These disorders occurred more than twice as often in males as females. They are attributed to prolonged vocal abuse (Boone, 1977). The organic changes on the vocal folds result from functional misuse of the laryngeal tissues in the form of excessive yelling, screaming, and a multitude of other abuses that are discussed later in this chapter.

When the vocal folds are irritated by abusive voice production, their delicate tissue is affected. The final stage of their reaction is the formation of tiny growths of extra tissue. These growths are benign (nonmalignant) and will not invade the muscular tissue of the folds. They have been compared with corns or calluses on toes and hands from excessive rubbing and physical abuse. They develop at the junction of the anterior and middle thirds of the vocal folds because that area constitutes the midpoint of vocal fold vibration where the most significant contact occurs during phonation.

Following the initial irritation and inflammation, the body's defense mechanisms attempt to fight against the abuse by providing extra layers of epithelium at the trouble point. As these layers stratify into fibroid tissue, a nodule (node) develops. This seems to be the process of pathogenesis of vocal nodules. Figure 4-1 is an artist's rendering of how the folds look before and after the development of vocal nodules.

The following voice characteristics are typical of persons who have developed vocal nodules:

Pitch Factors

The pitch of these individuals usually is too low, considering the age and sex involved. Early literature in speech/language pathology suggested lowering the habitual pitch level clinically (West, 1947). However, it now is rather universally recognized that vocal nodules cause the voice to lower because of extra mass of the folds, and further lowering is likely to contribute to the abuse. Some persons may attempt to compensate for the vocal nodules by increasing the tension in the folds, thus causing an increase in the pitch, but the typical pattern usually is found to be too low. This results from the increased mass on each vocal fold, which lowers the fundamental vibration frequency. The person with nodules usually is not attempting consciously to lower the pitch; it is happening likely because of the extra mass, but this must be determined clinically.

It is necessary to determine whether a lower level is a function of extra mass or a result of a habitual pitch that is too low. If it is a function of extra mass, the lower level is a byproduct of the disorder. However, if it is a reflection of habitual pitch level it is likely to be a contributing factor in causing the nodules. This is analyzed further in the section of etiology of vocal nodules.

Voice Therapy in the School System 125

Figure 4-1 Vocal Folds Before and After Nodules Appear

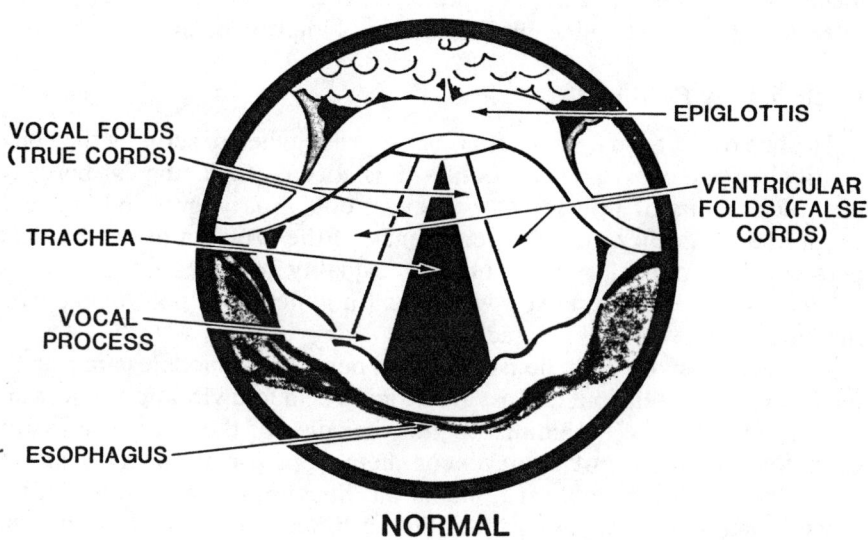
NORMAL

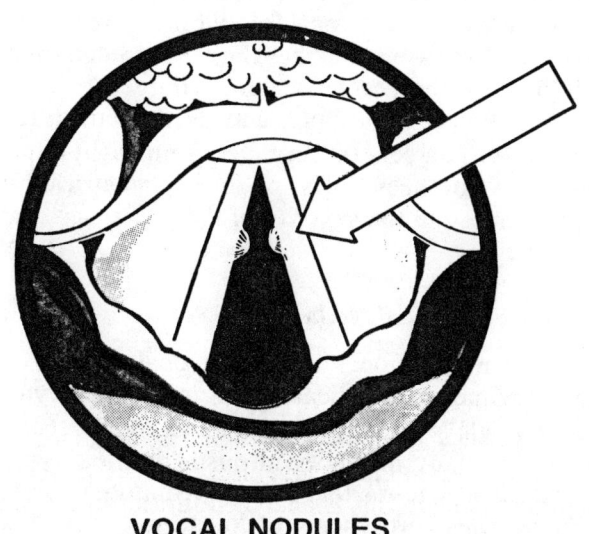
VOCAL NODULES

Pitch control and stability also are problems for persons with vocal nodules. Pitch breaks can occur at the onset of phonation in either an upward or downward direction. They reflect a highly unstable laryngeal mechanism. A decrease in pitch breaks at the onset of phonation constitutes one of the most noticeable indications of improvement under therapy.

Voice Quality Factors

The use of the term hoarseness is appropriate when describing the voice quality of a person with vocal nodules. It is not easy to distinguish between the voice quality of a person with a severe cold or laryngitis and one with vocal nodules, other than the persistency of the problem over time. The person with a cold or laryngitis finds voice quality improves as the infection subsides, whereas the person with vocal nodules does not change over time until abuses are eliminated.

The factors involved in hoarseness in a person with nodules are breathiness, excessive tension, and asymmetrical vocal fold vibration. There are two reasons for the breathiness. First, because of the nodular mass on each fold, they cannot achieve complete approximation. This allows excessive air to escape during phonation. Second, constant abuse of the voice structures produces irritation in the tissue, particularly around the arytenoid cartilages. This causes the person to avoid hard approximation of the arytenoid cartilages during phonation, which allows excessive air to escape and causes the voice to be breathy. The excessive tension factor is a functional attempt to exert increased effort to overcome the incomplete approximation of the vocal folds. This effort is the basis of the tension that is heard. The asymmetrical vocal fold vibration results from the fact that a nodule on one fold rarely matches the mass content of the nodule on the opposite fold. Therefore, each vocal fold vibrates in a different phase, i.e., asymmetrically, which contributes a negative element to voice quality.

The severity of hoarseness can range from slight to severe, depending mainly on the size of the nodules and the asymmetrical nature of each. An observable decrease in the severity of the hoarseness indicates improvement under therapy.

Etiology (Cause) of Vocal Nodules

The general cause of vocal nodules is vocal abuse, i.e., vocal behavior that harms or damages the delicate structures of the larynx. Nodules rarely result from a single instance of vocal abuse; rather, they develop from an accumulation of many instances of misusing the larynx. Vocal nodules also are identified by terms that define the nature of abuse involved, i.e., screamer's nodules, preacher's nodules, singer's nodules, and cheerleader's nodules. However, it is not merely screaming, preaching, singing, or even cheerleading that cause these nodules to develop, but specific and abnormal aspects of these activities that abuse the vocal folds.

The SLP working with a student with nodules must carefully investigate the pupil's vocal behavior to distinguish those behaviors that are abusive from those that are not. This is not easy. There are many forms of vocal abuse in addition to these just cited. Allergies and upper respiratory infections also are important factors in the development of vocal nodules. Senturia and Wilson (1968) find that in many children with vocal nodules, nasal secretions are present on the arytenoids and surrounding laryngeal tissues. They caution that inflammatory changes in the upper respiratory tract can be an important cause of nodules by increasing vulnerability to vocal abuse.

Each of the following is a possible cause of vocal nodules in children.

Playground Yelling. Many children when playing outside tend to express their emotions in an uninhibited manner. They yell directions at others, call across the field at their friends, compete for verbal leadership by having the loudest voice, argue over everything, scream loudly when being chased or caught, talk loudly at the same time other children are talking—the list seems endless. Anyone watching children play in these groups must wonder about their physical and verbal energy. Although not all children who play this way develop nodules, those who do often engage in such vocally abusive activities. Children with vocal nodules must be investigated carefully as to their specific vocal activities at play to determine whether they are causal factors.

Toy and Animal Noises. When children play, verbal dramatics often are important parts of the action. Bears growl, lions roar, monsters make weird noises, airplanes scream as they dive in combat, machine guns and rifles make sharp bangs, and bicycles become motorcycles with the help of the rider's voice. Numerous play activities seem to require children to mimic sounds, abusing the larynx. The SLP, when working with a child with vocal nodules, should explore these verbal activities thoroughly. Some children engage in many such activities, others in only one or two but often and routinely. For example, the child who makes only motorcycle sounds when riding a bicycle, but does so often, can abuse the larynx sufficiently to produce nodules even when good vocal hygiene is practiced in all other circumstances (Johnson, 1976).

Cheerleading. Perhaps the most classic example of vocal abuse in school is organized cheerleading. In most junior and senior high schools, students are encouraged to abuse their vocal folds physically to improve school spirit and support the teams. Many of these cheerleaders can be effective without causing vocal nodules or other voice disorder, but others cannot without abusing their larynges.

For several years, the author of this chapter and several graduate students in speech/language pathology have studied the effects of cheerleading on the voice and vocal folds. Several cheerleaders have been investigated longitudinally through the basketball and football seasons. An otolaryngologist periodically examined each one's vocal structures to determine whether cheerleading had damaged them. Each subject's voice was tape recorded at each medical examination. These recordings were analyzed by a team of SLPs, who judged the voice quality of each cheerleader. Voice spectrographs also were obtained from the recorded samples and analyzed by a speech scientist.

The results of this research confirm the notion that cheerleading can have a significant negative effect on the physical status of the vocal folds, resulting in abnormal voice quality. In one group of 36, 59 percent developed pathology on the folds attributed to the vocal abuse in cheerleading. Much of the pathology noted was in the form of vocal nodules (Case, Thome, & Kohler, 1979).

Since many cheerleaders are likely to develop vocal nodules, it is important to identify specific factors that can determine whether a given one will be affected:

- cheering without good abdominal breath support
- yelling with tension in the neck and larynx
- hard and abrupt onset of voice (coup de glotte)
- cheering during colds, infections, or severe allergy attacks
- yelling at an inappropriate pitch level (too high or too low)
- excessive individual yells beyond the organized squad cheers

Inappropriate Habitual Pitch Level. Data are not available regarding the pitch characteristics of persons before they developed vocal nodules. However, clinical experience shows that speaking at too low a habitual pitch level is a common cause of the disorder. Once nodules develop, the voice is found to be pitched too low because of the extra mass on each vocal fold, but this *is not a causal factor*. Only when the pitch is too low before the extra mass develops is it considered a causal factor.

A person who speaks at a too-low habitual pitch level puts considerable tension on the larynx in order to maintain adequate loudness at such a low tone. Cooper (1973), who has reviewed the literature on pitch and reported on his own clinical experience, has determined that vocal pathology resulting from abuse is likely to be based on a lower rather than a higher habitual pitch. A child can abuse the vocal folds by screaming at a high pitch level, but this occurs only periodically, and such a pupil rarely speaks habitually at that same level.

When a child has vocal nodules, the habitual pitch level often is not stable. Mattson (1980), in a report on the pitch changes over ten months of a single subject (a cheerleader) with vocal nodules, finds significant fluctuation of habitual pitch. These changes occur between morning and night voice, before and after cheerleading, and particularly the day following extensive cheerleading. On one occasion, this subject's pitch changed from a habitual pitch level of A_4 (220 Hz) to F_3 (174 Hz) overnight as a result of the cheerleading the previous night. Many similar pitch fluctuations were revealed during the ten-month span.

Aggressive Personality Factors. The personalities of children who develop vocal nodules have been found to differ from those who do not. Several papers at American Speech and Hearing Association conventions indicate that children with nodules have a tendency to be more aggressive, verbally repressed, with greater feelings of inadequacy, poorer relationships with parents, greater difficulty controlling themselves in verbal relationships, and greater withdrawal and antisocial feelings (Glassel, 1972; Mosby, 1967; Wilson & Lamb, 1973). These findings have been verified in many respects by clinical experience. The most prominent personality feature the authors have noted is that children with nodules tend to be more active verbally than those who do not. This finding also has been reported by Toohill (1975).

Evaluation Processes for Vocal Nodules

When a student is screened or referred as having a possible voice disorder, the SLP first determines the nature of the problem and identifies possible causes and effects. The only information provided is that the child has a hoarse or raspy voice. The etiology of the disorder is not known until a medical inspection has been conducted. That process should begin as soon as it has been established that persistent voice disorder—hoarseness—exists. As noted at the beginning of this chapter, medical referral requires the support and active involvement of parents. To gain this support, it is important that the SLP meet with the parents and student to explain voice disorder and why it is necessary to have the medical information. This process is explained at the beginning of this chapter.

Once the medical confirmation of vocal nodules has been obtained, the formal evaluation of the student can proceed. The first step is to explain the disorder and its cause (vocal abuse) by showing slides and playing tape recordings of persons with nodules. This should be more thorough than the parent orientation procedure.

Once the disorder is understood, the SLP questions the student to identify all forms of vocal abuse in the pupil's behavior. The SLP can begin by asking whether the student engages in any of the following vocally abusive behaviors: yelling loudly to friends, making strange noises such as motorcycle sounds or machine gun rat-a-tats, clearing the throat often, talking or singing loudly, talking in a noisy place, talking while angry, calling from room to room in the home, cheerleading, grunting during exercise, and so on. Each of these should be explored in detail to determine whether modification is needed. So as not to overlook any forms of abuse, the SLP should ask the student to give a detailed account of a typical school day and weekend day from awakening to bedtime. This often will reveal potential abuse categories that can be analyzed further.

To elicit information about the development and stability of the voice disorder, the SLP can ask such questions as these:

- When did the voice disorder begin?
- How consistent has the voice disorder been since it first began? Does it change much from day to day, week to week?
- Does voice quality seem related to how much talking is done in a day, or how happy or sad the state of the student's mind, or whether the student is under stress or pressure.
- Does the student have allergies that cause nasal congestion and throat irritation? Is medicine taken for such conditions? If yes, what specific medicines?
- How concerned is the student about the voice disorder?
- What aspects of the voice are most distressing: Pitch? Loudness? Quality? Durability?

These questions often provide information that can be used clinically to understand the individual. It is important to realize that it is not a voice disorder that is being evaluated, but a person with a voice disorder, and the more the SLP knows about that individual the better. For example, such questioning might reveal an attitude that the student is not at all concerned about the quality, pitch, or duration of the voice. If so, the SLP must help the student understand why concern is necessary or the therapy is likely to fail. Motivation to change is fundamental to successful voice therapy.

Following the case history part of the evaluation, the voice characteristics of the student must be analyzed on the parameters in Exhibit 4-2. After listening to the student and rating these factors, the SLP obtains a baseline recording to compare voice quality from therapy session to session. The following format is recommended in the recording:

Exhibit 4-2 Voice Characteristics Analysis Form

Pitch: (Use musical tones or numerical fundamental)
  Habitual pitch level:_____Optimal pitch level:_____
  Basal pitch (lowest):_____Ceiling (highest):_____
  Diplophonia noted:_____Pitch breaks noted:_____
Quality: (Check aspects appropriate to the student)
  Aphonia?_____Whisper only?_____Breathiness?_____
  Tension?_____Spastic (stoppage)?_____Hoarseness?_____
  Combination of breathiness and tension?_____
  Rate the voice quality in terms of most prominent negative feature on the following ordinal scale of severity. Feature that is rated:_____ (Slight) 1 2 3 4 5 (Severe)
Loudness: (Check loudness aspects appropriate to the student)
  Excessively loud voice:_____
  Normal loudness of voice:_____
  Inadequate loudness of voice:_____
Laryngeal Efficiency: (Identify factors indicating voice efficiency)
  Ease of voice initiation:_____
  Breathy initiation of voice:_____
  Audible inhalation of air:_____
  Sustain /s/ in seconds:_____Sustain /z/ in seconds:_____
  S/Z ratio:_____ (Pathological larynx makes it difficult to prolong /z/ as long as /s/.) (Boone, 1977)
Muscular Aspects of Voice:
  Neck tension during phonation:_____
  Larynx movement during phonation:_____
  Mouth and jaw muscle tension during phonation: _____
Miscellaneous concerns noted: _____
_____

The student should state name, date, time of day, sustain the sound /a/ for five seconds, count from 1 to 20, and read a few lines from a paragraph.

It is important to obtain a quality recording in this baseline and future tapings since recurrent analysis provides important information about improvement (or lack of it). When distortion and excessive tape noise are present, this comparison is more difficult to evaluate.

The final evaluation procedure is to teach the student how to use the vocal folds to produce a hypofunctional type of voice. Inasmuch as vocal nodules result from hyperfunction of the laryngeal mechanism (vocal abuse), it is important to teach the student to use the larynx with less effort, less tension, less abruptness of voice onset, less loudness—i.e., less vocal abuse. The initial target voice quality is slightly breathy and is temporary. This type of voice production is incompatible with vocal abuse. The purpose of this temporary pattern is to break the tendency to use a hyperfunctional manner of voice production. It should be taught by modeling from the SLP. When the student can approximate the hypofunctional manner, the individual should be directed to use it in all communication for the next few days.

Teaching hypofunctional production is not a recommendation to rest the voice nor to whisper. That is a highly controversial procedure that is not advised as treatment for most voice disorders, including vocal nodules. Although voice rest is necessary for a brief period following surgery on the vocal folds, SLPs and laryngologists often use it unwisely, with serious negative results. Aronson (1980) provides a good description of these negative effects.

Summary of Evaluation Procedure

The purpose of the evaluation session is to obtain general case history information, identify specific forms of vocal abuse, analyze and rate the student's voice on several factors, obtain a quality baseline recording of the individual's voice, provide information on vocal nodules, and teach a hypofunctional method of voice production to be used for a few days. It should be clear to the SLP reading this chapter that the evaluation procedures recommended become therapy or modification procedures by the end of the session. When all this has been accomplished, the SLP makes an appointment with the student to begin the process of eliminating systematically the vocal abuse forms identified in this evaluation session.

Individual Therapy for Vocal Nodules

Therapy for children with vocal nodules becomes a natural extension of the evaluation procedures. The individual therapy procedure involves identifying all forms of vocal abuse and systematically eliminating them from the student's communication patterns. This sounds rather straightforward and easy to accomplish, but any SLP who has attempted it must realize how difficult this process can become. Communication patterns are so intertwined with personality and self-concept that it is difficult to foster change in style without influencing personality. To accomplish such behavioral modification requires understanding of the personality of the student as a whole person. To view the therapy process as merely one of eliminating vocal abuse from someone's larynx is to invite failure.

The following procedures are recommended in the first two therapy sessions following the evaluation process.

Session #1

The SLP reviews briefly what was discussed and decided during the evaluation, including the success of using the hypofunctional voice taught then. The SLP asks whether there were many instances of forgetting to use the hypofunctional voice, what difficulties (if any) were experienced in using a more relaxed form of voice production, and how those difficulties were handled.

Another voice recording is made on the same tape as the baseline, using the same format. The SLP and the student then listen to both the baseline and current recording to determine whether any noticeable changes in voice quality, efficiency, and pitch have occurred. Sometimes a slight positive change is noticeable after only a few days of less intense vocal behavior. When this gain can be demonstrated, it is easier to motivate the student to continue working hard for even greater improvement.

The process of choosing identified abuse forms to be modified then begins. Using the factors identified in the evaluation, the SLP establishes a hierarchy of abuses ranked from most common and significant to least common. The student ranks the abuse forms according to ease of elimination, with the easiest at the bottom of the hierarchy. For example, a student may feel it is easy to stop making toy and animal noises but difficult to stop shouting and yelling on the playground. These differences should be reflected on the list.

Two or three of the more significant and common abuse forms that the student feels are easy to eliminate (low on the hierarchy) should be chosen as targets during the first few days, with total elimination by the next therapy session as the goal.

As an important motivating factor, the student should be taught datakeeping and accountability as abuses are eliminated. By listing the occurrences of a target abuse on a 3" × 5" card (Boone, 1977), awareness of the abuse is heightened and elimination is facilitated. It is common to see such a data card reveal a high incidence on the first day, with gradual reduction in succeeding days. If the datakeeping is reliable, this day-by-day reduction of abuses indicates progress. It is helpful to obtain information from an additional source such as a parent or teacher regarding the reliability of the abuse data on the card.

During this first therapy session, it also is important to establish a speaking voice that is normal in terms of effort. For the previous few days, the student used a hypofunctional voice in most, if not all, communication. Now the individual must be taught to speak in a voice without tension, extra effort, or breathiness. The student is told to try the voice likely to be used when speaking with a friend in a quiet place. The SLP should demonstrate and model the target voice. Once it has been established, the student is directed to use only that voice during the therapy process and to count any departure from it as an abuse.

It is important in teaching the student to speak with normal vocal effort to direct attention on eliminating abrupt voice onset. This abruptness is called coup de glotte, or hard glottal attack, and must be eliminated. The SLP should demonstrate the difference between the coup de glotte and an easy voice initiation. A slight aspiration such as in the production of the /h/ sound is helpful in teaching this concept. Practice will help the student master this element by drilling on such phrases as

- (h) open the door
- (h) ask me about it
- (h) kick the ball
- (h) tell the truth

After it is obvious that the presence of the /h/ sound before the word helps eliminate the coup de glotte, the student is told to merely think about the /h/ without actually using it as voice is initiated. This helps soften the onset of voice and eliminates another form of vocal abuse.

Some students find it difficult to motivate themselves to change vocal habits. Having a voice with better quality and efficiency is a rather hazy goal, particularly in view of the difficulty of the effort needed to effectuate the change. Systematic reinforcement for making such an effort often is necessary and helpful in the clinical process. Principles of behavioral modification using techniques of operant conditioning are utilized in the treatment of vocal nodules by a number of authorities, including Wilson and Rice (1977) and Johnson (1976). Their programs include procedures for identifying and reducing abuses with tight reinforcement schedules for either reducing the abuse or counting the target behaviors accurately. By choosing the proper reinforcement, whether it is money, a token economy, verbal praise, opportunity to perform activities the student enjoys, or whatever, the individual is motivated to count and eliminate abusive verbal behaviors. The precision with which behaviors are counted, charted, and reinforced distinguishes programs that are based on truly operant conditioning from those that merely involve reward or reinforcement. It is a good idea to include the concept of reinforcement for following therapy suggestions, however precisely this is done. Before the end of the first session, the SLP should determine the role of reinforcements, select specific ones toward which the student will work, and establish criteria for attaining them.

After reviewing the activities in Session #1, an appointment is made for the next therapy session.

Session #2

The format for this session is essentially the same as for the first. The student is asked about the previous few days, how easy it was to avoid the target abuses, what progress had been made, and how parents and others reacted—all to establish a general feeling for how well the individual responded to the therapy assignments. The data are checked to determine whether target abuses were reduced significantly and whether reinforcement was given when criteria were met. A new voice recording is made and compared with the previous recordings, additional abuses on the hierarchy are targeted, strategies are discussed to eliminate these while maintaining control over the previous target factors, and an appointment is made for the next therapy session.

Additional Sessions

Additional sessions follow the same format. Each time a recording is made and analyzed. Each session should reveal improvement in voice quality and voice efficiency, i.e., efficient voice onset without pitch breaks and breathiness. When there is no improvement, there usually is an identifiable reason such as overlooking or not controlling some significant abuse. Considerable time should be spent in therapy sessions discussing the significance of vocal nodules as deterrents to good voice quality and efficiency.

The SLP should help the student identify factors in everyday living that make it difficult to control vocal abuses such as sibling contention, forgetfulness under social pressure, or peer influence. Some of these factors are easy to correct, others are not. The SLP must take time to listen and understand how difficult it is to change deeply rooted behaviors. If siblings or peers are involved in the lack of control, the student should invite them to therapy sessions so the process can be explained. Often a brother, sister, or peer who does not have a voice disorder and who is involved in the therapy process can be extremely helpful by serving as a gentle reminder to the student about good vocal hygiene.

When vocal nodules are large enough to affect voice in any significant way, it takes usually about three months of careful control to allow the body to heal itself and the nodules to disappear. After three months of therapy, it is a good idea to have the student return to the otolaryngologist to determine the status of the larynx. It should not be a surprise to find significant improvement has occurred in the physical status of the vocal folds even when there is a residual voice quality pattern indicating nodules still are present. Several times the author of this chapter has sent students back to the physician for visual inspection of the vocal folds and received reports that the nodules were gone even when slight voice disorders still could be heard.

Group Therapy

A number of students with vocal nodules often constitute a homogeneous population for group therapy. Even though each student might have different vocal abuses, the general cause is the same. Students can spend time discussing difficulties in eliminating the abuses and strategies for dealing with them, encouraging each other when voice improvement is heard, and generally helping everyone realize they are not unique individuals because of having vocal nodules.

Telephone Therapy

The SLP can provide support between therapy sessions by either telephoning the student to discuss how assignments are going or by having the individual call in at regular intervals. These calls can occur before, during, or after a period of particular difficulty for the student. A call reminding the student to be aware of certain difficulties can be most supportive. Often telephone calls to parents or other persons important to the problem can provide support for the student and information to the SLP regarding progress at home.

Teacher Participation in Therapy

Classroom teachers function just as well as therapy associates in treating children with vocal nodules. They are with the students much of the time and are in constant verbal interaction with them. When provided with information about vocal abuse and general principles of therapy, teachers (with student approval) can report to the SLP about a pupil's vocal behavior, watching for vocal abuse in the classroom, on the playground, during lunchtime, and immediately after school. These teachers are overloaded with work and must not be expected to be responsible in any primary way for monitoring the child but rather can act as support persons to the SLP and the student.

The SLP should alert the classroom teacher as to activities from which the student with vocal nodules should be excused during the therapy. Cooperation should be sought to ensure that the teacher will limit or stop a student from participating in plays, singing, and recitations that might be vocally abusive. Teasing from student peers can become a problem and a cooperative teacher can thwart such tactics quickly. In coping with the oral or verbal communication that is such an important part of daily classroom activities, an understanding teacher can help a student with vocal nodules control target behaviors. It is the responsibility of the SLP to solicit such support and to demonstrate appreciation when it occurs.

Modification of Coughing and Throat Clearing

Coughing and clearing of the throat can be a most abusive laryngeal activity. Anyone who has viewed the movements of the vocal folds and surrounding laryngeal tissues during coughing when captured in high-speed cinematography will recognize the dynamics involved. Moore, Frazer, and von Leden (1962) provide such a record. However, these actions often occur under conditions of upper respiratory infection or allergic attack and control is nearly impossible because of the reflex nature of the processes involved. Coughs can occur without warning; even when a warning is provided, little can be done to eliminate them. Throat clearing usually is controlled more voluntarily, and much of it is unnecessary. The student with vocal nodules should be taught the difference between coughing and throat clearing that is reflexive and that which is not. With instruction, reflexive coughing and throat clearing can be modified to be less abusive, and nonreflexive occurrences can be eliminated.

Zwitman and Calcaterra (1973) describe a means of modifying coughing—the "silent cough" method that involves forcing more air out of the lungs in blasts while attempting to keep the vocal folds as much apart as possible during the cough. This process helps move mucus from the laryngeal valve without the explosive contact that becomes abusive. The person should cough as much as possible without voice, using only blasts of air. A similar process can be used to clear the throat of mucus.

Other Approaches to Therapy for Vocal Nodules

Several SLPs have described methods of management of students with vocal nodules that are helpful in dealing with this difficult clinical disorder. Aronson (1980), Wilson (1979), Boone (1977, 1980), Johnson (1976), Wilson and Rice (1977), and Holbrook, Rolnick, and Bailey (1974) all are excellent references for the SLP seeking complete information on vocal nodules.

Case Example of Vocal Nodules Management

N.M., an 11-year-old male student, was screened by the school SLP because of a weak voice. He was referred to a local otolaryngologist who identified bilateral vocal nodules and generalized swelling of the vocal folds. The otolaryngologist also was concerned that N.M. had an aggressive personality and wondered whether referral to a psychologist would be necessary.

The youngest of four boys in the family, N.M. found it difficult to compete in daily activities. He was large for his age and interested in all sports. He often took a leadership role in sporting activities. He had one close friend, Joe, with whom he seemed to be in constant conflict.

After the initial screening and referral to the otolaryngologist, the SLP set up a meeting with N.M., his parents, his brothers, and Joe to explain vocal nodules and to solicit their support in the therapy process. Following the orientation, time was spent evaluating N.M.'s voice, which was analyzed as being high pitched and extremely tense, with slight breathiness. When he began phonation, often no voice was present, just a tense breathy approximation. It seemed apparent that his high-pitched voice was a result of an effort to compensate for poor vocal efficiency.

Several specific abuses were identified by N.M. and the others. They are listed here without regard for order of severity:

- intense verbal interaction with siblings, especially the brother just older than N.M.
- intense verbal interaction with friend Joe
- yelling and screaming on the playground and during athletic activities
- phonation while in an angry and tense state
- hard glottal attack
- constant clearing of the throat in an abusive manner
- miscellaneous verbal activities of an abusive nature

A quality recording was made of N.M.'s voice as a baseline. This was analyzed later for specific pitch information. His habitual pitch was found to be F_4. No attempt was made to establish an optimal pitch because of the severity of his voice quality. He was able to sustain /s/ for 11 seconds and /z/ for only 7, indicating vocal inefficiency. His s/z ratio was computed as $-.64$.

Toward the end of the first session, N.M. was shown how to phonate with less effort in a hypofunctional manner. He then was asked to use this method for the next three days and to keep a record on every instance of forgetting by marking on a 3" × 5" card. N.M.'s parents then decided that each week his data and voice recordings indicated that he was making a strong effort to modify his vocal abuses, he would be allowed to attend a professional baseball game with his friend, Joe. When his nodules were eliminated as confirmed by medical inspection, N.M. would receive the new baseball glove he desired.

After three days, N.M. returned to therapy. His voice was recorded again and his data card analyzed. He had recorded 13 instances of forgetting to use his hypofunctional voice the first day after therapy, 9 the next day, and 3 the day after. N.M. reported that Joe had been helpful in reminding him to talk "softly."

Two forms were chosen from the list of vocal abuses: yelling on the playground and hard glottal attack. It was decided that during the next few days he would make a special effort to eliminate these and keep data to verify his control. He also was told to begin talking in a voice that was not as breathy as his hypofunctional voice and time was spent teaching him how to do it. He was told that the SLP would call him every evening about 5 o'clock to ascertain how he was faring.

Therapy proceeded in essentially the same manner as in previous sessions until N.M. had worked his way through the list of abuses. Each week his voice was recorded and analyzed. After two weeks, the recordings demonstrated that his voice was becoming more efficient. For example, when he initiated voice, the breathy onset seldom occurred. His vocal tension and general breathiness decreased markedly. His pitch lowered to $C\#_4$, a drop of two whole tones. His pitch level was then appropriate for a boy of 11 who had not begun puberty. His overall voice quality was quickly becoming normal.

Two and a half months after enrolling in therapy, N.M. returned to the referring otolaryngologist, who reported that the laryngeal tissues appeared normal and vocal nodules were absent. The boy received his baseball glove. It was decided to have him return for periodic checkups on voice quality and vocal behavior. Each time he came in, his voice was recorded and analyzed. At the time of this writing, the SLP had seen N.M. for seven checkups, with three weeks between visits. No relapse had occurred on his abnormal voice quality and it was assumed that his laryngeal tissue remained normal.

Summary of Vocal Nodules

Vocal nodules constitute an interesting voice disorder in which organic change on the vocal folds (nodules) results from functional misuse. Treatment for vocal nodules involves the identification and eliminating of all forms of functional misuse, i.e., vocal abuse. When this is done, the organicity of nodules is replaced by healthy tissues and voice quality and efficiency improve.

DISORDERS OF RESONANCE

Hypernasality

Hypernasality is a general term with several synonyms in the literature, i.e., nasality, hyperrhinolalia, hyperrhinophonia, rhinolalia aperta, and assimilated nasality. The condition involved is one of excessive resonance in the nasal cavity during voice production. It does not involve voice functions at the vocal fold level but merely the influence of nasal resonance on the sound generated by vocal fold vibration. Of the many terms available to describe this condition, hypernasality is used in this chapter.

The speech articulation structure that regulates the extent of nasal cavity participation in the resonance of voice is the velopharyngeal mechanism, i.e., the soft palate (velum) and pharyngeal muscles at the same level. Under normal conditions, the velopharyngeal mechanism provides an open port for nasal breathing and for resonance of the nasal consonants /m/, /n/, and / ŋ /. The port closes for all other speech sounds and swallowing functions so there is complete separation between the oral and nasal cavities. Under closure conditions, no nasal resonance can occur. However, when the soft palate does not close completely against the pharynx, a gap is created that allows sound to get into the nasal cavity. When this occurs, the voice will have a nasal quality to it. The degree of nasality can vary from slight to severe. It is this condition of nasal voice quality that is referred to here as hypernasality.

Hyponasality

Hyponasality is the opposite of hypernasality. It is a vocal quality that occurs when the nasal cavity has some condition that prevents it from participating normally as a resonance chamber. The English consonants /m/, /n/, and / ŋ / require nasal resonance for normal production. When these sounds are used in speaking, the soft palate opens away from the pharynx and allows sound to enter the nasal cavity and resonate. Hyponasality also is called denasality.

Several conditions in the nasal cavity can cause hyponasality: allergies of the nose and throat, upper respiratory infections (URI), large adenoid tissue, nasal polyps, and other growths. Hyponasality occurs under these conditions because resonance space is occupied by the congestion produced by the abnormality. It is not caused by abnormal functioning of the velopharyngeal mechanism but does occur when that mechanism opens normally to allow sound to enter the nasal cavity and proper resonance does not result because space is restricted by one or more of the conditions mentioned.

Therefore, it is the author's opinion that hyponasality is a medically based disorder that does not require the services of the SLP other than to refer for medical attention. When a child is evaluated as having a hyponasal voice, medical referral is the only action to take. The physician will treat the child to improve or eradicate the congestion in the nasal cavity and, when this has been done, the voice quality will be normal.

Degrees of Hypernasality

Normal oral-nasal resonance occurs when there is complete velopharyngeal closure on all sounds in the English language except the nasal consonants /m/, /n/, and / ŋ /, which require velopharyngeal opening. When there is some dysfunction of the velopharyngeal mechanism so that complete closure cannot or does not result, nasality will be perceived in the voice quality when it should not be present. The person has a hypernasal voice. Sometimes hypernasality is apparent only when words are being spoken that contain the nasal consonants /m/, /n/, or / ŋ /. The vowel sounds that fall immediately in front or back of a nasal consonant are influenced by it and become excessively nasalized. This process of a nasal consonant's influencing an adjacent vowel is called assimilation nasality.

Assimilation nasality can be caused by either borderline organicity of the velopharyngeal mechanism or functional influence of regional dialects. When borderline organicity is present, the soft palate opens for the nasal consonant and is slow or incomplete in its closure process after it completes producing the nasal consonant. Continuously running speech sounds slightly hypernasal because of the common occurrence of nasal consonants. Only upon careful evaluation does it become apparent that the nasal quality is a result of the influence of normally produced nasal consonants. Inspection of the velopharyngeal mechanism during speech is likely to reveal a slight gap between the soft palate and the pharynx when complete closure is being attempted.

When assimilation nasality results from regional dialect, the student sounds similar to most of the others reared in the area. The hypernasality occurs only in the phonetic contexts explained above, but is of little clinical consequence unless the student desires to sound different from other persons in the region. This is an individual choice. Any SLP working for a significant period in a given location becomes aware of the unique characteristics of the regional dialect. Decisions regarding whether a pattern of assimilation nasality requires clinical attention can be made easily.

When nasality occurs on all vowel sounds regardless of adjacency to a nasal consonant, a significant voice disorder exists. This is apparent to most people rather immediately and is recognized as a deviation in voice quality. It requires clinical attention. The vowels are not distorted in any way other than by the nasality. Intelligibility of sound production is not affected. Consonants are not distorted. It is a disorder of nasal voice quality, i.e., hypernasality on vowels only.

A more severe form of hypernasality involves excessive nasal resonance on vowel sounds as well as distortion of many consonants. Consonants thus distorted are those that require intraoral breath pressure as part of their formulation. There are 16 English consonants with such characteristics: /s/, /z/, /tʃ/, /dʒ/, /ʃ/, /ʒ/, /p/, /b/, /t/, /d/, /f/, /v/, /k/, /g/, /θ/, and /ð/. If a student attempts to articulate one of these high-pressure consonants when a large gap in the velopharyngeal mechanism exists, air pressure involved in the sound production escapes out the gap and through the nose. A nasal snort of air is released as the consonant is articulated. When the hypernasality is this severe, all the vowels are nasalized and many of the consonants are distorted. Speech intelligibility is affected. The wider the gap in the velopharyngeal mechanism, the greater the speech distortion and the poorer the intelligibility (Bzoch, 1979).

The following are etiological or causal factors in the development of various degrees of hypernasality:

Cleft Palate

When a child is born with a cleft involving the secondary palate, velopharyngeal closure is affected even after surgical repair. The soft palate can be deficient in tissue and immobile in function, making effective velopharyngeal closure difficult. It also should be realized that surgical closure of such a palatal cleft does not occur until the child is between 9 and 30 months old. The influence of the unrepaired cleft during early formative months of speech development cannot be overestimated.

Submucous Cleft

The soft palate is composed of muscles covered by mucous membrane. These muscles are attached in a complicated manner to the midline structures of the soft palate as well as to the bony structures of the hard palate. There frequently is a defect in the muscular tissues of the soft palate that is masked by the presence of normal mucous membrane. There also could be a notch or deficiency of bony structures on the posterior aspect of the bony hard palate also covered by normal mucous membrane. Either condition, or both, is known as a submucous cleft. Such a cleft often is difficult to detect because of the normal mucus covering. When a submucous cleft is present, velopharyngeal closure usually is abnormal and insufficient to support normal voice and speech production. Hypernasal voice and sometimes distorted articulation of pressure consonants result from these submucous clefts (Bradley, 1979).

Neurological Abnormalities

The movements of the soft palate against the pharyngeal structures during speech are rapid and complex. It is no wonder that many individuals have difficulties with them. The neurological bases of these movements also are complex. The velopharyngeal structures are innervated by the pharyngeal plexus nerves of the peripheral nervous system as coordinated by the central nervous system. Any disease or traumatic condition that disrupts these nerves causes dysfunction of the velopharyngeal structures. Such disorders as cerebral palsy or congenital suprabulbar paresis can seriously affect the coordination of the muscles involved in velopharyngeal closure. Many of these disorders also have components of laryngeal as well as velopharyngeal dysfunctions (Aronson, 1980).

Postadenoidectomy

Velopharyngeal closure for speech often is aided by the presence of extra tissue in the posterior nasopharyngeal cavity. This is the special lymphoid tissue normally present in children and is called the adenoids. In some children, adenoid tissue is excessive. When it is, it masks potential physical abnormalities of the velopharyngeal mechanisms. Closure of these structures occurs because the soft palate contacts the adenoid mass rather than the pharyngeal wall. This added support for closure causes no problems so long as the adenoid tissue remains. However, it often is necessary to perform an adenoidectomy to remove this tissue when it becomes diseased. Only then is the velopharyngeal insufficiency unmasked. The child's voice suddenly is hypernasal because the soft palate no longer can contact the pharyngeal wall completely.

Structural Abnormalities

A variety of structural abnormalities can negate the proper functioning of the velopharyngeal mechanisms. Some of the more common include a deep pharynx; a short, soft palate; a short, hard palate; congenital palatal webbing; or unusual origin and insertion of the soft palate muscles. In recent years, a problem has developed in velopharyngeal closure as a result of surgical advancement of the maxillary bone to correct facial and maxillary abnormalities (Witzel, Munro, and Chir, 1977).

Evaluation of Resonance Disorders

The first concern of an SLP when evaluating a student suspected of having a voice disorder related to abnormal resonance is to determine whether hypernasality or hyponasality exists. The physical status of the structures involved in resonance disorders should then be determined. The structural bases of resonance disorders can be evaluated with complex instrumentation such as motion picture x-rays (cineradiography) or pressure airflow measurement. However, these are of value only when performed with good clinical understanding of the procedures involved coupled with an ability to relate findings to the practical aspects of human communication.

Often it is necessary to make clinical judgments about resonance factors without these complex instruments because they and the expert personnel required to use and interpret their results are not always available to the SLP in the school system. Judgments must be made on the basis of speech behavior alone. The evaluation procedures described in this chapter involve analysis of speech and voice without elaborate instrumentation. The SLP who seeks information about more elaborate forms of evaluation is referred to Bzoch (1979), Cooper, Harding, Krogman, Mazaheri, and Millard (1979), and Fletcher (1978).

Hypernasality vs. Hyponasality

A SLP may listen to a student's voice and detect a "nasal factor" but have difficulty determining whether it is hypernasality or hyponasality. This is not an easy decision in some cases. There are instances when both factors are present. For example, a student can have velopharyngeal insufficiency that allows nasal resonance to occur but because of nasal congestion from an allergy or cold there is insufficient nasal resonance on the consonants /m/, /n/, or /ŋ/.

The best method for discriminating between hypernasality and hyponasality is to have the student read words or phrases that are either loaded with or lacking nasal consonants. For example:

NASAL PHRASES

My mom can be mean
Many times a man can
May I plan my menu?

NONNASAL PHRASES

See what I do to it
If you see what I did
Carry it to the truck

By listening carefully to how these phrases sound, the SLP can judge whether the voice quality heard is hypernasality or hyponasality. The student who is hypernasal sounds excessively nasal on the nonnasal phrases and rather normal on the nasal phrases, depending on how severe the condition is. The hyponasal student sounds nearly normal on the nonnasal phrases but manifests the hyponasality most obviously on the nasal phrases. The /m/ phoneme takes on the resonance and articulation characteristics of a /b/, the /n/ of a /d/, and the / ŋ / of a /g/. Stated succinctly, a student who is hyponasal manifests the disorder when reading phrases highly loaded with nasal sounds, whereas the hypernasal one shows it when reading phrases devoid of nasal sounds.

The child with mixed hypernasality and hyponasality evidences these same differences, but the discrimination process usually is more difficult. Hypernasality is heard on the nonnasal phrases, but not noticeably so. Hyponasality is just as apparent in its pure form as it is in a mixed state, i.e., the nasal consonants do not sound nasal.

It is important to determine how easily a student with resonance disorder can breathe through the nose. If sufficient nasal congestion is present to restrict airflow through the nose for respiration, it is likely that nasal resonance for the nasal consonants also will be dampened. The SLP can have the student run in place for a minute or so until slightly out of breath, then have the individual sit down and attempt to achieve normal breathing cycles using only the nose. If the child has considerable difficulty and must open the mouth to catch up on breathing, it is reasonable to expect a nasal congestion factor sufficient to produce a hyponasal voice quality. When this test is performed, it is a good idea to determine whether breathing is better through one nostril than the other. Congestion on only one side still is sufficient to generate hyponasal resonance.

Hypernasality also can be detected by producing a cul-de-sac resonance. Cul-de-sac resonance is a form of closed tube resonance and occurs in humans when the nostrils are pinched together as a vowel sound is produced and prolonged. Under these conditions, the student emitting an /i/ sound as the nostrils are pinched experiences a sudden change in the nature of the sound. An extention of this is the nasal flutter test (Bzoch, 1979). It is performed by alternately pinching and releasing the nostrils as the child prolongs the vowels /i/ or /u/. The rapidly alternated pattern makes the changes produced by cul-de-sac resonance more noticeable. If no such change is heard, there is no excessive or hypernasal resonance.

One of the most helpful devices available for detecting hypernasal or hyponasal resonance is the nasal listening tube (Figure 4-2). It is a rather simple device constructed of rubber tubing with glass or plastic tips on each end that can be placed in either a nostril or an external auditory

Figure 4-2 Subject Using Nasal Listening Tube

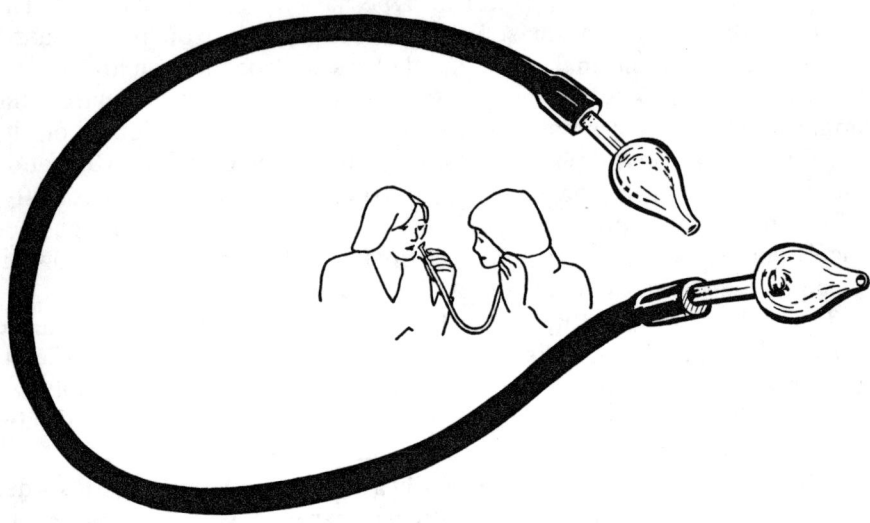

meatus. When one tip is placed into the student's nostril and the other tip into the SLP's ear, amplified sound is heard when present in the nasal cavity. Hyponasality is detected by having the child alternate saying a /b/ and an /m/ sound in a consonant-vowel-consonant (CVC) phonemic relationship. For example, /bib/, and /mim/ alternated do not sound that different through the listening tube when hyponasality is present. However, hypernasality is detected easily no matter how slight its presence. It also is possible to discern easily when air is escaping into the nasal cavity on the pressure consonants. The nasal listening tube can be helpful in evaluation as well as therapy by allowing the SLP and the student to detect the presence of abnormal nasal resonance.

When analysis of the student's voice reveals a pattern of excessive nasal resonance during speech, it is imperative to determine whether the reason is a structural abnormality in the velopharyngeal mechanism or whether it is a functional disorder. A complete evaluation of the structures involved should be carried out, including an oral inspection of the mechanisms. An x-ray study of velopharyngeal function also is important. Until a functional etiology for the hypernasality can be determined, and an organic basis eliminated, prolonged voice therapy to modify hypernasality is inappropriate.

Oral Examination of Velopharyngeal Structures

It is important to keep in mind that when a student is being examined to determine the adequacy of the velopharyngeal structures, the position of the head should be as upright and normally positioned as possible. It should be held in a way that compares favorably with the head position during normal speech production. When the head is extended or flexed in any abnormal way, it is easier for velopharyngeal closure to result (McWilliams, Musgrave, & Crozier, 1968). The student should be positioned so the examiner can inspect the structures from a direct front view in a horizontal plane. Inspection of soft palate movement also should be done under normal speech production conditions.

The SLP should not have the child extend the tongue to assess velopharyngeal functioning since such excessive protrusion alters normal anatomical and physiological relationships and restricts full motion of the soft palate. The mouth also should not be opened excessively during this examination. The SLP should ask the student to open the mouth slightly as an /a/ vowel is prolonged. By shining a light directly into the oral cavity during this normal speech effort, the SLP should be able to view the palatal movements. If not, the student should be instructed to continue prolonging the vowel as the mouth gradually is opened more until the structures can be viewed easily.

In normal velopharyngeal closure, although the processes vary from person to person, they essentially are sphincteric in nature. The soft palate does not merely move up against the posterior pharyngeal wall, it moves up and back, the lateral walls of the pharynx move medially, and the posterior wall of the pharynx moves forward to completely close the port between the oral and nasal cavities (Skolnick, McCall, & Barnes, 1973). It is difficult to analyze these sphincteric movements from direct oral inspection, particularly since closure occurs above the level of the palatal plane. However, direct oral inspection is the only means readily available to the SLP, and care must be taken to determine that it is done as efficiently as possible.

Considerable information can be gained by visual inspection of the velopharyngeal structures' tissue color. When the color of the soft palate midline is blue or purple, a possible submucous cleft is indicated. The midline attachments of the soft palate muscles may be directed abnormally toward the posterior border of the hard palate rather than at the palatal raphe. This abnormality can affect the functions of the velopharyngeal structures significantly. A submucous cleft of the soft palate also should be suspected when a split or bifid uvula is noted. A bifid uvula and submucous clefting have been shown to be highly correlated (Bzoch 1979).

The SLP should inspect the velopharyngeal mechanisms to determine whether any obvious abnormalities exist by noting the length, color, pharyngeal depth, and movement patterns. These observations should be correlated with judgments about voice quality and articulation accuracy. A decision then can be made as to whether further diagnostic procedures need to be instituted or whether therapy to modify aberrant speech patterns can be started.

A complete oral examination format has been provided by Mason (1980) and Dworkin and Culatta (1980). By following either of these formats while keeping in mind the suggestions of this chapter, the SLP can make the necessary judgments about the status of the velopharyngeal structures that support voice and articulation. Should such judgment indicate further diagnostic evaluation is necessary, a referral might be appropriate for cineradiography or aerodynamic analysis. Information regarding the use of these techniques of velopharyngeal assessment can be obtained by reading Bzoch (1979) and Skolnick et al. (1973).

Therapy for Resonance Disorders

Therapy procedures differ for hyponasality and hypernasality. For hyponasality, as previously mentioned, traditional speech remediation is neither required nor appropriate. The SLP's only course of action is to refer the student to a medical specialist who can improve the physical condition of the nasal cavity so it can function properly as a voice resonator. Such conditions as allergies causing nasal congestion, enlarged adenoid tissue, deviated nasal septum, and growths in the nose can cause hyponasality and must be corrected before voice quality can improve. Attempting to help the child modify this voice quality without such correction only generates frustration and disappointment for both student and SLP.

Therapy for hypernasality must be preceded by a complete evaluation of the physical structures involved in velopharyngeal closure, as previously indicated. It is important to determine whether they are insufficient or merely incompetent in function. If insufficient, physical management usually is necessary; if incompetent, therapy is effective in producing the desired change in voice quality. Too often, a medical/physical evaluation involving cineradiography and aerodynamic analysis occurs only after several months of unsuccessful therapy. It is as though this long therapy period is needed to justify the time, effort, and expense of a complete evaluation. The SLP should take the opposite view. Even when it is necessary to travel afar to a large city to obtain such an evaluation, the effort is worth it. Once the evaluation is made and any recommendations for physical management completed, therapy will proceed more successfully.

Articulation Therapy and Hypernasality

When a student has both hypernasality and nasal distortion of pressure consonants, therapy should begin with the consonants. Articulation distortions from velopharyngeal dysfunction should be corrected before attempting management of the voice quality of hypernasal resonance. Correction of articulation has improved nasal resonance without direct attention to the nasality. The opposite has not been found when nasality treatment takes precedence over articulation distortions. Articulation does not improve as a function of improved resonance.

The specific processes involved in articulation correction are well outlined in the chapters on articulation—Chapters 1, 2 and 3. However, a few specific procedures directed at the student with nasal distortion of consonants must be considered: articulation placement, light contact of articulation, and quick contact of placement.

Placement. Careful attention must be directed at correction of any abnormal placement errors. Children with velopharyngeal closure difficulty often make compensatory movements in articulation placement, supposedly to help facilitate the closure process. The placement compensations, whether they are too far forward or backward of normal placement, produce sound distortion and can reduce intelligibility. By analyzing placement and correcting any abnormalities found, an important first step can be taken in improving the student's speech.

Students who have confirmed velopharyngeal insufficiency that is scheduied to be corrected physically at some future time should have abnormal placement errors corrected as soon as they are identified. Correction of the velopharyngeal insufficiency is not necessary in order to correct the placement errors.

Light Contact of Articulation. Since air leakage out the nose occurs in children with velopharyngeal insufficiency or incompetency, it is important to teach principles of articulation that decrease the probability that such emissions will occur. One compensation is the tendency to produce pressure consonants with hard contact of articulation. Children who manifest these problems, for example, often push the tongue tip hard against the alveolar ridge in making a /t/ or /d/ sound as though the hard contact will help them build the pressure needed to articulate the sounds involved. In actuality, the hard contact merely increases the likelihood that pressure in the sound will escape out the nose rather than past the point of articulation. Teaching a lighter articulation touch allows the child to form the sound and release it orally with sufficient pressure for proper sound recognition. This is an important principle to keep in mind when working with the articulation distortions in children with velopharyngeal abnormalities.

Quick Contact of Articulation. Everything mentioned in the previous section on light contact pertains to quick contact of articulation. When the contact involved in producing the sound is extended excessively, the probability that pressure will escape out the nose is increased. For example, Klatt (1974) indicates that normal duration for the /s/ phoneme is about 120 milliseconds. Should a child with velopharyngeal insufficiency hold this sound much longer than that, air pressure can be released through the nose rather than orally. The SLP need not attempt to measure this duration factor but merely should encourage the student to keep the sounds as short as possible to eliminate this problem. A combination of teaching a student to produce pressure consonants with a light and quick touch at the proper place of articulation can improve speech intelligibility significantly.

Voice Therapy for Hypernasality

Voice therapy for hypernasal vowel resonation should begin only after all articulation errors related to velopharyngeal dysfunction are corrected. At that point, the following approach to correcting the nasal voice quality on vowels is recommended.

The nasal listening tube inserted into the student's nostril can be used to evaluate and rate the nasality heard on each vowel sound. The nostril into which the tip is inserted should be the one through which breathing occurs most easily should a difference in the two exist. The SLP should rate each of the following vowels: /i/, /ɪ/, /e/, /ɛ/, /æ/, /a/, /o/, /ʊ/, /u/, /ʌ/, and /ɚ/. The following ordinal scale can be used to rate each vowel:

0 = Normal, no nasality heard
1 = Slight nasality
2 = Moderate nasality
3 = Severe nasality

When the vowels have been rated, the listening tube can be used to help students identify their own hypernasality. By inserting the listening tube into their own ear as they produce the vowels, they can differentiate between those that the SLP judges to be normal or only slightly nasal and those that are more severe. When students can discriminate those differences, it is appropriate to begin modification of the moderately and severely judged vowels.

The SLP can take the following steps in teaching the student to produce voice devoid of hypernasality:

- The student says monosyllabic words in consonant-vowel-consonant relationships (CVC), beginning with vowels rated as normal (0) or only slightly nasal (1). The student listens with the tube to these sounds, then produces vowels rated as moderate (2) or severe (3) in the same CVC relationships so the contrast can be heard between the mildly nasal and the more severely nasal. The student then should be drilled to produce the severely nasal vowels in the CVC relationships until they are like the mild or normal vowels. This should be done by pairing the contrasting CVCs together, e.g., /tat/ (1) with /tit/ (3).
- Once the student can produce monosyllabic words or CVC relationships without nasality using the nasal listening tube to discriminate, the SLP begins drilling on other words and phrases that do not contain nasal consonants while maintaining the normal or only slightly nasal rating of (0) or (1).
- Nasal consonants are introduced into the phrases by ending them on a nasal consonant, e.g., see the ice cream, put up the beam, etc. If the student can maintain a lack of moderate or severe nasality even with the presence of a nasal consonant, the SLP should begin to scatter a few nasal consonants in other word positions in the phrases, e.g., some of us care, I am at my school, etc. The presence of the nasal consonants should not have a significant effect on the vowels in the phrase, which should remain nonnasal.
- When the student is able to say these phrases without excessive nasality on the vowels while listening on the tube, the tube is removed to determine whether that action affects monitoring ability: can the pupil tell when the voice is nasal or nonnasal without the tube? If the student can, and also can eliminate the excessive nasality, the SLP should continue work on short phrases without concern for nasal consonants, then longer ones, then context reading, and finally conversation. At each increase in task difficulty, the SLP should determine that proper discrimination and production of voice without nasality is occurring by spot checking with the nasal listening tube rather than using it constantly.
- Negative practice is helpful at any of these steps. The SLP should have the student speak the sound, word, phrase, or sentence with excessive and deliberate nasality. When the student learns to handle the resonance voluntarily in either a negative or positive manner, the carry-over into everyday voice production is more likely to occur because the individual is in control of the process—the process of hypernasality is not controlling the student.

A Case Example of Hypernasality and Articulation Distortion

P.B., a 16-year-old female, was identified by teacher referral as having a severe speech and voice disorder. The SLP determined through case history that she had been born with a unilateral complete cleft of her primary and secondary palates. Early surgeries to close her clefts were performed in Canada and she could not report any details on them.

Language testing by the SLP revealed normal encoding, decoding, and usage of language symbols. Hearing testing showed normal auditory functioning in both ears. Articulation testing produced several errors, including abnormal placement and distortion of /t/, /d/, /s/, /z/, /k/, /g/, /dʒ/, /tʃ/, /θ/, and /ɚ/. P.B. was intelligible only when the context was understood. Her distortions were a function of abnormal placement and excessive air leakage through the nose.

An oral examination revealed teeth that were being managed orthodontically and were nearly corrected. There was excessive scar tissue on her bony hard palate and there was a rather large fistula (hole) through her palate just behind her maxillary central incisors. Her velopharyngeal mechanisms were hard to evaluate because of indistinct landmarks. It was apparent that she had had a pharyngeal flap operation to help facilitate velopharyngeal closure (Bzoch, 1979). Velopharyngeal closure occurred around the flap but was more complete on the right side than the left. The SLP decided that P.B.'s articulation distortions probably were a function of the fistula in the anterior part of her oral cavity and possible velopharyngeal insufficiency, particularly on the left side of her flap. She was referred to a plastic surgeon, who closed her anterior fistula.

P.B. also was judged to have hypernasal resonance on all vowel sounds. All of her vowels were judged as (2) or (3) except the /a/, which was (1). These judgments were determined by the SLP using a nasal listening tube.

It was decided that articulation therapy should begin as soon as the anterior fistula had been closed surgically. Directions were given to P.B. regarding proper placement for the distorted consonants. Therapy for placement involved the SLP's using a tongue depressor to touch the point on the palate or soft palate that was normal for the target sound. The SLP touched the spot for the sound, then P.B. placed her tongue in the same spot while articulating the sound in a CV relationship. For example, for the /t/ sound, the SLP touched P.B's palate just anterior to the former fistula (near the palatal rugae), then asked her to say /ta/ several times while monitoring in a mirror. This procedure was repeated for all consonants that involved placement error. This was done without concern as to whether air was emitted through the nose—the only thought was proper placement.

After four weeks of therapy, P.B. could articulate all of the consonants with proper placement in words and phrases. Constant monitoring in the mirror was necessary. It then was decided to determine whether modification of the nasal air emission was possible. By using proper placement and light contact of articulation, while monitoring through the nasal listening tube, P.B. could eliminate air emission through the nose on all consonants in monosyllabic words. The tendency to produce consonants with nasal air emission had occurred primarily because of the fistula rather than the velopharyngeal insufficiency suspected on the left side of her flap. Even when proper placement occurred on the consonants and no air emission was noted, it was obvious that P.B. remained hypernasal on the vowels. Most vowels were produced with a (2) or (3) rating.

Several additional weeks of therapy were spent improving her articulation placement and air pressure control. As P.B. used her improved articulation techniques in conversation, her intelligibility improved significantly. No longer was it necessary to know the context in order to understand her speech. As of this writing, P.B. had achieved remarkable control over placement and nasal airflow and was beginning to work on controlling her hypernasality on the vowel sounds.

SUMMARY

Voice therapy can be an enjoyable facet of the SLP's activities in treating communication disorders in the school system. It requires an understanding of the anatomical, physiological, and psychological correlates of voice production as well as clear concepts of voice management. Effective management of voice-disordered students requires cooperation with numerous specialists such as otolaryngologists, pediatricians, psychologists, and classroom teachers. Cooperation of parents and family members also is important. To attempt to remediate a student with a voice disorder without such cooperation is to invite frustration and disappointment.

The purpose of this chapter has been to provide the working SLP with the practical essentials of voice evaluation and therapy. Disorders commonly found in schools have been detailed. Several less common disorders (or those found primarily in adults) have been excluded. However, it is hoped that sufficient detail has been given on the evaluation and treatment of the disorders covered here to allow easy utilization of these processes in any type of voice anomaly.

REFERENCES

Aronson, A. E. *Clinical voice disorders: An interdisciplinary approach.* New York: Thieme-Stratton, Inc., 1980.

Boone, D. *The voice and voice therapy* (2nd ed.). Englewood Cliffs, N.J.: Prentice-Hall, Inc., 1977.

Boone, D. R. *The Boone voice program for children*. Tigard, Oregon: C.C. Publications, Inc., 1980.

Bradley, D. Congenital and acquired palatopharyngeal insufficiency. In K. R. Bzoch (Ed.), *Communicative disorders related to cleft lip and palate* (2nd ed.). Boston: Little, Brown and Co., 1979.

Bzoch, K. R. (Ed.). *Communicative disorders related to cleft lip and palate* (2nd ed.). Boston: Little, Brown and Co., 1979.

Case, J., Thome, J., & Kohler, S. *A longitudinal study of vocal abuse among cheerleaders*. Paper presented at the American Speech-Language-Hearing Association national convention, Atlanta, 1979.

Cooper, H. K., Harding, R. L., Krogman, W. M., Mazaheri, M., & Millard, R. T. *Cleft palate and lip: A team approach to clinical management and rehabilitation of the patient*. Philadelphia: W. B. Saunders Co., 1979.

Cooper, M. *Modern techniques of vocal rehabilitation*. Springfield, Ill.: Charles C Thomas, Publisher, 1973.

Daniloff, R., Schuckers, G., and Feth, L. The physiology of speech and hearing: An introduction. Englewood Cliffs, N.J.: Prentice-Hall, Inc., 1980.

Dworkin, J. P., & Culatta, R. A. *Oral mechanism examination*. Nicholasville, Kentucky, Edgewood Press, Inc., 1980.

Fletcher, S. G. *Diagnosing speech disorders from cleft palate*. New York: Grune & Stratton, Inc., 1978.

Gillespie, S. K., & Cooper, E. B. Prevalence of speech problems in junior and senior high schools. *Journal of Speech and Hearing Research*, 1973, *16*, 739–743.

Glassel, W. L. *A study of personality problems and vocal nodules in children*. Paper presented at the American Speech and Hearing Association national convention, San Francisco, 1972.

Holbrook, A., Rolnick, M. I., & Baily, C. W. Treatment of vocal abuse disorders using a vocal intensity controller. *Journal of Speech and Hearing Disorders*, 1974, *39*(3), 298–303.

Johnson, T. H. *Vocal abuse reduction program*. Logan, Utah: Utah State University, Department of Communicative Disorders, 1976.

Klatt, D. The duration of /s/ in English words. *Journal of Speech and Hearing Research*, 1974, *17*, 51–63.

Mason, R. M., & Grandstaff, H. L. Evaluating the velopharyngeal mechanism in hypernasal speech. *Speech, Hearing Services in Schools*, 1971, *4*, 53–61.

Mattson, P. *Vocal abuse from cheerleading: A case study*. Unpublished master's project, Arizona State University, 1980.

McWilliams, B. J., Musgrave, R., & Crozier, P. The influence of head position upon velopharyngeal closure. *Cleft Palate Journal*, 1968, *5*, 117–124.

Minifie, F. D., Hixon, T. J., and Williams, F. *Normal aspects of speech, hearing and language*. Englewood Cliffs, N.J.: Prentice-Hall, Inc., 1973.

Moore, P., Frazer, D., & von Leden, H. Ultra-high speed photography in laryngeal physiology. *Journal of Speech and Hearing Disorders*, 1962, *27*(1), 165–171.

Mosby, D. *Predominant personality characteristics of 25 children with voice disorders*. Paper presented at the American Speech and Hearing Association national convention, Chicago, 1967.

Senturia, B. H., Wilson, F. B. Otorhinolaryngic findings in children with voice disorders. *Annals of Otology, Rhinology, and Laryngology,* 1968, *77,* 1027–1041.

Silverman, E.M., & Zimmer, C.H. Incidence of chronic hoarseness among school-age children. *Journal of Speech and Hearing Disorders,* 1975, *40*(2), 211–215.

Skolnick, L. M., McCall, G. N., & Barnes, M. The sphincteric mechanism of velopharyngeal closure. *Cleft Palate Journal,* 1973, *10,* 286–305.

Toohill, R. J. The psychosomatic aspects of children with vocal nodules. *Archives of Otolaryngology,* 1975, *101,* 591–595.

West, R., Kennedy, L., & Carr, A. *Rehabilitation of speech* (Rev. ed.). New York: Harper and Brothers, 1947.

Wilson, F. B., & Lamb, M. M. *Comparison of personality characteristics of children with and without vocal nodules on Rorschach protocol interpretation.* Paper presented at the American Speech and Hearing Association national convention, Atlanta, 1973.

Wilson, F. B., & Rice, M. *A programmed approach to voice therapy.* Austin, Texas: Learning Concepts, Inc., 1977.

Wilson, K. D. *Voice problems of children* (2nd ed.). Baltimore: The Williams and Wilkins Company, 1979.

Witzel, M. A., Munro, I. R., & Chir, B. Velopharyngeal insufficiency after maxillary advancement. *Cleft Palate Journal,* 1977, *14.* 176–180.

Zwitman, D., & Calcaterra, T. C. The "silent cough" method for vocal hyperfunction. *Journal of Speech and Hearing Disorders,* 1973, *38*(1), 119–125.

Chapter 5
Psychogenic and Neurogenic Voice Disorders in Adults

This chapter is designed to provide the speech/language pathologist (SLP) with practical information and strategies for improving management of adult clients with psychogenic and neurogenic voice disorders. Many of the considerations in Chapter 4 on voice disorders among school children may or may not apply to adults, and an attempt is made to clarify the distinctions. The language describing the voice symptoms of these adults is the same as in the previous chapter—terms such as hoarseness, breathiness, laryngeal tension, spasticity, aphonia, hypernasality, and hyponasality. The methods of pitch evaluation outlined can be applied easily to adults, and where adjustments are necessary they are provided. The concept of habitual and optimal pitch evaluation is even more critical in adult voice management than it is with children, and these pitch considerations receive elaboration in this chapter as well as in Chapter 6 on vocal abuse among adults.

Most therapy with adults who have psychogenic and neurogenic voice disorder occurs in a hospital, speech and hearing clinic, university training center, or private practice. The interaction necessary between the SLP and the medical community is more readily available for adults than for school children but the same practical concerns about physician relationships and medical referral persist. It is even more critical in many respects that adults with laryngeal disorder have a medical inspection. The vocal symptoms of cancer of the larynx do not differ significantly from many other laryngeal disorders but treatment procedures are radically different. If the SLP does not have medical clearance before managing adults with laryngeal symptomatology, the client may have a disease such as laryngeal cancer. Not to recognize this possibility is to invite a malpractice suit for the SLP and perhaps death to the client.

PSYCHOGENIC VOICE DISORDER

The larynx is a well-organized and stable biological structure that maintains separation of the respiratory and digestive tracts. The reflexes involved in such critical separation work well even under trying circumstances such as emotional and physical duress. However, the laryngeal mechanisms do not seem to be so stable in producing voice or phonation for communication and are highly vulnerable to breakdown under stress conditions. Consider the example of a major league baseball manager who had been dismissed. At a press conference to announce his departure, partway into his message this highly verbal manager had to stop and walk away. He could not control his emotional state sufficiently to speak.

Many persons have had similar experiences under even less traumatic circumstances when voice could not be produced, when speech was stopped or, if not stopped, certainly affected negatively so the emotional state could not be hidden or masked. Whether the emotional state is one of fear, fright, anger, or happiness, the human voice generally communicates the condition. It is indeed almost impossible for individuals to mask their emotional state from this delicate structure of voice. The biological functions of the larynx are not affected, since swallowing water or some other liquid or food does not jeopardize the integrity of the protective valving mechanisms.

All of this vocal symptomatology involving stress, fear, fright, anger, or happiness is experienced by everyone and is normal. However, in many individuals these vocal effects are the standard, not the emotional exception. Such persons have psychogenic voice disorder (Aronson, 1980). The symptoms are varied, ranging from a slight but rather consistent quiver or tremor in the voice on one extreme to complete aphonia on the other. The common factor in each disorder is the absence of any physical basis that can be identified to explain the voice symptoms. A laryngoscopic examination reveals normal structural aspects—only the voice function is abnormal.

Case Example of Psychogenic Voice Disorder

L.H., a 56-year-old female, was referred by an otolaryngologist who found a severe dysphonia with no organic or physical basis. Indirect laryngoscopy revealed normal vocal structures. The case history revealed nothing of consequence as to emotional factors that might be the basis of her phonation disorder. Her voice was characterized as manifesting severe tension to the degree of completely stopping her from phonating periodically as she spoke. Tension was present constantly in her voice. She seemed a remarkedly well-adjusted woman who said she enjoyed life each day and spent much time fishing and relishing nature.

Therapy for L.H. involved a rather direct symptomatic approach that focused on her vocal tension. No further attempts were directed at uncovering any underlying emotional basis for her voice disorder. However, after two weeks of therapy, L.H. mentioned to her SLP that her voice disorder began when her husband divorced her and ran off with a younger woman. Knowing this fact did not change the nature of her voice therapy, but it certainly facilitated understanding why her dysphonia had occurred. L.H.'s case example illustrates the close relationship between emotional states and the development of psychogenic voice disorder. She was terminated after five weeks of therapy with a normal voice.

Vocal Symptoms

When the functional stability of laryngeal voicing is affected by some psychological factor, the symptoms can vary on a continuum from aphonia (hypofunction) to spasticity (hyperfunction). Although Moses (1954) proposes that psychological states of neurosis can be diagnosed by vocal symptoms, few practicing SLPs have found success in such attempts. It is entirely possible that similar dysphonic voice patterns result from quite varied psychological states of the mind.

Voice symptoms can also occur in pitch and resonance as well as hypofunctional or hyperfunctional laryngeal valving. The pitch of the voice may be excessively high or low, or the vocal tract may be significantly constricted, preventing full resonance. The loudness of the voice can be affected by psychological states so the person speaks in a very soft voice. Some adults present abnormal pitch inflections as a symptom. All of these voice dimensions can interact in subtle ways to produce a complex of symptoms of underlying psychological disorder.

One unique characteristic of psychogenic voice disorder is the variability of its symptomatology. Within one voice sample, the trained SLP usually can detect vocal hyperfunction, vocal hypofunction manifested as breathiness, and even instances of normal vocal fold vibration. These symptoms occur randomly during a communication utterance. Patterns of symptomatology can be so unusual that no organic condition would affect the larynx in such an extreme and variable manner.

Excessive muscular tension in the extrinsic and intrinsic laryngeal structures usually is present even when the primary vocal symptoms involve hypofunction such as breathiness or aphonia. Tension can be detected in the masseter, sternocleidomastoid, and mylohyoid muscles. Most other laryngeal muscles manifest similar tension but these specific ones are easier to palpate. The hyoid bone and thyroid cartilage rise excessively during phonation attempts. The SLP should not be confused by these seemingly incompatible symptoms of hypofunctional voice patterns accompanied by hyperfunctional laryngeal structures.

Laryngoscopic examination of the laryngeal structures may reveal slight swelling or reddening of the vocal folds, giving the impression that an organic or structural basis for the voice disorder exists. However, it should become apparent that the severity and extreme variability of vocal symptoms is inconsistent with the slight organic factor. The swelling or reddening most likely results from the general hyperfunctional nature of psychogenic voice disorder and can be considered as a slight vocal abuse factor.

Evaluation Procedures

Before proceeding into the management of an adult suspected of psychogenic voice disorder, the SLP should be sure the client is evaluated medically by an otolaryngologist, just as is recommended with children. Organic conditions of a neurogenic nature produce voice symptoms similar to psychogenic voice disorder, so medical referral is necessary to diagnose the etiology properly. Aronson (1973) reports a case diagnosed as having "functional aphonia" that actually was based on a disease called myasthenia gravis, a myoneuronal junction disease that can affect laryngeal, swallowing, and palatal muscle functions. Only after case-history examination and endurance speech testing was the vocal deterioration noted, prompting the neurological testing necessary for the diagnosis.

When a medical examination has eliminated organicity as the basis for the voice disorder, the SLP should begin the evaluation by taking a thorough case history. Questions should explore background and general aspects of life style to identify possible interpersonal or environmental sources of stress and conflict. In a general and nonthreatening manner, the SLP should explore with the client such areas as family and marital interpersonal relationships, employment stress factors, attitudes about self-worth and self-acceptance, financial concerns, and general life style considerations. Many of these areas are private, emotionally laden, difficult to express, embarrassing to the client, and in general highly sensitive. It is not necessary to probe deeply into the individual's private life as this would be inappropriate for the SLP whose purpose is to manage voice disorder. Instead, a general atmosphere of communication encouragement and acceptance is appropriate.

The SLP should begin something like:

"It has been found that persons with voice patterns similar to yours are experiencing conflicts and stresses that might be affecting the voice. Is anything happening in your life that might be important for us to understand? What about your family life? Your marriage? Job? Financial concerns? What do you think?"

An encouraging attitude from the SLP can stimulate communication about those areas. The adult at first may deny any such conflicts, but time and rapport in an encouraging atmosphere usually provide the forum for the client to communicate about these sensitive concerns.

The case history also helps the SLP determine whether there is a significant disparity between the emotional or psychological state of the adult and the degree of vocal symptomatology. Therapy to eliminate abnormal voice symptomatology usually is effective only in removing voice patterns that are extremely disparate from the emotional or psychological state. This information also may reveal that the client's psychological or emotional state is so critical that immediate referral to a psychologist or psychiatrist is necessary rather than a professional effort by a speech/language pathologist directed at eliminating the person's voice symptoms.

By the end of the evaluation process, it should be clear that the significant aspects of the client's voice disorder are psychogenic in nature. Medical evaluation should have produced a diagnosis of functional or psychogenic dysphonia and the SLP should expand on it with an analysis of the vocal symptoms. Therapy then can begin to remediate the dysphonia. The therapy procedures recommended in this chapter involve removal of vocal symptoms found to be abnormal in the evaluation, a process Boone (1977) calls symptomatic voice therapy.

Therapy for Psychogenic Voice Disorder

The prognosis for removing abnormal symptoms in psychogenic voice disorder depends on several factors. One of the most important is the latency between the onset of vocal symptoms and the initiation of therapy. The sooner the SLP is consulted after the voice disorder begins, the better the prognosis for improvement. However, several months or even years may elapse before the client seeks help and under such conditions it is more difficult to eliminate the abnormal symptoms because they become more resistant to removal as time passes.

Another prognosis factor is the severity of the symptoms. The more extreme the symptoms, whether hypofunctional or hyperfunctional, the better the prognosis for improvement, particularly when managed soon after onset. Aphonia, whispering, or extreme tension that produce spastic stoppage in phonation all are easier to modify than slight quivering or tremor in the voice.

Symptomatic voice therapy with an adult with newly developed and extreme patterns of voice production can be managed in a direct and straightforward manner. One of the most effective facilitators in a client who is aphonic or only whispering is to use a simple coughing pattern of voice initiation. Adults with psychogenic voice disorder with primarily hypofunctional symptoms do not seem to realize that the sound heard in a cough involves the same valving and vibration principles as true phonation. The sound of the cough is the sound of vibrating vocal folds. When asked to cough, the aphonic adult produces "voice" without realizing it. By extending the cough phonation into normal vowel production, normal phonation is facilitated. Once the person can cough and prolong it into a vowel, the SLP can suggest the cough be dropped while holding onto the vowel. The individual may have trouble doing that without dropping the cough phonation. If that is the case, the SLP should suggest the adult think of beginning to cough without actually doing so. The client should feel the "set" of a cough without actually coughing, then prolong the set into a normal vowel.

A suggestion to grunt as though lifting something heavy can produce the same valving action of the vocal folds as heard in coughing or normal phonation. This form of voicing then can be prolonged into a vowel in the same manner as the coughing method. The adult can be asked to demonstrate a forceful hum. This can facilitate phonation in the person with aphonia or hypofunctional voice disorder.

The coughing, grunting, and humming all are techniques of distraction. The client suddenly is producing voice without being aware of it. Whichever technique is used, it is important that the SLP move the adult quickly through steps leading to normal voice usage in communication:

1. coughing or similar technique
2. prolongation into a normal vowel without the cough
3. production of all vowels
4. monosyllabic words
5. any word
6. simple phrases
7. oral reading
8. simple conversation
9. conversation about anything and with anyone in the clinic setting
10. generalization to everyday communication

Since a number of suggestions or techniques are workable, a word of caution should be given regarding how to proceed. Before trying any particular technique such as coughing or grunting, the SLP should make a general statement such as:

"You have not lost your voice. You have merely lost the ability to make it work. We are going to try a variety of things to help you regain this ability. Let's see how they work. Let's begin by having you . . ."

The SLP is not setting the stage for one powerful technique to work in an "I command you to be healed" manner. Such a general statement permits one technique to be attempted and, if it fails, another can be tried without discouraging the individual.

Once the adult can communicate with voice in the therapy session, it is important to move as quickly as possible into conversation by following the steps established previously. When the aphonia or hypofunctional problem has been of rather short duration, the client often can move quickly into a conversation mode without the voice disorder. The SLP should accept such rapid change and say something such as:

"There, your voice is back. You have done the right thing(s) to get it back, and you do not need to worry that you will ever lose it again."

The SLP should continue the conversation mode until convinced of vocal stability, then set up an appointment for a checkup in a few days. When rapid and successful change occurs, the SLP should remember that only the symptom of psychological disturbance has been removed. The client may need to be referred to a psychologist or psychiatrist for professional help with unresolved conflicts, but the SLP may have confidence that the vocal symptom is not likely to return nor be replaced by some other symptom.

Case Example of Aphonia

The following example illustrates the therapy approach recommended for psychogenic voice disorder when the emotional conflict or trauma is of rather short duration and the voice symptoms have been manifested rather recently.

R.T. was an 18-year-old female who was referred because of a severe voice disorder of recent duration. She was a victim of a robbery while working as an attendant at a local self-service gasoline station. It was late at night and the robber held a knife to her throat and told her to empty the cash register. After she complied, the robber took the money but before leaving ran the knife across R.T.'s throat, making a superficial cut across the larynx. She was taken to the hospital and examined for possible laryngeal damage. Nothing of consequence was found other than a superficial cut of external tissue—there was no laryngeal damage. However, R.T. could produce only a weak and breathy voice even several days after the incident.

At the time of her appointment, the SLP decided that no long case history about her emotional status was necessary since it seemed rather obvious that she suffered from hysterical aphonia. R.T. reported, and her mother confirmed, that she had had no voice problems before the robbery.

The approach chosen by the SLP was symptomatic voice therapy. R.T. was instructed to cough. She gave a loud and abrupt cough. She then was instructed to cough again and prolong it into a vowel /a/, which the SLP demonstrated. R.T. accomplished this without difficulty. Several other vowels were attempted in the same manner and the cough was eliminated. Next, she was asked to repeat several words from a list, then to count from 1 to 20. Following the counting, she was asked to name the days of the week, months of the year, items that could be purchased in a department store, how to scramble eggs, and finally what her plans were for the next few days. She explained in clear and strong voice that she was planning a wedding and that she was glad to have her voice back before her wedding day.

After a few minutes of conversation about her wedding plans, the SLP was convinced that R.T.'s voice was entirely normal and no further therapy would be needed. An appointment was made for her to return in three days for a checkup. The SLP also mentioned that she might experience some horror memory from the robbery and that it might be helpful to see a psychologist or psychiatrist even though her voice had returned. She was not sure how she felt about that but said she would consider it. When the time came for her next appointment, her mother called to say that because of the wedding pressures, R.T. did not want to come for the checkup and that her voice was entirely normal. The case of R.T. clearly represents successful voice therapy.

SPECIFIC TECHNIQUES OF THERAPY

Many forms of psychogenic voice disorder are not as easily managed as the case of R.T. For example, when considerable time has passed between the development of the voice disorder and the initiation of therapy, the prognosis for significant change or improvement is diminished. When the adult has had the voice symptoms for several months or even years, it is as though they become an integral part of coping strategies of everyday conflict. The voice pattern seems to become part of the client's communication personality and, as a result, much more resistant to easy modification. This should not discourage the SLP because such resistance to easy change is more typical of the everyday clinical experiences in communication disorder. Quick and easy management is the exception rather than the rule in any therapy, so why should voice therapy be different?

With patients who have experienced long-term psychogenic voice disorder, a simple cough, hum, or grunt technique will not produce significant change or improvement. That will come only when the client learns the processes of voice production, how the vocal folds work to produce voice, how various dimensions of voice such as tension, pitch, loudness, and quality can be regulated, and how stress affects these factors. The adult must become informed and aware that although personality, emotion, and voice are highly intertwined, considerable conscious control can be exerted over the vocal system. This control will not develop easily but with careful instruction and therapeutic direction, vocal stability can be achieved by those who really seek such improvement.

Several techniques have been reported in the literature as clinically effective in achieving control over long-term psychogenic voice disorder. Most of these are directed at reducing the hyperfunctional aspects of voice production in persons with psychogenic voice disorder. When tension exists and the voice manifests such tension, it is not enough to suggest that if the person could relax when talking the voice would improve. Rather, the individual must be taken through systematic stages of control over the muscles involved in the hyperfunctional basis to phonation. The following techniques have been used to accomplish this control.

Progressive Relaxation

Jacobson proposed a method of training persons to master tension by learning to contrast states of tension in the body with its elimination through progressive relaxation. In the fifth edition of his book, Jacobson (1978) suggests a series of steps of muscle isolation to identify and eliminate tension:

> We call the relaxation "progressive" in three respects: (1) The subject relaxes a group, for instance the muscles that bend the right arm, further and further each minute. (2) He learns one after the other to relax the principal muscle groups of his body. With each new group he simultaneously relaxes such parts as have received practice previously. (3) As he practices from day to day, according to my experience, he progresses toward a habit of repose—tends toward a state in which quiet is automatically maintained. (p. 161)

The specific method of obtaining muscle relaxation in the person with psychogenic voice disorder is not as critical as focusing on the laryngeal mechanism once general body relaxation has been achieved. As Boone

(1977) states, "The clinician who chooses to use relaxation methods with particular patients should remember that these methods are usually best combined with other facilitating techniques designed especially for producing a better voice" (p. 152).

Biofeedback

Clients have been helped in eliminating specific areas of body tension by receiving information of excessive muscle contraction fed back through visual or auditory means. Prosek, Montgomery, Walden, and Schwartz (1978) report success with three of six patients with hyperfunctional voice disorder by means of biofeedback. Biofeedback methodology differs from system to system but generally uses information from muscle or brainwave activity as a reflection of the biophysical state of the body. When muscle activity is being monitored, a process called EMG (electromyography) is used. EMG electrodes are placed in surface contact with the muscle being monitored so contractions can be detected, amplified, and fed back to the client as visual or auditory signals. When the adult is made aware of the contraction of the monitored muscle(s), efforts can be directed to the muscle to relax. EMG techniques also have been developed that introduce electrodes into the muscles of the larynx to monitor contractions during phonation, but such efforts have involved basic research rather than clinical modification of speaking patterns.

A therapy approach using biofeedback as an adjunct to vocal management could develop as follows. Assuming the SLP understands the technology of operating the biofeedback instrumentation, or is working with someone who does, the client is instructed to concentrate on monitoring the signal that detects excessive contraction of the muscle(s) being analyzed. A stable baseline of biofeedback tension or contraction is thus established. The person is directed to think about relaxing activities while maintaining awareness of the signal. The purpose is to have the client use the relaxing thoughts to help eliminate the muscular tension. The signal provides the feedback necessary to indicate whether the process is working.

In gradual hierarchical steps, the adult is directed to concentrate on more stressful and anxiety-provoking situations while attempting to keep the biofeedback signal at low levels. When the client's self-projection into imagined images or situations is achieved, reality is introduced by having the person actually produce voice by humming, prolonging a sustained /a/, or a similar task while maintaining biofeedback control. As the task of phonating without triggering the biofeedback sensors is established, the level of difficulty is increased from phonemes to words, to phrases, to reading, and finally to conversation. At each stage, it is necessary to allow the client to adapt to the biofeedback signal for a period of time before task escalation.

The adult soon should be able to determine when relaxation has been achieved without the biofeedback signal. When this has been accomplished, generalization of the control should be attempted by having the person speak in more natural settings away from the clinic under the SLP's careful supervision. Each time the client undertakes a speaking venture it should be followed by a therapy time for discussion as to the success of the task.

Digital Manipulation of Phonation

Although it is difficult for the typical adult with a hyperfunctional voice disorder to understand, normal phonation should be an easy process. The SLP should demonstrate that the larynx does not work efficiently under conditions of tension but does its best when little or no effort is involved. Easy, relaxed phonation should result in the client's not feeling much vibration in the larynx. The voice vibration should be felt more in the resonance chambers above the larynx rather than in the larynx itself. Most of the vocal energy during phonation should be felt diversely in the oral and nasal cavities, referred to by music teachers as the mask of the face. This balance of resonance in the mask of the face can be demonstrated by having the client feel the vibrations in the SLP's face during normal phonation. The person should place one finger lightly on the side of the SLP's nose, another finger on the face around the lips, and another lightly on the side of the larynx around the thyroid laminae. As the SLP phonates an /m/ sound, the adult should be able to detect a balance of vibration in all three areas, with most of the sound concentration felt in the mask of the face around the lips. The client then can phonate an /m/ sound and personally feel the results in the same manner. In addition to the balance of resonance felt in the mask of the face, the client should experience a tingling sensation generally throughout that area and around the lips. If this is felt, chances are excellent that the larynx is being vibrated efficiently without excessive tension. The SLP should point out how phonation in this manner seems devoid of significant vibration happening in the larynx. This concept is supported by Boone (1977) and Cooper (1977) and is strongly recommended by the author of this chapter as an effective method of monitoring normal phonation in clients with hyperfunctional voice disorder.

Case Example of Hyperfunctional Voice Disorder

J.B., a 46-year-old clergyman, referred himself for a voice evaluation because of vocal difficulty that was interfering with his ministry. He said that for several years he had found it more and more difficult to preach effectively and to deal with the numerous problems presented by members of his congregation. He also reported having considerable difficulty with his daughter, whom he called a "free spirit." He noticed that at the beginning of the day his voice was quite clear but as he faced problem after problem he felt it grow tighter and tighter until he was unable to speak. He recently had seen an otolaryngologist who found nothing wrong with the structures of his voice and that the disorder was nonorganic. J.B. indicated that he understood that nonorganic was a euphemism for psychologically based.

His voice examination revealed a pattern characterized by excessive tension during most phonation efforts and periodic spastic stoppages. It also was weak in loudness. Excessive contraction of muscles surrounding his neck (sternocleidomastoid, mylohyoid) and in his jaw area (masseter) supported the perception of vocal tension.

J.B.'s therapy began with a complete explanation of the larynx, how it worked, and what happened to it when used improperly, using pictures and models. The myoelastic-aerodynamic theory of phonation was explained simply. He also was shown how phonation could occur under variable amounts of tension in a continuum from hypofunctional control (breathiness), to normal phonation, to hyperfunctional control (spasticity). The purpose was to show him how much voluntary control over the voice was possible.

During the next few sessions, J.B. was given instructions on progressive relaxation and taken through the steps necessary to achieve voluntary relaxation. After he had learned to consciously relax most of the muscles of his body, including his extrinsic laryngeal ones, he was instructed to take a deep breath and let the air escape from his lungs in an easy, relaxed manner. After a few cycles of relaxed respiration, he was told to add a breathy sigh as he released air. This showed him that voluntary control of the tension in his voice was possible. He repeated this breathy sigh process until he was able to exhale and phonate various vowels in the same breathy manner.

As J.B. was producing these breathy utterances on vowels, the SLP pointed out that when phonating with this easy manner he should not be able to feel anything happen in the larynx. All the vibration of voice production should be felt in the mask of the face. J.B. agreed that such was the case and said he was surprised how easy phonation could be.

At this point in therapy, negative practice (Boone, 1977) was introduced to show him the difference between hypofunctional and hyperfunctional phonation. The ability to shift into and out of tense phonation indicated that he had achieved voluntary control over the tension level of voice. J.B. then was directed to use his new voice, which was deliberately established at a slightly breathy level, in large articulation units, i.e., monosyllabic words, any word, phrases, short sentences, context reading, simple dialogue, and finally conversation. At each stage of escalation, negative practice was used to help him maintain the contrast of tension vs. nontense, normal phonation.

When J.B. was able to converse with the SLP about various topics with his new voice, a hierarchy was established that allowed systematic generalization to everyday communication. The hierarchy involved having J.B. rank specific situations that he felt caused stress and concern while communicating on a continuum from low stress to high stress. Some of the conversation situations he ranked low in the hierarchy were speaking with his wife early in the morning and offering personal and family prayers. The highest ranking involved leading a group counseling session among young people in his church. J.B. then was instructed to attempt as well as he could to control the tension in his voice when speaking in the situations ranked low on the hierarchy and gradually move up the list. It took him three weeks of constant effort to approach the higher situations.

At the higher levels, he began having difficulty controlling his voice. For example, J.B. reported that at times the tension level at the counseling sessions with the young people got so high that everyone felt it. It was in these situations that control of vocal tension was rather poor. He felt he was controlling the tension better than before therapy started but also felt there was room for improvement. After a few more sessions in which little progress was made, he terminated formal therapy. A checkup schedule was established to help him maintain the control he had achieved. Five checkups in a seven-month period revealed only minor setbacks in J.B.'s ability to control the tension in his voice.

SUMMARY OF PSYCHOGENIC VOICE DISORDER

The human voice is highly influenced by fluctuations in emotional and psychological status. When vocal symptoms become a symptom of psychological disturbance, or a constant aspect of coping strategies, symptomatic voice therapy is appropriate to remove the parameters of voice that are judged abnormal. This therapy can be conducted before, concurrent with, or following counselling or psychotherapy directed at helping the adult obtain better control over factors influencing the psychological state.

Some forms of psychogenic voice disorder are of a hysterical nature with rather dramatic onset. Other forms develop more insidiously and become part of a general coping strategy for handling environmental or interpersonal stress. The prognosis for successful treatment depends upon the factors of client cooperation, latency between the onset of the disorder and the initiation of therapy, the clinical skill of the SLP, and the application of appropriate clinical management procedures. The cooperation of other professionals is an important part of this management process.

SPASMODIC (SPASTIC) DYSPHONIA

It often is difficult to discriminate symptomatically between some forms of psychogenic voice disorder previously described and one known as spasmodic (spastic) dysphonia. Earlier literature considered spasmodic dysphonia as having a significant psychogenic basis. For example, Murphy (1964) states that the onset of spasmodic dysphonia "may be sudden—following an emotional shock of some kind—or of longer duration. And, although it is usually a hyperkinetic phenomenon, hypokinetic conditions have been observed. We are probably dealing with hysteria in such cases. The disorder may be regarded psychodynamically as a somatization developed unconsciously as a defense against the recognition of unacceptable urges" (p. 71).

Few professionals today consider spasmodic dysphonia a psychogenic voice disorder. Rather, it is classified more as having a neurogenic etiology with possible psychogenic byproducts. It is clear to most who work with clients with spasmodic dysphonia that the vocal symptoms are varied, capricious, affected by emotional states, and often absent during laughter, singing, or unusual vocal efforts. These factors give the impression that the disorder is affected significantly by psychodynamics but such evidence does not solve the issue of etiology directly. A brief review of recent literature more clearly communicates the neurogenic theory of etiology.

In a study involving 12 spasmodic dysphonic patients, Aminoff, Dedo, and Izdebski (1978) find no evidence of psychiatric symptomatology. Ten males and two females were evaluated by a team of specialists representing neurology, psychiatry and otolaryngology. No evidence of psychiatric or laryngeal disorder was found to justify the voice symptoms. However, eight of the patients were found to have coexisting neurological disorders, including postural tremor, buccolingual dyskinesia, blepharospasm, and idiopathic torsion dystonia. The authors conclude that spasmodic dysphonia should be regarded as a focal tremor of the laryngeal musculature. Perhaps the most striking aspect of this study, and one that can support generalization, is that not one of the 12 patients demonstrated evidence of the psychogenic basis considered historically to be the cause of spasmodic dysphonia.

Vocal Symptoms in Spasmodic Dysphonia

The vocal symptoms of spasmodic dysphonia can be classified in the hyperfunctional range of voice disorders. Symptoms of tension, vocal strain, vocal strangle, and vocal squeeze are described by Aronson (1973, 1980). In some patients, the symptoms begin rather suddenly although in the majority they appear more gradually (Aminoff et al., 1978). Once symptoms stabilize, there is little variation in the vocal patterns except under conditions of fatigue and emotional lability. The voice patterns can become so severe as to produce occupational disability and social maladjustment. Depression is not uncommon among these clients since there is so little relief from the vocal symptoms.

One of the most striking aspects of spasmodic dysphonia is that therapy generally is unsuccessful in improving the voice condition. Most adults can improve and control the vocal symptoms in small units of voice production such as monosyllabic utterances but rarely in contextual speech. The poor prognosis for remediation is one of the most significant symptoms of this voice disorder.

Surgical Considerations in Spasmodic Dysphonia

Because of the poor prognosis reported by most SLPs working with spasmodic dysphonia clients, an alternative treatment method has been developed involving surgical disruption of the innervation to one vocal fold. Dedo and Shipp (1980) report a procedure that involves surgically sectioning the recurrent laryngeal nerve unilaterally to produce a paralysis of the vocal fold on the side sectioned. When this occurs, the paralyzed vocal fold remains fixed in a position just off midline in the paramedian or intermediate position, making spastic valving of the vocal folds difficult or impossible. The voice quality is usually hypofunctional rather than spastic. Inasmuch as this procedure is not reversible, care must be taken to ensure that vocal improvement will result. This is accomplished by injection of an anesthetizing substance (lidocaine) in the nerve to be sectioned, producing a temporary paralysis of the vocal fold innervated by that nerve. During the temporary paralysis, the client's voice can be taped and evaluated for potential benefit from the surgical procedure.

The results of this surgical procedure are varied and not free from controversy. Whereas Dedo, Izdebski, and Townsend (1977) report success on 200 patients, others find that after a few months several of the adults sectioned experienced spasmodic relapse. Wilson, Oldring, & Mueller (1980) report that in one case in which the female patient's voice symptoms improved considerably following surgery, the spasmodic dysphonia returned nine months later. Inspection of her laryngeal tissues and nerve fibers revealed an intact recurrent laryngeal nerve, presumably from nerve regeneration. Aronson (1980) recommends careful follow-up on clients receiving this or similar surgical procedures in order to evaluate the long-term results as well as to provide therapeutic support.

Therapy for Spasmodic Dysphonia

Whether or not surgical procedures have been used in a client with spasmodic dysphonia, several approaches can help eliminate or reduce the symptoms. Techniques recommended for the hyperfunctional voice patterns in psychogenic voice disorder include relaxation, biofeedback, digital manipulation, and hierarchical analysis. These are used in a manner similar to that described earlier in this chapter.

Case Example of Spasmodic Dysphonia

N.K., a 27-year-old female graduate student majoring in psychology, was seen for an evaluation of her voice. She was concerned that her effectiveness as a psychologist was hindered by the voice tension that was present rather constantly. She was found to have spasmodic characteristics. She was referred to an otolaryngologist, who diagnosed her voice as spastic dysphonia. The otolaryngologist found her vocal folds during phonation were in a tightly adducted position sufficient to stop vibration.

N.K.'s case history revealed nothing of significance with regard to social or psychological maladjustment. She was in the final stages of her Ph.D. in clinical psychology and had worked successfully in an institute for the criminally insane. Her only complaint was the tension in her voice. She had experienced such tension for several years and was not sure when it started other than that it had had a rather gradual onset.

Voice analysis indicated that her pitch was appropriate, loudness adequate, breath support adequate, and resonance (oral/nasal) normal. The primary vocal symptom was laryngeal tension, which was marked by periodic spastic stoppage of phonation. When spasticity occurred, it was momentary. She would stop and breathe, then begin speaking again with tension.

Therapy for N.K. consisted of (1) an accurate yet simple description of the mechanisms of voice production with emphasis on the fact that vocal efficiency did not require extensive effort, (2) drill to demonstrate voluntary control over the amount of voice tension by having her produce a vowel sound first in a whisper, then with breathiness, then with slight tension, and finally with such tension as to stop phonation, and (3) drill on vowels and words utilizing a slightly breathy phonation pattern.

N.K. was able to control the laryngeal spasticity on a sound and word level so long as she kept her voice breathy. When she tried to produce voice with normal vocal fold approximation, spasticity occurred. She next was introduced to a technique that facilitated an open glottis at the onset of phonation by eliminating a hard glottal attack. By teaching her to initiate voice with a preceding consonant /h/, the onset of phonation was less tense. This technique is explained by Boone (1977). Drill using this silent /h/ technique included having N.K. say phrases such as the following with an /h/ sound at the beginning:

/h/Open the door
/h/I'm in here
/h/Ask me about it

With this technique, she could phonate without the vocal folds' becoming spastic and tightly closed. After practicing several phrases with the /h/ at the beginning, she was instructed to imagine an /h/ as she began to speak so she could approach phonation with less tension.

After several sessions of therapy directed at teaching N.K. to voluntarily control the tension in her body and laryngeal mechanisms during phonation, an attempt was made to gain control in conversations in her "real" world. This was done by means of hierarchical analysis. She made a list of typical examples of communication difficulties and ranked them from low stress (low voice symptom occurrence) to high stress (high voice symptom occurrence). She then was given assignments to work her way up the hierarchy systematically.

N.K. succeeded in achieving significant control in the communication situations ranked low on the hierarchy, but experienced poor control in the more difficult situations. One of the most difficult involved frequent meetings with her faculty and graduate student peers, at which she was unable to gain any significant control over her vocal tension.

After a semester and a half, N.K. terminated therapy. She said it was unlikely that she could achieve further gains in learning to control her vocal tension in the difficult speaking situations. She expressed pleasure about the gains she had made but complete frustration about why she was not able to master her voice. The last communication from N.K. indicated she was considering the surgery (Dedo & Shipp, 1980) mentioned earlier in this chapter to see whether that would help.

SUMMARY OF SPASMODIC (SPASTIC) DYSPHONIA

Although the etiology of spasmodic dysphonia remains unclear, it constitutes one of the most perplexing voice disorders to professionals working with persons who have it. The rather poor prognosis for improvement should not discourage the SLP from attempting to modify the vocal symptoms involved with this disorder since some adults can attain substantial control. This takes considerable patience and understanding on the part of both client and the SLP. Several techniques have been described that can foster improvement when properly applied by the SLP. Even when surgical management is attempted, the SLP should work with the client to help facilitate optimal usage of the improved valving mechanism of the larynx. Several authors have described techniques for working with clients who have spasmodic dysphonia, and the reader should explore these (Boone, 1977; Aronson, 1980; Cooper, 1977).

NEUROGENIC VOICE DISORDER

The neurological basis of human phonation is complex and yet stable as a biological process. The larynx must function well in its valving processes to keep food, liquid, saliva, and other substances from entering the delicate respiratory system. As an insurance against such a threat, the larynx receives innervation from both cerebral hemispheres of the brain in rich supply. As a result of both ipsilateral and contralateral innervation from the brain, damage to one cerebral hemisphere sufficient to paralyze a person's body on one side (arm, leg, facial muscles, etc.) will not result in laryngeal paralysis of either sensory or motor functions. The innervation received from the nondamaged hemisphere is sufficient to maintain laryngeal function.

Notwithstanding this stability, numerous diseases, surgical procedures, and specific traumas can disrupt the neurological integrity of the laryngeal system for both biological valving and phonation. This section elaborates on those common neurogenic factors and provides evaluation and remediation considerations for the SLP treating clients with such a voice disorder.

Review of Laryngeal Innervation

The peripheral nervous system that supports the sensory and motor functions of the larynx is primarily the X cranial nerve, called the vagus, with assistance from the XI cranial nerve, the accessory. The accessory enters the vagus prior to any laryngeal branch and therefore the vagus is considered the primary nerve of laryngeal control. The vagus innervates many of the visceral organs of the body, including the cardiovascular and digestive systems. Specific branches of the vagus exit the main trunk of the nerve to innervate the larynx.

The first branch off the vagus that has laryngeal function is the superior laryngeal nerve, which immediately divides into two branches—internal and external. The internal branch is sensory in function and is responsible for providing the brain with information regarding the sensory status of the laryngeal structures above the level of the vocal folds. Any foreign substance that touches the mucous membranes of the larynx above those folds stimulates the internal branch at its sensory nerve endings. This stimulation is passed to the brain for a motor response. The external branch is motor in function and is responsible for the innervation of the cricothyroid muscle on the side of the larynx served by the nerve. The cricothyroid muscle is important for laryngeal adjustments necessary for pitch control of the voice.

The second branch off the main trunk of the vagus that innervates the larynx is the recurrent laryngeal nerve. The left recurrent laryngeal nerve exits the vagus below the larynx, courses under the aortic arch, then passes in a superior direction along the trachea to enter the larynx. The recurrent laryngeal nerve is both motor and sensory in function: motor to all intrinsic laryngeal muscles (thyroarytenoid, posterior cricoarytenoid, lateral cricoarytenoid, and interarytenoid) except the cricothyroid; sensory to the mucous membranes of the larynx from the vocal folds to the inferior margins of the larynx.

The right recurrent laryngeal nerve functions in the same way except that it exits the vagus nerve at a point higher than the left and has a more direct course to the larynx. Therefore, all motor functions of vocal fold abduction and adduction are innervated by the recurrent laryngeal nerve and motor functions for pitch control by the external branch of the superior laryngeal nerve.

The right vagus with its laryngeal branches innervates the right side of the larynx, including the right vocal fold, and the left vagus with its laryngeal branches the left side and the left vocal fold. Sensory functions are shared by the recurrent and superior laryngeal nerves. The clinical significance of these divided nerve functions cannot be overemphasized (Zemlin, 1981).

When the innervation of the larynx is abnormal for some etiological reason, the functional aspects of voice and laryngeal valving are affected either unilaterally or bilaterally in terms of adduction or abduction of the vocal folds or in terms of elongation of the folds. The functions disrupted depend on the location of neurological damage. For the larynx to be affected bilaterally, damage to innervation processes must occur before the vagus nerves exit from the brain stem of the central nervous system. When damage occurs in the central nervous system (CNS) sufficient to have laryngeal effect, it is likely to produce functional disruptions in other structures of oral and laryngeal processes such as swallowing, articulation, velopharyngeal valving, and respiratory control for phonation. Such widespread neurological disorder is labeled dysarthria and has been reviewed extensively in all its manifestations by Darley, Aronson, and Brown (1975).

An extensive review of neurogenic voice disorder has been provided by Aronson (1980), and does not need to be duplicated here. However, the more common neurogenic voice disorders are presented in terms of specific symptomatology, evaluation, and remediation considerations.

It is important for the SLP to have medical information on the status of the laryngeal structures before any significant clinical management of clients with neurogenic voice disorder. The specific information includes:

1. the etiological factors involved in the client's voice disorder
2. the movement potential of the larynx to support phonation without aspiration
3. the physical status of the laryngeal mechanism and whether it is static, deteriorating, or improving
4. the position of the involved vocal fold(s) under phonation attempts
5. the medical clearance to begin voice therapy
6. the additional information the reporting physician may think is necessary for the SLP to understand the client's voice disorder

With this information, the SLP is ready to evaluate and begin treatment.

Vagus Nerve Lesions Affecting the Larynx

Any lesion along the branches of the vagus nerve innervating the larynx produces a clinical effect on phonation. The specific aspects of the disorder depend on the site of the lesion. One of the most common neurogenic voice disorders occurs when trauma, disease process, or surgical error disrupts the recurrent laryngeal nerve. The left recurrent laryngeal nerve is particularly vulnerable because of its long and wandering course to the larynx. Because of that nerve's adjacency to the aortic arch, the thyroid gland, and other structures close to the larynx, it is common for surgery on these structures to involve error that sections or traumatizes the nerve, resulting in disrupted innervation to the left side of the larynx and paralyzing the left vocal fold. The vocal fold is paralyzed in a position just off midline, usually the paramedian position, and does not adduct or abduct from that position. The voice disorder resulting from this paralysis involves vocal fold vibration. Since the paralyzed vocal fold is off midline, incomplete approximation of the folds occurs when phonation is attempted. The voice sounds breathy and its capacity for loudness is reduced. Tension often is heard most likely because of effort to obtain better adduction of the vocal folds during phonation.

In addition to the vocal symptoms of this condition of unilateral paralysis, it is common for the adult to experience difficulty with inhalation. Noise is heard as air is inhaled into the lungs because of the incomplete abduction of the vocal folds. The uninvolved fold abducts completely for inhalation but the paralyzed one remains nearly closed. The noise heard is called laryngeal stridor and is a form of phonation on inhalation.

Aspiration of food and liquid is another common complaint of such clients. Incomplete approximation of the vocal folds for phonation can occur also during swallowing. Because the protective valving mechanisms close incompletely, aspiration may occur. The more abducted the static position of the involved vocal fold, the greater the possibility of aspiration, and the worse the vocal symptoms. The more adducted the static position of the vocal fold, the less the possibility of aspiration and the better the voice, but the worse the stridor during inhalation. This is a well-understood reciprocal state of relationship between stridor, dysphonia, and aspiration.

Many of the vocal symptoms in an adult with unilateral paralysis are diminished when the person raises pitch, because the superior laryngeal nerve with its external and internal branches is intact when just the recurrent nerve has been damaged. Therefore, innervation to the cricothyroid muscle on both the normal and paralyzed sides remains functional, making vocal fold elongation possible in a normal manner. As the vocal folds are elongated during phonation, the pitch rises and the longitudinal tension generates better approximation (adduction) of the folds, even the paralyzed one. Therefore, not only is the pitch raised by this action but the quality of vibration is less breathy.

Case Example of Recurrent Laryngeal Nerve Paralysis with Masked Symptoms

The following case illustrates the voice disorder resulting from unilateral lesion of the recurrent laryngeal nerve. It also illustrates how cricothyroid contractions can mask the severity of the voice disorder.

M.S., a 29-year-old male, was referred by a fellow employee who was a SLP. M.S.'s main vocal concern was the voice pitch, which he felt was too high. His case history revealed that six years previously, he had had cancer of the thyroid gland that required surgical removal of much of the gland. During the surgery, his left recurrent laryngeal nerve had been accidently severed, after which he reported he "hardly had a voice at all." In the ensuing years, M.S. experienced gradual improvement in the strength and quality of his voice. His only concern at the time of his evaluation was that his pitch seemed too high and that he often was mistaken for a female on the telephone.

An evaluation of M.S.'s voice revealed essentially normal voice quality, indicating adequate approximation of his vocal folds at midline. However, his habitual pitch was found to be F_3 (174 Hz), which was typical of that of a mature female. He also experienced pitch breaks into the falsetto range.

Indirect laryngoscopy revealed a paralyzed left vocal fold as expected from the case history, but with normal midline approximation of the vocal folds when phonating at his habitual pitch level of F_3. It was hypothesized that the midline approximation occurred because of extensive contraction of his cricothyroid muscles. This also accounted for his high-pitched voice. It was hypothesized further that by lowering his pitch to a normal male level, the compensation mechanisms would be eliminated and his paralytic dysphonia would be unmasked.

Therapy during the next three weeks was directed at lowering his pitch from the F_3 to B_3 (123 Hz). When this had been accomplished, the quality of M.S.'s voice became breathy and lost loudness. Indirect laryngoscopy confirmed that a significant space (chink) existed between his vocal folds when he attempted phonation at the lower pitch level. His true paralytic dysphonia had been revealed. He then was referred to an otolaryngologist, who injected Teflon paste in three places lateral to his paralyzed vocal fold, displacing it closer to midline. M.S. tolerated the procedure well and upon recovery from the surgery had an appropriately pitched voice (C_3, 130 Hz) with normal vibration quality and loudness function (Case & Cleary, 1976).

Lesion of the Superior Laryngeal Nerve

A unilateral lesion of the superior laryngeal nerve primarily affects the elongation potential of the vocal fold on the side of the lesion. A sensory disorder also is manifested but this does not result in dysphonia. Normal adduction and abduction of the vocal folds remain. The cause of such a lesion affecting the superior laryngeal nerve usually is surgical error or trauma (Aronson, 1980). A bilateral lesion affecting both superior laryngeal nerves, although rare, affects severely the pitch regulating the voice potential. A slight breathiness is likely to be heard as well, inasmuch as bilateral cricothyroid dysfunction causes a bowing of the vocal folds as a result of the diminished longitudinal tension.

Central Nervous System Lesions Affecting Phonation

The nature of laryngeal innervation from the cortex to the vagus nerve nuclei in the brain stem is such that a lesion in the higher cortical centers of the central nervous system rarely affects the larynx unilaterally. If a lesion occurs on the cerebral cortex in one hemisphere at a location on the motor strip that innervates the larynx, no contralateral paralysis occurs because of the ipsilateral innervation it receives from the nondamaged cortex. Therefore, most lesions in the CNS that affect the larynx occur in the brain stem area where the vagus nerve nuclei are located. Such lesions do not produce the flaccidity of muscle function found in peripheral nerve lesions; rather, they do produce symptoms of spasticity, leading to vocal symptoms of tension and abnormal pitch control. More likely than not, the vocal symptoms are accompanied by dysarthria of a general nature, including sluggish articulation, hypernasality, and imprecise elements of speech prosody. A lesion is unlikely to be so specific in the brain stem as to affect only the cranial nerve nuclei innervating the larynx.

Medical Treatment of Vocal Fold Paralysis

When the innervation to the larynx is affected in such a way that abduction and adduction of the vocal folds cannot occur, considerable improvement to laryngeal valving can be produced through a procedure that involves injecting Teflon paste lateral to the paralyzed vocal fold (Dedo, 1973) as in the case of M.S. earlier. This paste has the effect of displacing the mass of the paralyzed vocal fold toward midline—the position of each fold during phonation. With the paralyzed vocal fold fixed at midline, and the uninvolved fold able to open and close properly, nearly normal phonation is possible. This procedure is especially effective when the paralyzed fold is positioned in the paramedian or intermediate position as compared with a widely abducted one.

When the laryngeal paralysis involves a unilateral condition in which the vocal fold is widely abducted and there is a difference in the horizontal planes of the two folds, a surgical procedure described by Isshiki, Massehiro, & Masaki (1978) involves transposition of the pars recta fibers of the cricothyroid muscle to the arytenoid that is immobile from the paralysis. Since the cricothyroid is the only intrinsic laryngeal muscle to receive innervation from a nerve other than the recurrent laryngeal nerve, it remains functional even when all other muscles of abduction and adduction are paralyzed. With fibers from the cricothyroid connected to the paralyzed arytenoid, when the arytenoid is contracted, it tilts toward a midline position and voice quality is improved.

Therapy for Vocal Fold Paralysis

The most standard and common therapeutic procedure SLPs use with adults who have unilateral paralysis of a vocal fold involves pushing or lifting during phonation. This technique is described by Boone (1977). The patient with paralysis is instructed to sit in a chair that the client can grasp underneath by both hands. When the adult lifts up on the chair in a futile effort to raise it off the floor, the entire laryngeal valving mechanisms are brought into an adducted state. The paralyzed vocal fold is brought closer to midline by passive constriction of the surrounding structures. The uninvolved vocal fold usually adducts across the midline plane to better approximate the paralyzed fold.

The client is instructed to phonate while lifting in this manner. The sound of the voice is recorded and analyzed by the adult and the SLP to determine whether such effort improves its quality. If such is the case, the process is continued as less and less lifting is done while the client attempts to maintain the improved quality. The goal is to have the person internalize the physical effort involved in lifting to produce the desired approximation of the vocal folds. This lifting technique can be attempted as soon as medical clearance to begin therapy is obtained, and can be performed whether or not physical management such as Teflon laryngoplasty or arytenoid adduction has been introduced.

Case Example of Laryngeal Paralysis

L.T., a 60-year-old female with a fourteen-year history of dysphonia, was diagnosed as having a paralyzed left vocal fold with unknown etiology (idiopathic). Four years after the diagnosis, she underwent Teflon laryngoplasty. She reported improved voice quality but her improved quality gradually diminished. She sought the help of another laryngologist who discovered "scar tissue, beads of Teflon extending into the glottal space from the left vocal fold, and a paralyzed left vocal fold." L.T. underwent surgery to remove the Teflon beads. Following recovery, she was seen by an SLP for a voice evaluation and possible therapy.

L.T.'s voice was judged as breathy, lacking in intensity, monotone, and diplophonic. Her diplophonic voice was the most striking aspect of the disorder. Her diplophonic pitch levels were G_3 (196 Hz) and $F\#_4$ (355 Hz). She also manifested an intermittent hoarse quality that sounded as though she had considerable phlegm on her vocal folds. Tension also was present, seemingly to compensate for her weak vocal intensity.

Therapy was directed at improving her vocal quality by controlling the diplophonia. With a tape recorder running throughout the therapy sessions, L.T. was instructed to phonate an /a/ sound at various pitch levels. She also was told to lift slightly on her chair as she phonated at the various pitches. Intermittently, a voice could be heard that lacked the diplophonia and had improved quality. When this was heard, the recorder was stopped and the voice sample played until L.T. had in her mind the target voice. Soon she was able to make the laryngeal adjustments to eliminate the higher pitch (F#$_4$, 355 Hz), leaving her with a habitual and optimal pitch of G$_3$, 196 Hz.

She then was directed through therapy steps at the target pitch and improved quality from the /a/ to words, phrases, sentences, oral reading, simple conversation, and finally normal conversation in the clinic. Once she was able to sustain her voice in therapy sessions in the clinic, a hierarchy was established for her to begin control in real life situations. After four weeks of therapy, L.T. was using her new voice in every situation. She still reported her voice was weak and inadequate in noisy situations such as restaurants and public places but appreciated the quality in most of her communication. As she stated, "I have not experienced this kind of voice quality for 14 years."

MISCELLANEOUS NEUROGENIC VOICE DISORDERS

The complex and delicate nature of laryngeal function makes the larynx highly vulnerable to abnormalities resulting from numerous diseases. In addition to the disorders already mentioned, several disease processes involving more generalized body functions can have a deleterious effect on the larynx. A common example is amyotrophic lateral sclerosis (ALS)—the so-called Lou Gehrig's disease. The specific etiology is unknown but generally involves progressive degeneration of both the corticospinal tracts in the cerebral hemispheres as well as the lower motor neuron nuclei for all motor functions, i.e., cranial and spinal nerve motor functions. In addition to the more general functional breakdown of ambulation, motor coordination of arms and legs, visceral functions of digestion and waste elimination, specific speech mechanisms are affected, sometimes early in the degeneration process. The cranial nerve nuclei innervating the tongue, soft palate, lips, and larynx can be affected severely.

The voice disorder manifested in ALS becomes part of a more general dysarthria affecting articulation and resonance. Consonant articulation is imprecise, causing diminished intelligibility. Hypernasality of vowels and nasal air emission of pressure consonants are common. The voice can be either weak and breathy in some patients or tense and strained in others. A "wet" hoarseness is common in ALS patients as a result of inadequate oral management of salivation.

At this time ALS is considered a terminal disease. However, when voice and speech symptoms appear early in the pathogenesis, support to maintain the integrity of articulation and phonation processes is important to help such patients maintain communication with people around them. Should the disease weaken speech and voice processes sufficiently to make verbal communication impossible, the SLP should give support to facilitate nonverbal communication. Excellent references for providing such assistance to nonverbal patients with ALS and similar disorders are provided by Silverman (1980) and Johns (1978).

Another common disease with associated speech and voice symptoms is myasthenia gravis. This affects the myoneuronal junction and is caused by a lack of production of the neurotransmitter, acetylcholine. The symptoms are progressive and rapid fatigue of the muscles affected. In some patients, the disease is widespread and most motor systems are affected; in others, it is specific to such systems as the articulation and phonation structures. When affected by myasthenia gravis, voice and articulation processes deteriorate rapidly with use.

In addition to this deterioration, weak, monotone, and breathy voice qualities are common symptoms of myasthenia gravis. These vocal symptoms range in degree from slight to severe but always are manifested under conditions of prolonged usage. It is this change in communication pattern as the structures are used that should alert the SLP that myasthenia gravis must not be ruled out as an etiology of communication disorder. Without being aware of the specific symptoms of this disorder under conditions of prolonged usage, it is possible to overlook it as an etiology of voice and articulation disorder. Aronson (1973) reports one such case in a patient with myasthenia gravis who was diagnosed incorrectly as having a functionally based voice disorder. The rapid breakdown in speech function provided the stimulus for diagnostic testing which identified the true etiology.

When a client is suspected of having a disorder caused by myasthenia gravis, it is important to determine whether continued usage of the speech and voice structures produces rapid deterioration. This can be done by having the client begin to read orally while recording the voice. Should a progressive breakdown in articulation, precision, oral-nasal resonance balance, and laryngeal quality be noted, and the patient's physicians are not aware of the breakdown, the adult should be referred to a neurologist or general physician for a reconsideration of the diagnosis.

SUMMARY OF NEUROGENIC VOICE DISORDER

Because the neurological control of phonation is complex, and the anatomical and physiological processes that support it are highly intricate, it is not unusual for breakdowns to occur. Numerous traumatic conditions, disease processes, and degenerative disorders have been discussed. To effectively manage the client with suspected neurogenic voice disorder, the SLP must have a clear understanding of the anatomical, physiological, and neurological bases for normal voice. The association and cooperation of other professionals such as neurologists and laryngologists are essential for proper management. Consultation with these professionals must occur before therapy is initiated. Every effort must be made to determine whether physical management of laryngeal disorder can be effectuated. When everything possible has been done to improve the physical status of the larynx but a voice disorder remains, specific strategies can be used to improve the valving potential of the vocal folds in order to provide better voice production.

REFERENCES

Aminoff, M. J., Dedo, H. H., & Izdebski, K. Clinical aspects of spasmodic dysphonia. *Journal of Neurology, Neurosurgery, and Psychiatry*, 1978, *41*, 361-365.

Aronson, A. E. *Psychogenic voice disorders: An interdisciplinary approach to detection, diagnosis and therapy*. Philadelphia: W. B. Saunders Co., 1973.

Aronson, A. E. *Clinical voice disorders*. New York: Thieme-Stratton, Inc., 1980.

Boone, D. *The voice and voice therapy*. Englewood Cliffs, N.J.: Prentice-Hall, Inc., 1977.

Case, J. L., & Cleary, K. *Psychogenic falsetto associated with surgically induced vocal fold paralysis*. Paper presented at American Speech and Hearing Association national convention, Houston, 1976.

Cooper, M. *Modern techniques in vocal rehabilitation*. Springfield, Ill.: Charles C Thomas, Publisher, 1977.

Darley, F. L., Aronson, A. E., & Brown, J. R. *Motor speech disorders*. Philadelphia: W. B. Saunders Co., 1975.

Dedo, H. H. Intracordal injection of Teflon in the treatment of 135 patients with dysphonia. *Annals of Otology, Rhinology, and Laryngology*, 1973, *82*, 661-667.

Dedo, H. H., Izdebski, K., & Townsend, J. J. Recurrent laryngeal nerve histopathology in spastic dysphonia. *Annals of Otology, Rhinology, and Laryngology*, 1977, *86*, 1-7.

Dedo, H. H., & Shipp, T. *Spastic dysphonia: A surgical and voice therapy treatment program*. Houston: College-Hill Press, 1980.

Isshiki, N., Massehiro, T., & Masaki, S. Arytenoid adduction for unilateral vocal cord paralysis. *Archives of Otolaryngology*, 1978, *104*, 555-558.

Jacobson, E. *You must relax*. 5th Edition. New York: McGraw-Hill Book Company, 1978.

Johns, D. F. (Ed.) *Clinical management of neurogenic communicative disorders*. Boston: Little, Brown and Co., 1978.

Moses, P. J. *The voice of neurosis*. New York: Grune & Stratton, Inc., 1954.

Murphy, A. T. *Functional voice disorders*. Englewood Cliffs, N.J.: Prentice-Hall, Inc., 1964.

Prosek, R., Montgomery, A., Walden, B. E., & Schwartz, D. EMG biofeedback in the treatment of hyperfunctional voice disorders. *Journal of Speech and Hearing Disorders*, 1978, *43*(3), 282-294.

Silverman, F. H. *Communication for the speechless*. Englewood Cliffs, N.J.: Prentice-Hall, Inc., 1980.

Wilson, F. B., Oldring, D. J., & Mueller, K. Recurrent laryngeal nerve dissection: A case report involving return of spastic dysphonia after initial surgery. *Journal of Speech and Hearing Disorders*, 1980, *45*(1), 112–118.

Zemlin, W. R. *Speech and hearing science: Anatomy and physiology*. Englewood Cliffs, N.J.: Prentice-Hall, Inc., 1981.

Chapter 6

Vocal Abuse in Adults

The purpose of this chapter is to provide the speech/language pathologist (SLP) with information for evaluating and remediating adults with voice disorder resulting from vocal abuse.

CONTACT ULCERS

Commonly found primarily among adult males is an organic voice disorder termed contact ulcers. They are caused by functional misuse of the delicate structures of the larynx. These ulcers form in the posterior aspect of the vibrating vocal folds, particularly at the junction of the posterior and middle thirds where the tips of the vocal processes of the arytenoid cartilages are located.

Pathogenesis in contact ulcers typically occurs as follows:

The adult engages in a vocal activity over a considerable length of time that abuses the larynx. The abused tissues become sore and irritated. When the abuse continues, the delicate tissues break down (tissue necrosis) and the ulceration process begins. The abnormal and abusive contact of the arytenoid vocal processes causes the surrounding tissues to be damaged.

Several specific causes of contact ulcers have been identified, with most categorized as vocal abuse:

- speaking at a habitual pitch level that is too low
- speaking with excessive laryngeal tension
- initiating phonation with sudden and abrupt onset (coup de glotte)
- speaking in a prolonged manner under conditions of loud noise
- producing voice with laryngeal tissues that are inflamed and tender from excessive smoking, alcohol consumption, allergy, or upper respiratory infection

- speaking in a loud and intense manner (adult yelling) such as at sporting events
- accumulating acidic secretions from the stomach and digestive tract around the arytenoid cartilages during sleep

Symptoms of Contact Ulcers

The symptoms of contact ulcers vary from person to person. Because the ulcers occur on the tips of the vocal processes of the arytenoid cartilages rather than on the vibrating muscular tissues of the vocal folds, the symptoms often are not dramatic, particularly in the early stages. However, many adults with contact ulcers have significant dysphonia manifested as an excessively low habitual pitch level that involves a vocal or glottal fry. Vocal fry is difficult to describe but easy to identify once it is understood. It sounds like corn popping and can best be approximated by speaking softly at as low a pitch level as possible so individual vocal fold vibrations can be heard. The voice often is breathy. Adults complain of pain during phonation, often a sharp pain that can be felt deep either in the larynx or felt (referred) in the ipsilateral ear. The breathiness is a likely result of the person's avoiding a tight contact seal of the arytenoid cartilages during phonation because of the pain it causes.

The most remarkable vocal symptom is the tension in the voice. Vocal tension is a significant etiological factor and remains even after the tissues have been ulcerated. Pitch breaks at the onset of phonation are common and occur because the person is unable to set the larynx properly with adequate vocal fold approximation. In summary, the typical voice profile of the adult with contact ulcers is low, breathy, and tense, characterized by vocal fry, pitch breaks, and pain.

Aronson (1980) characterizes contact ulcers in adults as psychogenic in nature. The reason is that men who develop contact ulcers tend to fit the same typical personality profile: in their early forties, highly vocal and dynamic in verbal interactions, hard-driving, and perfectionistic. Verbal aggression is typical. Verbalization is an important part of their profession—teaching, law, sales, or the ministry. It is easy to understand why a low-pitched voice is a common characteristic since most such males may find it a positive attribute.

Evaluation Procedures

In contact ulcer cases, it is important that the SLP obtain case history information to help identify background factors that require clinical attention. Information about the individual should be sought in the following areas:

- the nature of the work
- vocal characteristics associated with the profession
- noise levels in the typical speaking environment
- the onset of the vocal disorder and treatments obtained or sought
- personality characteristics in terms of attitudes about self, life style, social relations, ambitions, and achievement expectations
- relationships with friends, family, and colleagues

The purpose here is not to probe sensitive areas but to help the SLP gain insight into the adult's personality and general behavior to determine which factors need modification.

After the case history process, the pitch, loudness, quality, and vocal duration should be evaluated. It is important to determine the exact habitual, optimal, and basal pitch levels. The following is a format for determining these factors:

Habitual Pitch

The habitual pitch level is the modal pitch (the one most commonly used). To find it, the SLP should have the person count from 1 to 20 in a natural manner at a typical conversational pitch level. While listening, the SLP judges regarding whether the level seems typical of how the person sounded in the case history process. If so, the adult should repeat the counting process in a sequence of only three numbers such as "1-2-3, 1-2-3, 1-2-3" in a monotone followed by a humming sound at the same pitch: "1-2-3, 1-2-3, 1-2-3-mmmmm." The SLP determines whether the hummed pitch is the same as that heard in the counting. If so, the hummed tone should be matched on some instrumentation to obtain a musical or acoustic value, e.g., D_3 or 146 Hz. Once that value has been verified as reliable, the habitual pitch level has been found. The instrumentation can be a pitch pipe, piano, or some pitch-extracting instrument. Specific instructions for using a pitch pipe are provided in Chapter 4, on voice disorders in school.

Basal Pitch

The basal pitch is the lowest functional level the adult can produce. The person hums down the musical scale in whole tones until the tone reflects considerable tension and poor vocal efficiency, i.e., weak, raspy, and with vocal fry. The person then raises the pitch one tone, which effectively is the bottom of the range—the basal pitch. The tone value should be converted to the musical scale or acoustical fundamental, e.g., B_3 or 123 Hz.

Optimal Pitch

The level at which the larynx functions best and most efficiently is the optimal pitch. It is a judgmental rather than an absolute value level. The SLP and the adult judge various pitch levels to determine which sound best, which are easiest to produce, which facilitates the increase of voice intensity, and which can be produced with the least amount of effort. When the tone that represents these values is found, the optimal pitch level for that client has been identified. Usually the optimal pitch level is 3 or 4 whole tones from the basal. The process of finding the optimal pitch involves the adult's humming a tone close to the basal, then raising it in whole steps until reaching one that seems easy to produce and that increases slightly in intensity with the same amount of vocal effort. The person hums that tone as well as the ones just above and just below it to determine which seems optimal. A musical or acoustic value then is given to the tone obtained, e.g., E_3 or 164 Hz.

Optimal Pitch When Pathology Is on the Vocal Folds

Although in essentially every instance of voice disorder, the habitual and basal pitch levels can be found, it often is difficult and even inappropriate to attempt to determine the optimal level. When the mass and tissue structures of the vocal folds have been altered by pathology, they cannot vibrate at an optimal level. When the SLP evaluates a voice and finds considerable hoarseness because of the pathology, it is appropriate to determine the habitual and basal pitches. If the adult is using a habitual pitch one or two tones from the basal, it can be raised clinically approximately two tones without interpretation that the optimal is being used. Once the pathology on the folds has been eliminated or diminished significantly, the true optimal pitch can be determined.

Pitch Factors

Men who develop contact ulcers tend, consciously or unconsciously, to speak with a lower, more masculine and authoritative voice. If the habitual pitch level is only one or two tones from the basal, the laryngeal mechanisms are being used in a less efficient manner. This low level requires more vocal effort to maintain adequate loudness for communication. More often than not, this increased effort is translated into vocal tension. Tension occurs particularly when the adult uses language that involves considerable downward inflections, such as at the end of phrases or sentences. This downward inflection pattern places the pitch at the bottom of the range, which requires considerable effort and tension to maintain voice. Vocal fry often is heard in these downward inflections.

When a too-low habitual pitch level is being used by an adult who is attempting to maintain a dynamic and persuasive communication style, considerable tension is placed on the vocal structures, specifically on the vocal processes of the arytenoid cartilages. Substantial force is exerted by the muscles involved in vocal fold adduction. This force probably is the primary form of abuse contributing to the pathogenesis of contact ulcers, and the low-pitched voice is the factor responsible. Therefore, it is important that the SLP investigate the pitch characteristics carefully and be prepared to modify the contributing factors.

Loudness Factors

In evaluating loudness of the voice, the main concern should be to determine whether the adult uses too intense a level. This probably is the case. As noted, the man's personality typically is intense and dynamic, which usually is manifested in a rather loud voice. Loudness is not necessarily serious unless it occurs when the person is attempting to speak loudly at a low pitch level, in which case considerable abuse occurs. When this tendency is noted, it should be marked for modification.

Vocal Duration

One of the most distressing concerns of these adults is the rapid deterioration of the voice during the day. When the person is rested and the voice has not been used for some time, the quality is good and pain is minimal. But as the day progresses and vocal demands become great, the individual typically reports a rapid quality breakdown—the voice becomes more raspy, breathy, and weak. By the end of the day, it is not uncommon for the voice to be nearly aphonic unless considerable effort is used.

Therapy for Contact Ulcers

Since contact ulcers are caused by vocal abuse, it is necessary to identify all forms of that abuse and eliminate them systematically. The two most significant etiological factors are (1) hard glottal attack and (2) an inappropriately low-pitched speaking voice. Since the typical client is tense and rather hard-driving, it also is common to find extensive muscular tension in the laryngeal area during phonation. All of these factors must be modified.

Eliminating the Hard Glottal Attack

A hard glottal attack (coup de glotte) can be eliminated by having the adult initiate voice in a manner incompatible with an abrupt onset. The client is taught to aspirate slightly before voicing so the vocal folds are brought into contact gently and the arytenoid cartilages are not slammed together. The best way to aspirate is to have the person say an /h/ sound at the beginning of the utterance, e.g., /h/open the door, /h/up the stairs, /h/kick the ground, etc. This teaches the concept of gentle onset of voicing. For contrast with a hard attack, the adult alternates between hard and gentle onset:

Hard	Gentle
/h/out	*o*ut
/h/ask	*a*sk
/h/yell	*y*ell

This contrasting step should be practiced at each level of therapy to eliminate the hard glottal attack, i.e., in phrases, sentences, conversation, etc. The SLP should remember that the /h/ sound merely facilitates a gentle onset and should be used only to teach the concept that it is not necessary to have a hard and abrupt onset.

Changing the Pitch

One of the most challenging clinical tasks for many SLPs is to change an adult's pitch. This is explained in this chapter with the assumption that the SLP does not have elaborate instrumentation available and must rely on a simple pitch pipe and a trained ear. Using a pitch pipe, the SLP should blow the tone that has been found to be the client's optimal pitch, e.g., A_3. The person is told to hum or say /a/ at that pitch level. If the client can match the pitch pipe, and do so consistently, then the hum or vowel should be used as a starter as the individual is instructed to count, say the alphabet, or offer similar nonpropositional speech, i.e., hum (A_3) 1-2-3-4-5, hum (A_3) A-B-C-D-E-F, hum (A_3) Sunday, Monday, Tuesday, Wednesday, etc. The SLP must listen to ensure that the person is performing at the target pitch of the hum.

When sure the adult can hit the target pitch with the help of the hum and can maintain it while counting, etc., the SLP directs the client to say simple phrases such as "open the door" in a monotone. The target hum can be used intermittently if necessary to stabilize the pitch but it should be eliminated as soon as possible. The sequence can go something like this:

Hum (A_3) Open the door
Hum (A_3) Get the paper
            Tell the man
            Call me today
Hum (A_3) Forget it buster, etc.

The target hum can be used periodically to ensure the proper pitch is being voiced. Of course, the SLP should check the pitch periodically to assure correctness.

When the adult has mastered simple phrases in a monotone using the appropriate pitch, the next step is to ensure the ability to find that level without a target model and after a period of silence. This can be done by having the SLP discuss some topic while the client listens. Every few seconds the SLP should stop talking and signal the person to hum the target pitch, which can be checked for accuracy with the pitch pipe. When the individual is accurate in matching this pitch after an interval of not using it, the SLP can be assured it is stable in the client's mind.

In the next step, the client reads in a monotone at the target pitch. The SLP can test the ability to maintain the new level by having the person prolong vowels in the middle of reading so his or her pitch can be checked for accuracy. For example, the client reads the following paragraph from a newspaper or article and, on signal from the SLP, prolongs a vowel for a pitch check:

> A week later, a puff of steam and ash burst forth from the mountaintop, forming a crater. Sightseers flooded theeeeee (check pitch) area, eager for a glimpse of the peee (check pitch) -ak. Steam and ash eruptions, great in magnitude, were accompanied byyyyyyy (check pitch) more earthquakes and rumbles from the mountain.

When it becomes apparent that the person can read consistently in the appropriate monotone, variation around the new optimal pitch is introduced. The client is reminded that the new target is merely the central tendency of all pitches used in speech, and the voice will go up or down around this central level to add emphasis, style, and meaning to verbal expression. Through reading and conversation, the adult should practice pitch inflections around the optimal pitch under the supervision of the SLP, who should check constantly to ensure that the optimal remains the habitual level.

Carry-over of normal pitch inflections around the new optimal level into real-life situations can be accomplished by establishing a control hierarchy. When the person has reached and learned to control pitch in the highest situations on the hierarchy, it can be assumed the new behavior has been established clinically. The SLP must check the stability of the new pitch periodically.

Eliminating Muscular Tension

When the adult with contact ulcers has extensive laryngeal tension during voice production, it is necessary to modify that behavior as one part of the process of eliminating vocal abuse. This can be done using progressive relaxation, biofeedback, or other tension elimination procedures as explained in Chapter 5 on psychogenic and neurogenic voice disorders.

Case Example of Adult with Contact Ulcers

F.F., a 42-year-old insurance salesman, was referred by a laryngologist who reported the man had a contact ulcer on the left vocal process. A voice evaluation revealed a habitual pitch level of E_2 (82 Hz) and a basal pitch of D_2 (73 Hz). The optimal pitch level was found to be $G\#_2$ (104 Hz). It was obvious that F.F.'s habitual pitch was too near his basal pitch and was abusive. He spoke with considerable tension, which was apparent in his extrinsic laryngeal musculature. He manifested a loud, intense, and dynamic style of communication.

F.F. indicated that he was an emotional person, easily angered, easily upset, and became tense under those conditions. He also reported feeling considerable tension in his throat when he talked with people about emotional subjects. When speaking on the phone to a client about a topic that was upsetting, F.F. said he had a "tightness in the throat that almost chokes me." A hard onset of voicing (coup de glotte) was considered an important etiological factor.

Therapy for F.F. consisted of (1) raising his habitual pitch to $G\#_2$ (104 Hz) (his previous optimal level), (2) using slides and tape recordings to introduce him to the topic of vocal abuse and its consequences, (3) identifying all forms of vocal abuse in his speech, and (4) eliminating all abuses systematically, including excessive tension during phonation.

At the beginning of each therapy session, the SLP taught F.F. control over the tension in his body through relaxation training. The following is a transcript of a recording of the SLP's instructions on one such session:

Let's begin this session by relaxing as much as possible. First, I would like you to sit in the chair in a comfortable manner. Put your feet flat on the floor and your hands so they are resting on your legs. Now I want you to close your eyes and just listen to me. Follow my suggestions if you want to. Concentrate on the sound of my voice only. I will suggest that you focus your attention on various parts of your body to determine whether excessive tension is present. If it is, we will attempt to eliminate it until you are completely relaxed.

Now, first I want you to concentrate on your feet. Notice whether your toes are tight and curled at all. If they are, relax them . . . relax the feet muscles. Make them limp and relaxed. Any tension you feel in your feet must be eliminated. Now concentrate on your lower legs. Again, if you feel tension, eliminate it. Let your mind and body become totally relaxed. Your mind can control the tension you feel. (Pause of about 15 seconds.)

Now concentrate on your upper legs. If you feel tension, eliminate it. (Pause.) Now concentrate on your stomach area. Let your stomach muscles be as relaxed as possible. As you breathe in air, let your stomach muscles be relaxed so your breathing is deep and full. Let each breathing cycle make you more and more relaxed. Now concentrate on your chest muscles . . . let them be as relaxed as possible . . . .

The rest of the relaxation session continued in the same manner, with the SLP progressing up the body until all sections had been covered. Considerable effort was directed at relaxing the neck muscles since this area seemed to be the focus of tension.

This relaxation effort was included to some degree at the beginning of each therapy session. F.F. found it helpful in blocking out the tension he brought to the sessions. The SLP then worked on raising his pitch and eliminating his hard glottal attack, using the /h/ facilitator explained earlier.

After five weeks of therapy, F.F. was able to speak habitually at his new pitch level of G#$_2$. He also had eliminated some of the muscular tension in difficult speaking situations and most of the tension in less difficult ones. He was aware of voicing onset and learned to avoid the hard glottal attack. As a result of the therapy, he also became aware of various forms of vocal abuse such as yelling from room to room and shouting at sporting events and was able to eliminate many of these factors.

Two months after he enrolled in therapy, he was referred back to his laryngologist, who reported that the contact ulcer was gone. Three months after that medical inspection, F.F. reported he again was experiencing vocal tension. He had seen his laryngologist and there had been no change in his larynx but he felt the tension and wanted to get a handle on it before losing control. When he came in for a review session, he was found to be stable on pitch control and demonstrated continued control over the hard glottal attack but did seem tense in his neck region. He was given more relaxation help and it was suggested he return for evaluations every two weeks until he felt he had control of the tension. At the time of this writing F.F. had maintained his control for one year without relapse.

SUMMARY OF CONTACT ULCERS

Contact ulcers occur on the posterior surface of the vocal folds at the junction where muscle joins the vocal processes of the arytenoids. Vocal abuse causes the arytenoids to slam together with sufficient force to cause tissue breakdown at the point of contact. Several forms of vocal abuse etiology were identified. The therapeutic procedures involve identifying the abuses and eliminating them systematically. It is hoped that the evaluation and management procedures have been presented in such a way that the SLP can approach these clients with greater competency.

VOCAL NODULES IN ADULTS

Chapter 4, on voice disorders in schools, noted that a common result of vocal abuse was vocal nodules. It was explained that vocal nodules are tiny growths that form on the phonating edge of each fold at the junction of their anterior and middle thirds. They are the direct result of vocal abuse. The specific abuses mentioned were (1) excessive playground yelling, (2) abnormal toy and animal noises, (3) cheerleading, (4) speaking at an inappropriate habitual pitch level, all mingled with (5) a personality profile that involved a tendency to be loud, verbally aggressive, intense in interpersonal relationships, and more talkative than others.

The same factors occur in adults and can result in the same disorder—vocal nodules—with only slightly different forms of abuse. Whereas children yell on the playground, adults yell at football games and other sporting events; children enjoy toy and animal noises that are abusive and adults enjoy singing in styles and environments that foster vocal nodules; loud and aggressive children bully or intimidate other children verbally, and these same characteristics can be found in adults. When children grow into adults, they often enter professions with highly demanding verbal requirements: teaching, law, professional singing, sales, the ministry, etc. These nodules are also called singer's, preacher's, lawyer's, and (the more general term) screamer's nodes.

The pathogenesis of vocal nodules in adults is not different from that in children. The SLP's clinical responsibility is to help the adult identify and eliminate all forms of vocal abuse. When this is done, the body usually will heal itself and the nodules will be resorbed.

Often adults' vocal nodules become so large and fibroid that surgery is recommended to remove them. This surgery is somewhat controversial since removal of the nodular growth does not involve surgical removal of a disease but merely a symptom of vocal abuse. Strong and Vaughan (1971) recommend surgical removal of nodules of professionals who use their voice intensively only after three months of therapy have not produced improvement and the patients are not satisfied with their vocal quality. They report that 50 percent of their cases require such surgical intervention. They provide no data on actual numbers of cases nor on the vocal characteristics of the patients requiring the surgery. They also omit data on the vocal results of the 50 percent who did receive therapy and surgery. These data are needed to help professionals answer this important question regarding the use of surgery for removal of vocal nodules.

According to many SLPs, including the author of this chapter, surgery rarely is effective in eliminating the voice disorder of clients with nodules, with or without therapy. Surgical removal of tissue of a nodule that is large and fibroid may be necessary but it is most optimistic to expect the voice to be normal or near normal after healing. All too often, the postsurgical voice is no different from the presurgical one, and often is worse. One case, perhaps atypical, represents this concern:

Case Example of Surgical Management of Vocal Nodules

R.R., a female professional singer, was referred by a laryngologist who reported postsurgical return of vocal nodules. R.R. traveled with her husband, performing in lounges and private parties across the nation. During one extended tour through Florida, R.R. developed a prolonged hoarseness that interfered with her singing. A laryngologist diagnosed her as having singer's nodes and recommended surgical removal. Inasmuch as the singing couple had a one-week hiatus between jobs the surgery was scheduled.

R.R. reported she went to the hospital, checked in, underwent the necessary tests, had the surgery, and checked out the next day without ever seeing the physician who performed the operation. "He gave me no recommendations and I assumed the problem had been taken care of and I could resume my singing. I haven't been able to sing since," she stated. When R.R. arrived in Arizona, she contacted the laryngologist who had made the referral. He reported that she had large bilateral vocal nodules and generalized swelling of her entire vocal folds. Since she was still traveling across the nation with her husband, it was suggested that she obtain voice therapy for vocal abuses as soon as she would be available for help over several weeks. She indicated that would be nearly impossible in the foreseeable future. She left disappointed that there was no easy solution to her problem.

Perhaps this example is not at all representative of surgery for vocal nodules but without careful postsurgical management the results she experienced are not unexpected. Under any circumstances where surgery is being considered, it must be performed with as much postoperative control over patient behavior as possible. The surgeon can be aided significantly by an SLP who understands the recovery process and who can help the patient avoid abusing delicate tissues during that time. This provides the best opportunity for positive results from the surgery, but requires the closest of relationships between the physician and the SLP.

After surgery for vocal nodules, the physician must inspect the healing constantly and inform the SLP when progress is sufficient to allow therapy on phonation recovery. The SLP then can begin to introduce phonation gently in the recovery process. The SLP should start with a highly breathy and easily produced vocal effort. The first steps should be similar to soft sighs, mostly breathy with a little voice. This should be done only a few times, followed by a period of vocal rest. If possible, medical inspection of the vocal folds should occur after this first attempt to determine whether there were any negative results. If not, after a short rest, the same procedure can be repeated and somewhat expanded with a number of phonation efforts but without increasing the intensity of voicing, which should remain breathy and gentle as in a sigh. This procedure should continue with gradual increases in the number of phonation attempts followed by rest periods. Periodic medical inspection is an important part of this early therapy. With such medical support, the SLP can judge how quickly to move the patient toward normal phonation. Once the laryngeal tissue can withstand normal and nonabusive phonation, the therapy process should continue by systematic identification and elimination of all vocal habits that the SLP considers abusive. Without this postsurgical care, there is a great probability that within a short time the patient will suffer a relapse and nodules will develop again on the vocal folds.

Evaluation Procedures

The evaluation procedures for adult vocal nodules do not differ significantly from those used in contact ulcers except that a broader range of abuse etiologies must be considered. Where contact ulcers occur almost exclusively in adult males, nodules can develop in children and adults of both sexes.

The person suspected of having vocal nodules must be evaluated medically before any significant management by the SLP. The nodules' vocal symptoms do not differ significantly from the hoarseness that is the primary indication of cancer on the vocal folds. Therefore, the symptoms' etiology must be determined. If the SLP is the first professional to see the client, there must be a direct referral to a laryngologist or other physician who can inspect the laryngeal tissues to determine the etiology.

Abuses Causing Vocal Nodules

Once medical inspection has verified that the symptoms stem from nodules, the SLP can proceed to identify the vocal abuse factors. Most of this identification is done by careful case history questions on the client's daily vocal habits involving the following areas:

- yelling and screaming, primarily at sports or related events
- hard glottal attack
- singing in an abusive manner (professionally or as an amateur)
- speaking in a noisy environment
- coughing and throat clearing
- grunting as in exercising and lifting
- calling children or pets from a distance
- speaking or singing at inappropriate pitch levels
- speaking in an abusive manner during allergy or upper respiratory infection episodes
- vocalizing under conditions of tension
- smoking excessively (including marijuana) or speaking in a smoky environment
- speaking excessively or abusively during menstrual periods
- vocalizing excessively in any circumstance
- speaking with inadequate breath support
- laughing hard and abusively
- vocalizing while on medications such as antihistamines or any others designed to dry tissues

This list is not in any order of significance or importance to the development of vocal nodules but merely outlines categories the SLP should explore to determine whether the patient has been involved in vocal abuse. Most of the categories are straightforward but others may need some explanation as to how vocal abuse is involved. Therefore, each is discussed in the detail necessary to provide this understanding.

Yelling and Screaming

Adults, both males and females, become emotionally involved in sporting events to the degree that they assume a cheerleading role. They cheer favorable turns of events and boo unfavorable ones, each with gusto and lively enthusiasm. Players who are the children of adult clients add a factor of involvement. Parents scream at kids on the field, umpires, referees, coaches of opposing teams, and anyone else considered a threat to victory. Many adults become coaches of youth baseball or football teams and find themselves yelling constantly at the kids on the field. This is particularly noticeable in youth football programs, where the ears of the kids on the field are covered by helmets, making it even more difficult for coaches to communicate instructions. It is amazing to watch and to wonder why every coach of a youth team does not have vocal nodules or similar laryngeal trauma—especially the coaches of the losing teams. Regardless, when an adult has been referred for therapy because of vocal nodules, care must be taken to explore the possibility of these abusive behaviors.

Hard Glottal Attack

Even when nodules develop at the junction of the anterior and middle thirds of the vocal folds, it is not uncommon to find swelling and inflammation in the posterior region of the glottis around the arytenoid cartilages. Some of the trauma and inflammation could result from the slamming together of the arytenoid cartilages under conditions of hard glottal attack.

Singing in an Abusive Manner

One of the most vocally demanding professions is that of professional popular singer. Whether in the big-time recording and performing business or the small-time nightclub circuit, the demands for laryngeal effort are great. Tetter (1977) lists six common conditions leading to injury of the pop singer's voice:

- singing excessively high or low in pitch
- singing excessively loud
- using an exaggerated glottal stroke
- attempting to sing during respiratory infections
- using laryngeal irritants such as tobacco, alcohol, and other drugs
- singing despite lack of adequate voice training

Several other factors also must be considered. Duration of vocal performance is a major factor in the development of nodules. In the typical nightclub gig, the singer(s) must perform up to four sets of 40 to 50 minutes each, starting at 9 P.M. and ending at 1 A.M. During the breaks between sets, management often encourages the performers to mingle with the audience. This is wonderful for socialization and public relations for the management but deleterious to already traumatized vocal folds. The nightclub crowd typically is noisy, with constant chatter, background music from the jukebox, and clinking glasses. The performers must compete with that noise as they mingle and are forced to almost yell just to communicate when what they need most is vocal rest. The larynx is not given time to recuperate before another intense musical set begins. Often, these between-set conversations are more abusive than the actual singing, which may use amplifiers and loudspeakers that reduce the strain on the voice.

When a SLP is working with such a professional who has vocal or singer's nodules, the vocal pattern analysis must involve viewing the performer in action both onstage and off. Modification or elimination of behaviors that are not related directly to the performance can make a difference in the singer's durability. Abuses that are not part of the act are the only ones over which the singer has much control without taking away the means of employment. It is highly unlikely that the typical nightclub vocalist will have the talent or means to become a trained singer so as to advance to a better performance situation. It also is unlikely that a professional is willing to modify a singing manner to be less abusive if it means changing what the performer perceives as a true vocal style. By observing the singer in the actual work setting, the SLP often can discover abuses that can be modified rather easily but that can make a significant difference in vocal durability.

Speaking in a Noisy Environment

When a person is forced to speak in a noisy environment, several things happen to the larynx. First, a high ambient noise level makes it difficult to hear how loud the conversation is, so the individual is unlikely to eliminate the excessive vocal effort. Second, to be heard above the noise, the person generates greater lung airflow, to which the vocal folds respond with greater resistance. This resistance is the equivalent to what is perceived as laryngeal tension. Although the resistance is quantifiable and measurable, the instrumentation necessary to do so does not work well in the typical noisy environment such as a nightclub. However, it can be subjectively judged as being present and thus may be eliminated.

Coughing and Throat Clearing

Coughing occurs when the protective valving mechanisms of the larynx are stimulated by a foreign irritation. It is a reflex act and hard to control or eliminate without medicine. However, the manner of coughing can be modified when a person is taught to cough with less intensity and glottal explosion. Zwitman and Calcaterra (1973) recommend a method they call the "silent cough" that involves having the individual push excessive air from the lungs in blasts at the moment of coughing. The client must be taught to cough without producing voice. When no voicing is heard, glottal constriction is eliminated and vocal abuse is decreased.

Clearing the throat is less reflexive and more consciously stimulated. Much throat-clearing behavior is unproductive in terms of actually removing the stimulating mucus from the glottis. Swallowing after a quick air blast is more likely to clear the area of the mucus.

Grunting as in Exercising and Lifting

This is a significant form of vocal abuse and often is overlooked. Anyone who has been on the sidelines of a football game can attest to the grunting that goes on during blocking and tackling. Fortunately, the men engaged in this strenuous vocal activity are large and strong and their larynges no doubt are strong enough to resist the abuse involved. But many activities engaged in by the general population involve the same kind of laryngeal trauma as is heard at the line of scrimmage. Daily exercise and lifting involve glottal closure under pressure in order to contain air in the lungs to stabilize the chest cavity so skeletal muscles can function efficiently. Each push-up, pull-up, lifting of weights, hard tennis serve or volley, or jumping activity involves hard closure of the glottis. Vocal nodule clients should be informed of this potential form of abuse so they can analyze their behavior with regard to it.

Calling Children or Pets from a Distance

Men and women who develop vocal nodules often are surprised to discover how often they yell from room to room or yard to yard to communicate with their children and pets. It seems to be easier to yell than to walk closer for communication. However, walking—a simple activity— can eliminate significant abuse to laryngeal tissues and the SLP should encourage clients to do so.

Speaking or Singing at Inappropriate Pitch Levels

Considerable attention is given to pitch characteristics in the opening section of this chapter on contact ulcers. The same considerations exist for persons with vocal nodules. The SLP must evaluate the basal, habitual, and optimal pitch levels in such individuals, using the techniques outlined previously and modifying any significant disparity found between habitual and optimal levels for speaking.

With regard to pitch factors in singing, it is common for untrained but professional vocalists to attempt to use tones at the extreme limits of their pitch range, either too high or too low. The falsetto singer is common in current pop music. Falsetto singing does not need to be abusive but in pop music it often is. It actually is more falsetto screaming than singing, and it has affected many professionals adversely.

One of the first signs that a singer's larynx has been damaged is loss of control on high tones, including falsetto. However, singers usually do not try to change the pitch or range requirements of certain songs but rather work harder to achieve the target pitch. This effort is counterproductive to good vocal performance and abusive to the voice tissues.

Speaking in an Abusive Manner During Allergy or URI Episodes

When the delicate tissues of the larynx are inflamed by allergy or upper respiratory infection (URI), they are more vulnerable to vocal abuse. Even normal communication during these episodes can harm the tissues, but when it is intense, prolonged, at inappropriate pitch levels, or in any other way abusive, the negative effect is compounded. It therefore is important to determine whether such inflammations exist when the individual is evaluated. It requires a medical examination to distinguish between inflamed tissues resulting from allergies or from URI, but the client's own impression as to whether either is present can be helpful. In any case, when a client has a persistent allergy, medical treatment is necessary.

Vocalizing Under Conditions of Tension

Considerable attention has been given in this chapter to the counterproductive influence of excessive tension in the laryngeal areas during phonation. Although it is not easy to determine objectively the tension status of the intrinsic muscles of phonation, the SLP generally can determine whether excessive tension is present by palpating the extrinsic muscles (sternocleidomastoid, mylohyoid, sternohyoid, masseter, etc.). If tension is found in the extrinsics during phonation, it also is likely to be present in the intrinsic musculature. Such tension contributes to the overall pattern of vocal abuse.

Smoking Excessively or Speaking in a Smoky Environment

Several authors report on the abusive effects of smoking on the tissues of phonation (Cooper, 1977; Maccomb & Fletcher, 1967). The irritating effects of smoking, including even casual use of marijuana, on the vocal folds are so substantial that it is not unreasonable for the SLP to expect the voice client with nodules to significantly cut down or eliminate smoking to establish a good prognosis for therapy.

Speaking Excessively or Abusively During Menstrual Periods

Several authors report on the effect of menstrual cycles on vocal changes in women (Smith, 1962; Damste, 1967; Gould, 1972). Although these changes may be subtle, the SLP should alert the client of this possibility and advise caution about excessive vocalization. It may be necessary to document in a specific client whether changes in voice quality and pitch seem to be affected just before menstruation. If so, it would indicate that tissue edema is sufficient to establish a vulnerability factor on the effects of abuse on the vocal folds.

Vocalizing Excessively in Any Circumstance

It is not necessarily the amount of vocalization that becomes abusive, but the nature of it. However, when a person has vocal nodules it can be helpful to suggest the elimination of nonessential communication during the early weeks of therapy. Certainly, the SLP must judge whether such a suggestion would add such stress to the client as to be counterproductive, but the elimination of superfluous talking should at least be considered.

Speaking with Inadequate Breath Support

One of the benefits of formal singing or acting training is the realization of how important breath support is for proper laryngeal function, including specific instructions for proper breathing. When the larynx is supported well by proper breathing, it is as though vibration is occurring with little effort. Without such support, the larynx must be tense and work hard to produce the vibrations. It is important to evaluate clients with nodules to determine whether breath support for phonation is adequate. This is not a major etiological consideration in vocal nodules therapy, but the SLP should be prepared to evaluate a person who may have inadequate breath support. The following is a simple description of normal breath support for phonation.

Good breath support for phonation requires a sufficient, perhaps maximum, inhalation of air. This occurs with the abdominal muscles completely relaxed to facilitate the contraction of the diaphragm. The diaphragm is a muscle surrounding a central tendon that separates the abdominal cavity, which contains the stomach, intestines, and visceral organs, from the thoracic cavity, which contains the lungs and heart. When the diaphragm contracts, by virtue of its shape and skeletal attachments, it pulls itself downward and forward, expanding the vertical dimensions of the thoracic cavity and enlarging the lungs in that direction. This expansion draws air into the lungs and inhalation occurs.

For maximum inhalation, the diaphragm must be able to contract without excessive resistance. Resistance is less when the abdominal muscles have decreased tonicity. As the diaphragm contracts, its movements displace the visceral organs in a forward and lateral direction, distending the abdominal wall. The functions of the diaphragm during inhalation are complemented by musculature that lifts the rib cage to produce lung expansion in an anterior direction. In other words, deep and maximum inhalation requires that the stomach and visceral organs be displaced in a forward direction at the same time as the chest wall is expanding. If the client puts a hand on the stomach during proper inhalation, the hand should be pushed forward slightly. The deeper the inhalation, the farther the hand should move forward.

Following the inhalation cycle, the air is exhaled by essentially a reversal of these processes. The diaphragm relaxes and pulls itself back to its precontraction position, and the muscles that lifted the rib cage relax, allowing it to be lowered. These relaxation processes have the effect of decreasing the dimensions of the lungs, squeezing out their air through the open glottis. If phonation is to occur during this exhalation cycle, the glottis is closed and the exhaled air vibrates the vocal folds. The early stage of the exhalation is essentially passive, with tissues (diaphragm and rib cage) merely returning to their precontracted state. In the late stage of the cycle, the abdominal muscles increase their activity, compressing the visceral organs and displacing them up against the diaphragm. This compression has the effect of decreasing the vertical dimensions of the thoracic cavity and the lungs, causing more air to be exhaled.

Inadequate breath support for phonation occurs if the SLP notes whether:

- phonation is attempted before the client inhales adequately
- phonation is started when an exhalation cycle is nearly completed
- phonation is continued when the exhalation cycle is nearly completed

The items on breathing are directed at the typical client with vocal nodules or similar voice disorder such as contact ulcers. They are based on the assumption that breathing is essentially normal and devoid of pathology and merely needs to be maximized to support phonation. For an excellent description of both clinical and scientific aspects of human respiration, Hixon, Shriberg, and Saxman (1980) is recommended. For a solid reference the SLP can use when working with significantly abnormal patterns of breathing, Finnie (1970) and Johns (1978) are recommended.

Laughing Hard and Abusively

The SLP never wants to be accused of suggesting that a client eliminate the joy of a good laugh, but it should be pointed out that laughing is an altered form of phonation and that some of its forms can involve considerable abusive stroking of the glottis. This concern for laughing patterns usually is not a very significant item in the general scheme of vocal abuse, but some attention may need to be directed at modifying abusive laughter during the early weeks of therapy for vocal nodules.

Vocalizing While on Medication

Common medicines taken by persons with URI or allergies of the nose and throat are directed at drying their mucous tissues, including the larynx. Although in some cases the client does not specifically want to dry the laryngeal tissues, the medicine is not specific and selective enough to avoid it—it may dry the nose and throat as well as the delicate tissues of the larynx. When the mucous lining on the vocal folds is dried in this manner, the quality of phonation can be affected and vulnerability to vocal abuse can increase. The client should be warned that vocal effort when taking such medicines should be as nonabusive as possible.

SUMMARY OF ABUSES

The SLP should not consider this as a complete listing of potential vocal abuses that can be related etiologically to vocal nodules. Many other abuse forms are listed, and the SLP must encourage the client to elaborate on daily activities to help identify more elusive ones. This can be done by having the individual verbally describe a typical weekday and then a weekend day, including significant evening activities, to identify what needs to be explored to determine whether vocal abuse is involved.

PITCH EVALUATION IN VOCAL NODULES

Using the same procedures as described in the section on contact ulcers, the SLP should follow the case history interview to identify abuse forms and evaluate pitch characteristics. The habitual, basal, and optimal pitch levels should be determined. In some severe cases of nodules it is not possible to identify the optimal pitch because of the pathology on the vocal folds, but at least it should be determined whether the habitual pitch is at or near the bottom of the range. If so, the pitch must be raised two or three notes to eliminate the abuse factor of phonating too low. When the nodules have been eliminated or at least reduced, the true optimal pitch can be determined and stabilized.

VOCAL QUALITY IN PERSONS WITH VOCAL NODULES

The SLP then should judge the individual's voice quality and decide whether it is hoarse, raspy, breathy, and tense. Usually the voice quality heard in clients with nodules is a combination of breathiness, tension, and vocal roughness as a result of aperiodic (out-of-phase) vocal fold vibration. The breathiness results from incomplete approximation of the vocal folds because of the nodules. The tension probably is present because of the individual's attempts to compensate for the incomplete approximation. The aperiodicity occurs because the size and location of the nodule on one vocal fold rarely equals the nodule on the other fold and these mass differences cause the folds to vibrate out of phase.

In the voice evaluation, the verbal description the SLP uses is not as important as the actual acoustic characteristics as captured on high quality tape recording. This recording is most important for future comparisons in determining the effectiveness of therapy. The format should be simple, including (1) name of client, (2) date and time of recording, (3) voice sample of the individual counting to 20, prolonging an /a/ sound, and reading a short paragraph.

Particular attention should be directed at the efficiency of voice onset in the person with vocal nodules. Often there is an aphonic break in voicing accompanied by a sudden pitch break as the person begins to speak. This is important to note because a decrease or elimination of this inefficient voice onset often is the earliest indication that therapy is producing desired results.

In the next step, it is important that the client leave the evaluation session with a clear understanding of the nature of vocal nodules—what they are, how they are formed, what causes them, how they affect the voice, and what can be done to treat them. This information process should include slides or pictures of actual vocal nodules. Wilson and Rice (1977) provide an excellent kit that contains not only the appropriate slides but also audio recordings of adults and children with vocal nodules and other dysphonias.

The next part of the evaluation involves identification of the specific vocal abuses that need modification. From the list earlier in this chapter as well as any others that might have been identified, a list of abuses should be developed into a hierarchy. This hierarchy is a ranking of abuses, ranging from those the client feels are the easiest to modify to the most difficult. It is important to keep in mind that the opinion on the ranking is the client's, not the SLP's. Exhibit 6-1 shows a hierarchy of a hypothetical client, a university professor.

Each of these abuses must be eliminated if the body is to heal itself. Some of the abuses may be so difficult for the individual to modify that a separate hierarchy may need to be established. For example, changing the habitual pitch level to B_3 may be a great challenge to the hypothetical client who has heard himself speak at a different pitch for many years. Exhibit 6-2 presents a hierarchy for changing pitch that can be established in consultation with the hypothetical professor.

Exhibit 6-1 Hierarchy of Abuses in Vocal Nodule Cases

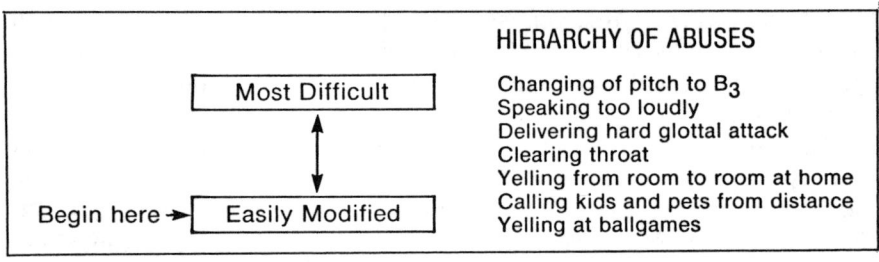

Exhibit 6-2 Pitch Change Hierarchy in Vocal Nodule Cases

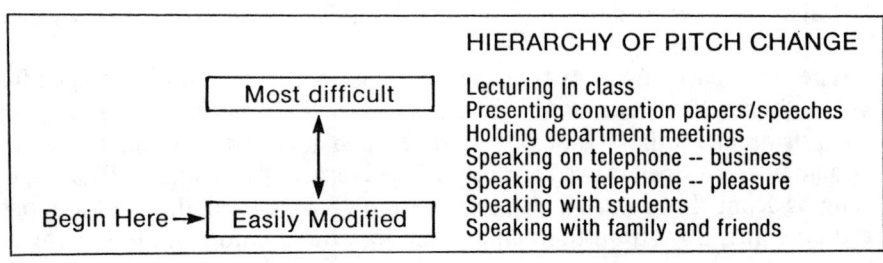

By the end of the evaluation session, the SLP and the client should have:

- a complete case history
- an identification of vocal abuses
- a ranking of abuses into a hierarchy
- a slide and audio presentation on the nature of vocal nodules
- an audio recording of the client's voice
- an analysis of pitch and quality characteristics of the voice

The client should be instructed to analyze vocal behavior in the next day or so to determine whether any other forms of vocal abuse might have been overlooked. An appointment is made for the first therapy session.

THERAPY FOR VOCAL NODULES

Therapy for vocal nodules in adults does not differ significantly from that for contact ulcers except that more factors of abuse contribute to nodules as compared to the ulcers. Essentially, the task in therapy is to identify and eliminate all forms of vocal abuse systematically.

At the beginning of each session, it is important to make a short tape recording of the client's voice. By comparing tapes from session to session, considerable information is obtained about the improvement (or lack of it) under the therapy. The most significant changes in dimensions of voice quality and efficiency usually will be heard during the first few weeks, followed by steady but continued slight improvements until the nodules no longer are present. When a medical opinion confirms that the nodules no longer are present or are significantly decreased in size, and all forms of vocal abuse have been eliminated, the person can be put into a checkup stage of therapy for periodic evaluations of voice quality and vocal habits. Once again, it is important to obtain a recording of the client's voice at each checkup for comparison purposes.

One final note about therapy with clients with vocal nodules is appropriate. This chapter has stressed the necessity for medical evaluation before any significant involvement of the SLP. It is easy for the experienced SLP to perform an indirect laryngoscopy and through it to identify vocal nodules. However, even when nodules obviously are present, medical evaluation is essential to rule out the possibility of a more serious disorder such as laryngeal cancer. The following case example communicates the concern expressed about medical evaluation.

CASE EXAMPLE OF VOCAL NODULES WITH SERIOUS COMPLICATIONS

J. A., a 62-year-old male, was referred for a voice evaluation because of severe dysphonia following surgical removal of vocal nodules. He was referred by a local laryngologist whose surgical report stated:

> Direct laryngoscopic examination of the epiglottis, true cords, false cords, ventricles, pyriform sinuses, and vallecula revealed normal tissue with the exception of the true and false cords which appeared to be chronically infected and had a peculiar nodular hypertrophy. The differences noted were thought to be secondary to previous surgery for nodular development and chronic irritation. There were nodules present at the anterior third of the vocal folds which were stripped bilaterally for pathological diagnosis. The pathology report revealed the biopsied tissue to be benign squamous epithelium with underlying hyalinization and vascular congestion.

At the time of J.A.'s voice evaluation, vocal parameters were judged with the following results:

Pitch: Normal (monotone) Habitual: B_3 (123 Hz)
Quality: Severe hoarseness with extreme tension and breathiness
Loudness: Voice weakness, but J.A. attempts to compensate with extreme effort to obtain adequate loudness

Case history questioning revealed a typically abusive pattern with the following characteristics: loud voice, history of talking over loud noise at work, frequent throat clearing, considerable yelling at sporting events (he considered himself at one time the Miami Dolphins' most intense football fan), and a general tendency to be intense in all interpersonal relationships, particularly when communication is involved.

Therapy goals included teaching him the consequences of vocal abuse, using slides and tapes, identifying all forms of it in his speaking including those cited in the case history, and systematically eliminating each abusive factor. Pitch did not need modification. It also was decided he needed considerable work in eliminating general body tension.

Therapy progressed well and J.A. responded in a more relaxed manner. He eliminated his throat clearing, yelling at sporting events and in any other situation, and competing with high levels of background noise. The most significant goal was to teach him to speak without tension by using a breathy, hypofunctional voice until his vocal folds had completely healed from the surgery. At that time an attempt would be made to have him phonate with normal approximation of the vocal folds with, it was hoped, improved voice quality.

After two months of this therapy, it was decided that sufficient healing more than likely had taken place to allow more vocal effort to eliminate the breathiness. He was referred back to his laryngologist for examination. Medical clearance was obtained to attempt to achieve a normal voice. No success resulted after two sessions of trying for better approximation of his vocal folds to eliminate the breathiness. Concern was expressed to J.A. about not accomplishing the vocal fold approximation. He decided to obtain a second medical opinion about the status of his vocal folds, particularly since he had not been feeling well recently.

J.A. was seen two days later by another laryngologist, who found deep squamous cell carcinoma (cancer) under several layers of benign tissue. The second laryngologist had decided to biopsy because indirect inspection had disclosed a paralyzed vocal fold. A total laryngectomy was performed two weeks later. Physicians were concerned about nodular masses noted in his lung x-rays but they were thought to be benign. A lung nodule was biopsied and found to be benign. However, approximately a year after his laryngeal surgery, J.A. developed lung cancer and died within four months (Case, 1981).

SUMMARY

Vocal abuse is common in adults. Two major clinical conditions in the larynx resulting from such abuse were presented—contact ulcers and vocal nodules. Evaluation procedures, case history questions, voice parameters, and strategies for therapeutic management have been provided. The need for medical clearance before working with these adults has been stressed. It is intended that the material in this chapter has been presented in such a manner that the SLP will find it helpful in working with these adult clients.

REFERENCES

Aronson, A. E. *Clinical voice disorders.* New York: Thieme-Stratton, Inc., 1980.

Case, J. L. Vocal nodules and laryngeal cancer. A case study. Paper presented at convention of the American Speech-Language-Hearing Association, Los Angeles, California, 1981.

Cooper, M. *Modern techniques in vocal rehabilitation.* Springfield, Ill.: Charles C. Thomas, Publisher, 1977.

Damste, P. H. Voice change in adult women caused by virilizing agents. *Journal of Speech Disorders,* 1967, *32,* 126–132.

Finnie, N. R. *Handling of the young cerebral palsied child at home.* New York: E. P. Dutton & Co., Inc., 1970.

Gould, W. J. Vocal cords can speak of hormonal dysfunction. *Consultant,* November 1972, pp. 101–102.

Hixon, T. J., Shriberg, L. D., & Saxman, J. H. *Introduction to communication disorders.* Englewood Cliffs, N.J.: Prentice-Hall, Inc., 1980.

Johns, E. F. (Ed.) *Clinical management of neurogenic communicative disorders.* Boston: Little, Brown and Co., 1978.

Maccomb, W. S., & Fletcher, G. H. *Cancer of the head and neck.* Baltimore: The Williams and Wilkins Co., 1967.

Smith, F. M. Hoarseness: A symptom of premenstrual tension. *Archives of Otolaryngology,* 1962, *75,* 66–68.

Strong, M. S., & Vaughn, C. W. Vocal cord nodules and polyps—The role of surgical treatment. *Laryngoscope,* 1971, *81,* pp. 911–922.

Tetter, D. L. Vocal nodules: Their cause and treatment. *Music Education Journal,* October 1977, pp. 38–41.

Wilson, F., & Rice, M. *A programmed approach to voice therapy.* Austin, Texas: Learning Concepts, Inc., 1977.

Zwitman, D., & Calcaterra, T. C. The "silent cough" method for vocal hyperfunction. *Journal of Speech and Hearing Disorders,* 1973, *38*(1), 119–125.

Chapter 7
Alaryngeal Phonation Therapy

Each year, thousands of persons lose their vital organ of voice—the larynx—to cancer or trauma. In the case of cancer, the patient is surgically laryngectomized to stop the spread of malignant cells in the hope of saving the person's life. In the case of trauma, the larynx is removed because it has suffered damage that has incapacitated the laryngeal valving mechanisms necessary to protect the respiratory tract from aspiration of food, liquids, or saliva. Regardless of why the larynx must be removed, life is altered significantly for the person, psychologically, sociologically, economically, and in particular communicatively. Laryngectomized persons do not necessarily experience difficulty in all of these areas, but many do. Many more experience maladjustments in at least some of the areas. The SLP working with a laryngectomee must understand the significance of the operation from both a communication point of view and from a more comprehensive point of view. This chapter seeks to provide this perspective, with emphasis on the role of the SLP in alaryngeal communication training.

SURGICAL ASPECTS OF LARYNGECTOMY

The specifics involved in surgical removal of the larynx are well described in the literature (Hinchcliffe & Harrison, 1976; English, 1976) and need not be repeated here other than from a general point of view. The SLP should understand the basic anatomical and physiological changes involved in this procedure (Figure 7-1). In a total laryngectomy, the larynx—including all cartilages, intrinsic muscles and membranes, and the hyoid bone—are removed. The upper tracheal rings usually are sacrificed and the exposed trachea is brought forward and provided with external attachment in the neck region just above the sternal notch. This external opening is called the tracheostoma, or stoma, and is the orifice for all respiration following the surgery. The stoma creates a permanent change for the patients, who will be neck breathers for the remainder of their lives.

Breathing through the stoma in the neck is necessary to maintain complete separation of the respirative and digestive tracts to prevent aspiration. This altered respiration path produces many significant changes: reduced olfaction, reduced sense of taste, increased respiratory irritation resulting in excessive coughing, reduced capacity to impound air in the lungs during lifting, defecation, or similar physical activities. It also has a major effect on voice and verbal communication. The larynx, the source of vibration in voice, has been removed and air from the lungs no longer passes through the oral or nasal cavities, making it impossible for the person even to whisper. The power to articulate sound remains for the patient who has had a total laryngectomy without involvement of oral structures, but there is no sound to articulate. The totality of communication loss is difficult to appreciate until experienced. Most laryngectomized persons report they were not prepared sufficiently for the experience of so totally losing their ability to communicate.

Figure 7-1 Profile Before and After Laryngectomy

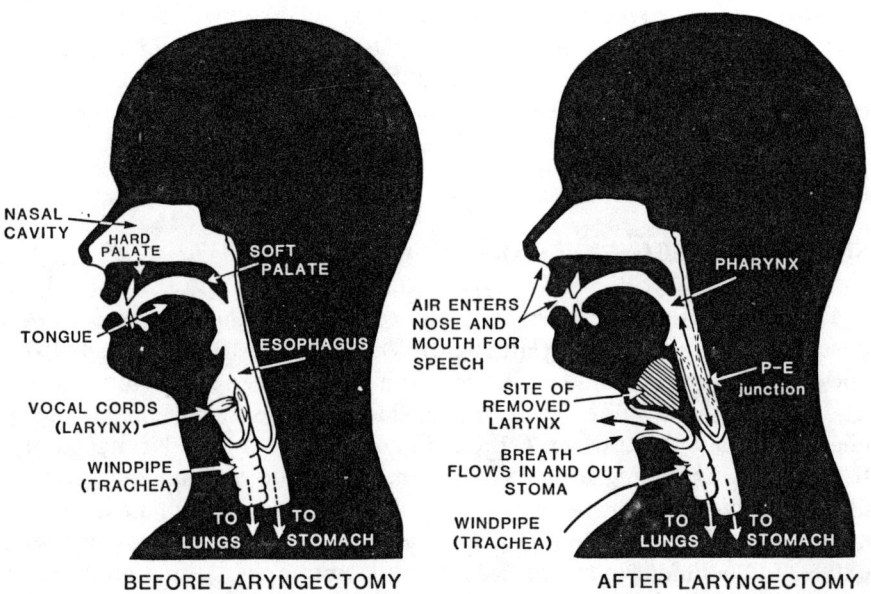

ROLE OF THE SLP IN LARYNGECTOMY REHABILITATION

The primary role of the speech/language pathologist in working with laryngectomized persons is to facilitate alaryngeal communication. Several options, divided into extrinsic and intrinsic alaryngeal sources of phonation, are available to help in this process. Extrinsic sources include devices that can produce a pseudolaryngeal sound. Examples are the battery-driven electrolarynx or the air-driven pneumatolarynx. Several manufacturers provide such instruments. Each type is discussed in some detail later. Intrinsic sources of alaryngeal phonation include generation of a sound source by tissue vibration in the buccal cavity, pharyngeal cavity, at the junction of the pharynx and the esophagus (P-E Junction), or by means of some surgically constructed shunt that connects the trachea to the esophagus and that can be used to vibrate sound.

The SLP must be comfortable with both extrinsic and intrinsic sources. Each of the available options has advantages and disadvantages, and this presentation provides the information necessary to understand these pros and cons. The criteria for judging the acceptability of a given option include (1) the ease of learning to use the method, (2) intelligibility of speech using it, (3) its limitations, and (4) the desire of the laryngectomized person to use it.

EXTRINSIC METHODS OF ALARYNGEAL PHONATION

The following are the commonly used extrinsic methods of producing alaryngeal phonation (sources are listed at the end of this chapter):

Cooper-Rand Electronic Speech Aid

This battery-powered electrolarynx is an intraoral device commonly used by the laryngectomized person. The device consists of a battery-powered pulse generator that is approximately 3" × 4" and fits nicely into a shirt pocket. The generator is connected by a wire to a hand-held tone generator—the alaryngeal voice. Connected to the tone generator is a plastic piece of tubing that fits into the oral cavity. The tone produced is channeled into the oral cavity for articulation purposes (Figure 7-2).

Many patients using the Cooper-Rand have difficulty at first coordinating the voicing with articulation. The placement of the tubing becomes a mild obstruction to the rapid movements of articulation until practice teaches the person proper positioning. Once the individual becomes used to articulating with the tubing in the oral cavity, good intelligibility is obtained. The lingual-velar consonants /k/, /g/, / ŋ / are not produced well

Figure 7-2 Three Types of Artificial Larynges

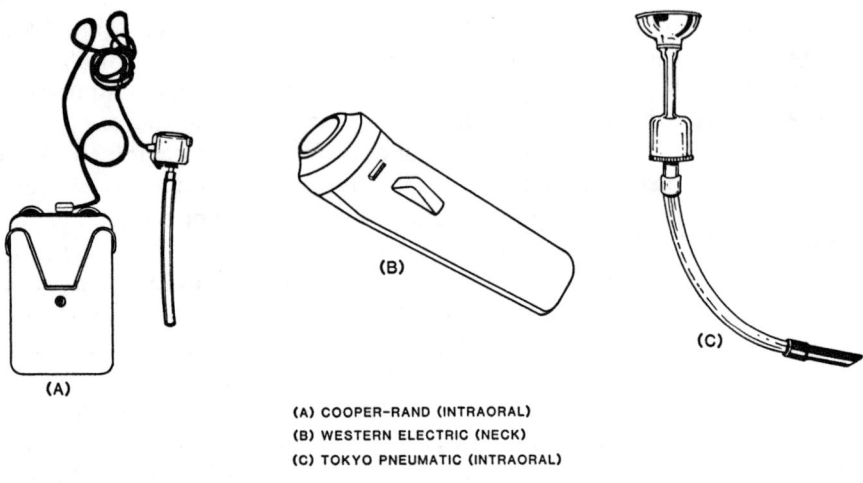

(A) COOPER-RAND (INTRAORAL)
(B) WESTERN ELECTRIC (NECK)
(C) TOKYO PNEUMATIC (INTRAORAL)

with this instrument because the tubing placement is not far enough back into the oral cavity to facilitate the stop portion of these consonants. Context usually is sufficient to produce intelligible speech even in the absence of these consonants.

One of the primary advantages of the Cooper-Rand is that it is an intraoral device. Since the surgery in most cases does not involve the oral cavity, the client can use the device immediately after the operation. Other extrinsic devices held against the neck could not be used at that point because of soreness and tissue healing. The Cooper-Rand is an excellent alternative to writing during the first few weeks of postsurgical rehabilitation and is used by many clients as a primary means of alaryngeal phonation.

Tokyo Artificial Larynx

The Tokyo Artificial Larynx is a pneumatic device driven by air from the stoma during respiratory exhalation. This is a rather simple sound source for the laryngectomized person, who merely places the mouthpiece end of the device against the stoma so air can be blown through it to vibrate a rubber "reed." The other end of the device is placed into the oral cavity so the sound generated by the vibrating reed can be articulated into human speech sounds. The Tokyo Artificial Larynx thus is also an intraoral device, but is driven by air rather than by a battery.

Weinberg and Riekena (1973) studied a single subject using the Tokyo and presented data on its acoustic and perceptual characteristics. They found 95 percent intelligibility with this subject, whom they cautioned might be extraordinary in ability. The Tokyo is an inexpensive option for alaryngeal phonation.

Western Electric 5A and 5B Electronic Larynges

The most commonly used electrolarynx probably is the Western Electric 5A (low pitch, male) or 5B (higher pitch, female). These are powered by battery.

The client holds the Western Electric device in one hand and places its vibrating head in contact with the neck. The person controls both the placement and the pressure exerted. The vibration generated by this device is transmitted into the vocal tract through the neck and the sound then is articulated into human speech. Neck placement is most important to avoid sound spillage that is not directed into the vocal tract. Pitch variation, within the limits of the specific device (5A or 5B), can be changed slightly by depressing a button on the handle. When used properly, the Western Electric electrolarynx is a highly intelligible sound source for alaryngeal communication.

Aurex Neovox Electronic Larynx

This is much like the Western Electric electrolarynges in that it is a hand-held neck device, battery driven, with limited pitch variability. It is more powerful, more expensive, and has a lower frequency response and therefore is more appropriate for males. One advantage the Aurex has over the Western Electric devices is that a battery charger can be purchased for rechargeable batteries.

Each of these devices (pneumatic, intraoral, and neck electrolarynges) can be used successfully by the laryngectomized person. The best results occur when an SLP works with the person to help facilitate intelligibility by proper placement and articulation. The SLP also can help decide which of the devices is best suited for the client or help choose one of the many modifications that also are available. The devices described here as well as many others are detailed thoroughly in a handbook by Salmon and Goldstein (1978). It provides specific costs of each device and an audio tape sample of each artificial larynx. Any SLP who works with laryngectomized persons should become familiar with this handbook.

INTRINSIC METHODS OF ALARYNGEAL PHONATION

Buccal Speech

This method of producing a pseudovoice is rather undesirable for a number of reasons. It involves pushing air through a constriction between the facial cheeks, lateral dental arch, and possibly the tongue in the buccal cavity area of the oral cavity. It is rather unintelligible except for a few sounds and words, probably because the tongue is involved in the site of vibration for voice and therefore is restricted in articulation movements. The SLP should recognize buccal speech when it occurs and eliminate rather than reinforce it.

Pharyngeal Speech

This is similar to the buccal method except the locus of vibration is more posterior in the oral-pharyngeal cavity. It is produced by forcing air through a constriction between the back of the tongue and the posterior pharyngeal wall. It is easy to accomplish and clients often generate this sound early in the therapy process when trying to obtain esophageal speech. It also is rather unintelligible but less so than in buccal speech. The likely reason for its relative unintelligibility is that the tongue is involved in both phonation and articulation. The SLP also should recognize pharyngeal phonation and not reinforce it. Once a person begins generating voice at a pharyngeal locus, it is difficult to correct. Therefore, it is better to avoid it at the outset rather than try to correct it once it becomes established.

Esophageal Speech

Most laryngectomized persons attempt to learn to speak again using the upper musculature of the esophagus as a vibrating site for alaryngeal phonation. Basically, to produce esophageal phonation, the person moves air, which is present in the hypopharyngeal space above the esophagus, into the esophagus below its constriction, then reverses the process so air is forced out of the esophagus under pressure. This movement of air under pressure causes the tissue of the upper esophagus to vibrate and produce alaryngeal voice. The frequency of this vibrating pseudoglottis varies depending on the tissue mass and tension, but it ranges from 52 Hz to 82 Hz (Aronson, 1980).

METHODS OF PRODUCING ESOPHAGEAL SPEECH

Besides frequency (pitch) variation in esophageal phonation, Diedrich and Youngstrom (1966) present data on the variability of the site of vibration in 27 esophageal speakers as revealed by cineradiographic analysis of vibrating tissue. They identify the locus of vibration as the variable pharyngo-esophageal junction (P-E junction) (Figure 7-1, supra). The subjects in this study are compared on various criteria such as speech proficiency, nature of the P-E junction, morphology of the hypopharyngeal and esophageal space, method of loading air for phonation, and surgical and radiotherapeutic factors. This reference is valuable for the SLP who seeks a thorough understanding of the interrelationships of these criteria.

Diedrich and Youngstrom and other researchers and clinicians such as Duguay and Shanks (1974), Aronson (1980), Lauder (1978), and Keith and Darley (1979) have described several methods of loading the esophagus below the P-E junction with air to be used in esophageal phonation. The following is a brief description of the more common methods:

Consonant Injection

Inherent in the voicing of many consonants, particularly stops and fricatives, is intraoral breath pressure that builds behind the place of articulation. This breath pressure can be used to force or inject air into the esophagus during the articulation of the sound. The quick movement of air into and out of the esophagus provides tissue vibration for voice. Thus esophageal voice is produced rather simultaneously with the articulation of the consonant.

To attempt voicing with this consonant injection method, the person is instructed to articulate sounds such as /p a/, /t a /, /k a /, /st a /, /tʃ a /, etc., and if the system works, esophageal voice is heard on the vowel sounds following the consonant. The greater the air pressure on the consonant, the greater the probability air will enter the esophagus. This method is effective for producing words that begin with the high-pressure consonants of the language: *pie, tie, kite, stop, scotch, scratch, skip, paper,* etc.

In a word such as *toothpaste,* there often are sufficient pressure consonants to load the esophagus for all the vowel sounds and the client can say the word without much effort by merely articulating it as though a larynx existed. This also is true of such phrases as "pick it up" or "pass it to me." Unfortunately, most languages have many words that begin with vowels or low-pressure consonants such as "I am here" or "roll your eyes." Consonant loading is not effective as a method of esophageal loading for such phrases but other methods are.

Glossopalatal or Glossopharyngeal Press

Air can be injected into the esophagus by using the tongue as a press or piston structure. The movements necessary to accomplish the task are essentially the same as those involved in the articulation of the stop consonants /p/, /t/, or /k/ except that the pressure is not released forward but is released or pushed backward into the esophagus. The movement forces the air that is trapped by the tongue past the P-E junction, loading the esophagus for esophageal voice. It is a matter of the tongue's squeezing the air into the esophagus.

As air is forced into the esophagus in a glossopalatal or glossopharyngeal press, a slight "klunking" sound of air moving into the esophagus can be heard. When the client hears this sound, the SLP immediately should instruct the individual to open the mouth and say some vowel such as /o/ or /a/. The attempted movements of vowel production usually generate enough pressure in the esophagus to force the trapped air out, thereby vibrating the tissue and producing voice for the vowel. This is one effective method the client can use when attempting to say a word or phrase that begins with a vowel sound such as "I am here" or "instead." The essential difference between the glossopalatal and glossopharyngeal presses is whether the tongue is primarily pushing against the hard palate or the posterior pharyngeal wall during the injection process.

Inhalation of Air into the Esophagus

Where the injection methods mentioned (consonant, glossopalatal, glossopharyngeal) involve action of the tongue that increases the air pressure above the esophagus to force air into it, the inhalation method is just the opposite. The person is instructed to inhale air into the esophagus simultaneously with the inhalation cycle of breathing air into the stoma. Just as negative pressure in the lungs draws air into them during inhalation, a similar negative pressure by the expanded esophagus draws air into it at the same time. This inhalation method loads the esophagus with air to be used in producing esophageal vibration.

If the inhalation method is to work efficiently, the esophagus must be as relaxed as possible. Under conditions of relaxation, air is drawn naturally into the esophagus during the inhalation cycles. Air moves into the esophagus when the negative pressure there is greater than the air pressure in the hypopharynx above the P-E junction.

To teach esophageal loading by the inhalation method, the SLP instructs the person to take a quick sniff of air while the esophagus is relaxed. This sniff of course draws air into the stoma, but it also should draw air into the esophagus. After sniffing, the client is told to open the mouth and say a vowel sound such as /O/ or / a /. The test of this method's workability is whether voicing is heard on the vowel utterance after several trials. To help relax the P-E junction as much as possible, the client can be instructed to open the mouth widely as air is inhaled into the lungs. Air also rushes into the esophagus past the relaxed P-E junction when this is done. This procedure can be repeated in practice until the client can inhale air into the esophagus when the mouth is open naturally.

Pseudoswallowing Method

The laryngectomized person who swallows air into the esophagus to produce esophageal voice is using what is called the pseudoswallowing method (Boone, 1977). Swallowing is such a common daily activity that the movements involved can be performed easily. In most clients, the mere act of swallowing pushes or presses some air into the esophagus; this air can be used to produce voice. However, Duguay and Shanks (1974) caution the SLP about using this method without some modification.

A true swallow is a rather slow and deliberate neuromuscular process that uses the tongue and pharyngeal muscles to move food or liquid through the esophagus and into the stomach. It is essentially a reflex movement. Its initial stages are voluntary and a certain amount of conscious control can be exerted. However, the latter stages, when food or liquid has entered the esophagus and moves toward the stomach, are involuntary. When the SLP instructs a client to swallow air, the individual usually attempts to complete the entire act of swallowing to merely load the upper esophagus with air. However, the result is that the stomach, rather than just the esophagus, is loaded with air, which is counterproductive to esophageal phonation.

If a laryngectomized client thinks it is necessary to swallow completely each time air is to be taken into the esophagus, there will be a considerable lag between the start of the act and the actual movement of air into the esophagus. Loading the esophagus for voice must occur rapidly in functional esophageal speech, and the swallowing process is too slow for that. To demonstrate how slow this reflex is, the SLP should swallow some saliva, then immediately try to swallow some more, then some more. It is obvious that successive swallowing does not occur rapidly. However, the SLP can use the concept of *beginning* to swallow to teach the person how to use the tongue to push air into the esophagus. Such movements, which represent the beginning stage of swallowing, do not involve the complete reflex and can be helpful in teaching the client.

SUMMARY OF METHODS OF ALARYNGEAL PHONATION

Several methods of producing alaryngeal phonation have been presented, including devices (electrolarynges, pneumatolarynges) and oral-pharyngeal-esophageal forms. The SLP has available many more methods not covered in this chapter. Diedrich and Youngstrom (1966), Salmon and Goldstein (1978), Duguay and Shanks (1974), Keith & Darley (1979), and Lauder (1978) identify most of the available methods. These references also cover the research foundations of each method, which are beyond the scope of this chapter.

REHABILITATION OF LARYNGECTOMIZED PERSONS

The successful rehabilitation of a laryngectomized person requires the competent efforts of many individuals. There is the medical team responsible for the physical care of the patient before, during, and after the surgery. There are other laryngectomized persons in social clubs organized under the auspices of the International Association of Laryngectomees, a branch of the American Cancer Society. There are friends and family who can offer such valuable support that successful rehabilitation is almost impossible without them. Psychologists and psychiatrists usually are available for counselling service. Finally, there is the SLP, who is the primary professional responsible for communication rehabilitation, a major concern to the person who has lost so much of that ability as a result of the operation. Each of these persons, professionals as well as loved ones, must function as a team working toward the successful adjustment and rehabilitation of the laryngectomized individual.

Presurgery Visit by the SLP

The role of the SLP in the rehabilitation process often begins before the surgery. Many physicians request a visit then from the SLP, who can be accompanied by a trained laryngectomized person who can provide a model of successful general and communication adjustment. Whether or not the latter is included, the visit must be planned carefully if it is to contribute successfully to the psychological well-being of the patient and family members.

The presurgery visit should start with advance notice to the client so family members who are interested can be present if the patient desires. This visit usually occurs a day or two before the surgery when the patient is in the hospital for testing. The SLP should realize that in many cases the patient is in a state of shock and confusion about the specifics of the surgery and the implications for the future, even when the physician has spent time explaining in detail the procedures and likely results.

In this visit, the SLP should discuss briefly the changes that will exist after surgery, particularly from a phonation point of view. The following dialogue is taken from a tape recording of a presurgery visit by an SLP the day before R.A. had a total laryngectomy:

SLP: I know Dr. R. has gone over the specifics of the surgery, but I wanted to review the implications of what the surgery will mean from a communication point of view. This diagram (Lauder, 1978) (see also Figure 7-1) shows the before and after surgery changes. The main point is that your larynx will be removed. Your larynx is important for two reasons: first, it is a valve which protects your airway to the lungs (trachea) from food, liquid, saliva, etc. Second, when air is forced through the valve during exhalation, the air vibrates the tissues of the valve and sound is produced. The tissues that vibrate are the vocal folds in the larynx. The sound of the vibration is what is known as the voice. You can feel the vibrations of the larynx when you are talking by touching here. (Demonstration.)

R.A.: I think I understand about that.

SLP: Good. Now, since the larynx must be removed, the protective valve will be gone and the tissue that produces voice will also be gone. To protect your airway, the operation will include bringing your trachea forward and attaching it to an opening in your neck. You will breath through this opening in your neck for the rest of your life . . . it is called a stoma. Do you understand that?

R.A.: Yes, I knew that.

SLP: So after your surgery you will breathe through the stoma and no longer will air go up through your mouth and nose, and you will no longer have a voice. You will not even be able to effectively whisper since whispering requires air movement. (Demonstration.) And that is why I am here. To help you regain the ability to communicate, to help you find new ways of producing voice. Any questions so far?

R.A.: Dr. R. said I should be able to talk within a few weeks after surgery, is that right?

SLP: My plan is to begin working with you as soon as possible. Dr. R. will have to tell me when you are ready. Then, when he gives me the green light, we will work as hard as possible to get you talking again. We have many options available to help you with communication. Some will be faster than others, and I want to go over some of those options now. First, many devices have been invented and are available to laryngectomized persons. Some of these devices are very effective in giving the laryngectomized person almost immediate communication. Let me demonstrate some of these. (The next few minutes were spent in demonstrating the Cooper-Rand, Aurex Neovox, Tokyo, and the Western Electric 5A.)

R.A.: Do you sell these?

SLP: No, but I can tell you where you can get one, and loaners are available until you can get your own, should you decide to do that. Most laryngectomized persons try to learn what is called esophageal speech, even when they are using one of these devices. What this involves is taking air that is always present in your mouth and throat down into your esophagus right here. (Shows diagram.) This air is then pushed gently up past this constriction and these tissues in the constriction are vibrated, very much like your vocal folds in the larynx are vibrated. This vibration produces a new sound, a new voice, and this sound is then resonated and articulated into the sounds of human speech. Because the esophagus is vibrating, it is called esophageal speech.

R.A.: You swallow air and I heard someone say it is belched up, is that right?

SLP: Not quite. You won't swallow the air because that would take it into the stomach, and we don't want it to go down that far; just a little ways into the esophagus, then it is brought back up to vibrate the tissue. There are many ways to get the air into the esophagus without swallowing it, and I will help you learn them when the time is right to begin. I want to play some tapes of people who have been laryngectomized who speak with esophageal speech. Some of these people are very good and others are more typical. Then later, after surgery, I will visit you again with a man who has been laryngectomized and speaks with esophageal voice. I think you will find his visit quite helpful. (Tapes are played and discussed.) I will leave these pamphlets (American Cancer Society) and this book (Lauder, 1978) with you. You and your family can look the material over. Here is my card with phone numbers. If you or any members of your family have questions, please call. Good luck on your surgery tomorrow. Dr. R. is an excellent surgeon and you could not be in better hands. I'll be in touch.

This is a typical example of how a presurgery visit can be handled. It is short, involves demonstrations and materials, involves the patient as well as family members, and is encouraging about the future of communication. It provides information but not in great detail. It offers an opportunity for the patient to ask questions. Most importantly, it establishes the professional relationship necessary for good communication rehabilitation.

Polemics of the Artificial Larynx

The artificial larynx is not without controversy in the rehabilitation of laryngectomized persons. Many laryngologists and laryngectomized persons have strong negative attitudes about the use of artificial devices for communication (Case & Holen, 1976; Salmon & Goldstein, 1978). Reasons for this attitude vary but generally the artificial nature of the sound generated is the basis. However, it is evident from the literature and clinical experience that many laryngectomized persons do not learn functional and intelligible esophageal speech (Diedrich & Youngstrom, 1966; Keith & Darley, 1979). A physician with a strong bias against the use of artificial devices can have such a strong influence on patients that they develop the same attitude.

This is unfortunate since so many persons fail to develop esophageal speech for a number of reasons. These individuals then have to turn to what is described as a crutch or a backup system because they could not learn the "best" method. A more reasonable attitude should be for all persons working with a laryngectomized person to have an open mind about all forms of alaryngeal phonation, expose the patient to each of them, and allow the individual to choose the form of communication after the surgery. The decision belongs to the patient, not to the physician, not to the SLP, and not to another laryngectomized individual who might be in a position to offer advice.

The SLP often provides specific instructions on the use of an electrolarynx before surgery. The Cooper-Rand or some modification of another type of device that involves intraoral sound generation is demonstrated and given to the patient to practice speaking. Then a few days after surgery, when the patient is out of intensive care and feeling stronger, the electrolarynx can be used in communication. A neck device such as the Western

Electric or Aurex is not appropriate at that point, nor is a pneumatic device. If an intraoral device is introduced, the SLP should visit the patient a few days after surgery to determine whether it is being used. Therapy can be given at that time to facilitate its use for immediate postsurgical communication.

An SLP who visits the patient should note in the hospital record the essentials of the call, i.e., whether an electrolarynx has been presented, questions answered, any specific instructions given about communication that the medical staff should be aware of. This also informs the physician that contact has been made.

Formal Alaryngeal Therapy

The SLP usually begins formal and regular therapeutic visits with the patient when the physician indicates the patient is ready. Diedrich and Youngstrom (1966) report therapy begins two to four months after surgery, but the actual time may vary. The time to initiate therapy depends on many factors such as recovery progress, whether radiation is to occur before therapy, and physician attitudes, but it should not begin until medical clearance has been obtained.

The initial therapy efforts should be directed at facilitating communication with artificial devices as well as with esophageal speech, assuming the patient has chosen those options. If the patient has been given an electrolarynx such as the Cooper-Rand before surgery and wishes to continue using it, the SLP should evaluate the effectiveness of mouth placement of the device as well as its articulation accuracy and intelligibility. If another device is desired, the SLP should help the patient learn to use it.

When a neck device is chosen, the SLP should provide direction with the following recommendations:

- The nondominant hand should be used to hold the device against the neck. This will free the dominant hand for writing, holding another object, or gesturing while talking.
- The placement on the neck is critical for proper transmission of sound into the vocal tract. Trial-and-error placement until the optimal spot is found should be under the SLP's direction.
- The patient should be able to place the device against the neck accurately without significant latency. This requires practice in moving the device to and from the neck in rapid sequence. This should be practiced before a mirror to help coordinate the process.
- The patient should be instructed in coordinating the activation of the electrolaryngeal tone with speech articulation. It is common for users

to turn the device on too early or too late for proper sequence with articulation. Patients also have a tendency to keep the device vibrating during speech pauses. Learning to turn the device on and off quickly and in concert with articulation is important and requires considerable practice.
- The patient should be encouraged to articulate with care and precision to distinguish between voiced and voiceless sounds, e.g., /t/ vs. /d/ and /s/ vs. /z/.
- The pitch and loudness controls can be altered easily on most devices and the patient should be encouraged to practice these changes to provide the inflections normally heard in speech.
- Practice on the telephone with the device is important. The patient must have confidence in the ability to communicate using the device for emergency and social telephone calls.
- The electrolarynx should be set on a low intensity level for most communication situations. It is disconcerting to the patient using a device in public when everyone can hear what is being said. When the patient is in a noisy place, the loudness setting can be increased.

To accomplish these steps will take more than one therapy session. Some part of each of the first few sessions should be directed at achieving excellence in the use of the artificial larynx.

During the first session, the patient also should be introduced to esophageal speech. The SLP should determine how technical the instructions should be. Most patients do not understand complex instructions regarding the anatomical and physiological bases of esophageal voice, so a behavioral approach is recommended. The SLP instructs the patient to do things that invoke esophageal voice without concern for whether the individual understands what is happening. Diedrich and Youngstrom (1966), Shanks and Duguay (1974), Boone (1977), Lauder (1978); Keith & Darley (1979) and the clinical experience of the author of this chapter indicate that a simple, rather direct approach is better during the first few sessions. It is better to tell the patient to say "/ta /" and determine whether esophageal voice occurs rather than to say something such as, "I would like you to put your tongue behind your upper teeth, build up some pressure, hold the pressure a little while until it has a chance to move down into your esophagus, then, when the air goes into your esophagus, bring it back up and that will cause the tissues to vibrate. That vibration will be your new voice and with it you can say /ta /." While the SLP was giving all those complex instructions (which more than likely would not be understood), the patient could have practiced several /ta / sounds.

With this concept of simplicity in mind, the following format for teaching a patient to produce esophageal voice is recommended. These steps are based on the work of many professionals already referenced as well as the clinical experience of the author of this chapter.

Step 1: Burp and Belch

The SLP asks whether the patient has experienced a burp or belch since the surgery. If the answer is yes, the patient is asked whether this can be produced again. If the patient is able to do so, the SLP asks for several repetitions. Next, the patient continues belching, but with the mouth shaped for an /O/ sound. The SLP should demonstrate the process. The mouth then is shaped for an / a /, then a /u/, and so on until all the following vowels have been attempted: / i /, /ɪ/, /e/ , / ɛ /, /æ/, / a /, / o /, /u/, /ʊ/, /ʌ /, and / ɝ/. Some vowels will be easier to produce than others. The patient should practice until each can be said intelligibly.

Step 2: Consonant Injection

If the method in Step 1 is not successful in stimulating esophageal voice, elicitation with a consonant injection should be attempted. The patient is instructed to say /t a /, /p a /, /k a /, /st/, / tʃ a /, /dʒ a / and all other stop and fricative consonants followed by a vowel that is produced with the tongue low in the mouth such as / a /. By having the patient attempt all of the consonants, the SLP can determine whether one is a better esophageal loader than another. If a specific one is, the patient should practice that consonant in combination with all of the vowels. For example, if the /t/ sound is found to stimulate a high incidence of esophageal voice when followed by an / i / vowel, the patient should say the /t/ consonant with all the vowels: /t i /, /t ɪ /, /t e /, /t ɛ /, /t æ /, /t a /, /t o /, /t u /, /t ʌ /, and /t ɝ/. It may be necessary to provide the patient with key words for each vowel such as /t i / as in *tea*. This drill can be practiced many times. The same process then can be attempted with another consonant until all stop and fricative ones have been tried.

Step 3: Inhalation

If the first two steps have not facilitated esophageal voice, the inhalation method should be attempted. This was explained earlier. It involves the patient's being told to relax the throat muscles as much as possible, open the mouth as though about to yawn, then quickly inhale air into the stoma and attempt to sniff air into the nose at the same time. The SLP should demonstrate this rather than describe it orally. If it works, as air is drawn into the stoma, it also will be drawn into the esophagus. The patient then is instructed to say /a /. If sound is heard on the /a /, the process should be repeated until consistent voice is demonstrated. The patient then can shape the mouth for other vowel sounds as the esophagus is loaded by this inhalation method. Consonants can be added to the vowels to form simple words such as *pie, tie, kick, I, above,* etc. In the inhalation method, it does not matter whether the words begin with a consonant or a vowel.

Step 4: Glossopalatal or Glossopharyngeal Press

If all these steps fail to stimulate esophageal voice, the SLP attempts to elicit it with a glossopalatal or glossopharyngeal press method, both of which are explained earlier. Essentially, these methods involve using the tongue to press or inject air into the esophagus in a piston-like fashion. The patient is told to put the tongue tip on the roof of the mouth just behind the incisor teeth, then pump it against the palate (glossopalatal) or palate and pharynx (glossopharyngeal) to squeeze air into the esophagus. The movements of either of these methods are similar to the beginning stage of swallowing, except that air rather than food or liquid is being moved.

As air is moved into the esophagus with these pressing methods, a slight noise (klunk) can be heard. This is the signal for the patient to push the air out of the esophagus to generate the voice sound. The voice then is shaped into sounds and words in a manner described in Steps 1, 2, and 3. The sequence is: inject . . . say /a /; inject . . . say / i /; inject . . . say / ɔ /. Later, after continued practice, the sequence is: inject . . . say *above;* inject . . . say *drink it,* etc. With this method of loading the esophagus, the patient can say sounds or words in any consonant-vowel (CV) or vowel-consonant (VC) combination.

The end result of these steps is to teach the patient to produce esophageal voice and speech. It is quite possible that the individual will learn to take air into the esophagus in a manner that does not exactly parallel any of those described. However voice is accomplished, if the patient can duplicate the process, and it is devoid of negative aspects in the judgment of the SLP, it should be reinforced. It also is quite possible that after the patient begins to put sounds and words together into functional speech, combinations of methods can be used to load the esophagus with air. There is no problem with this and it is more typical than atypical. Combinations are likely to occur without the patient's awareness as a consequence of the dynamic movements involved in alaryngeal voice and articulation processes.

Once alaryngeal voice is produced and used in monosyllabic words, the next task is to teach simple phrases. It is the SLP's responsibility to select phrases that are rather easy for most laryngectomees to use early in training. Lists of such phrases have been published by Lauder (1978) and Rosenstein (1977). The SLP also can have the patient practice words that are easy to say such as *pack, tack, stack,* and *pick* and put them into phrases such as "pack it, tack it, stack it" or "pack it up, tack it up, stack it up." The patient should articulate these phrases quickly. It is quite probable that esophageal voice, limited as it may be in this early stage, is sufficient to support the entire phrase.

Once a patient consistently and reliably produces esophageal voice and puts it into easy phrases, steady progress into functional communication occurs. It is important for the SLP to keep the patient functioning at a high percentage of success (80 percent or better) as task difficulty is increased. For example, if a patient is reading a list of phrases from Lauder's book, and 80 percent of them are intelligible, it is not necessary to be concerned about the 20 percent that are causing difficulty. The patient should pass over them after a single attempt. Often, on some future reading of the list, the difficult ones will be spoken clearly. It is counterproductive to become hung up on difficult tasks.

In addition to consistency and reliability of voice production, it is most important to work for esophageal speech that is intelligible. Strangers to the patient should listen as lists of words or phrases are spoken to determine whether the speech is intelligible. The SLP often becomes too familiar with the practice lists and thus is not a good judge of intelligibility. It is of some help if the SLP turns away from the patient as lists are read to determine whether they are intelligible without the conscious or unconscious help of lip reading. If a patient can be intelligible without the listener's having the benefit of lip reading, the SLP can be sure progress is being made toward functional alaryngeal speech.

Esophageal Speech Phrasing

Early in the esophageal speech training of laryngectomized persons, it becomes obvious that careful attention to phrasing is necessary. The patient soon learns that the capability has not yet been developed to produce sufficient voice to complete some long phrases, so the esophagus must be loaded with air again in order to continue. This loading process should be done at junctures that are natural to the flow of the utterance and must be practiced repeatedly. Long phrases can be marked at suggested junctures:

Open the door/ and bring/ the book to me./
Stay awhile/ but please/ don't awaken me./
Tell the doctor/ I'm not/ feeling well./

Another technique helpful in teaching phrasing is to tape-record a speech sample as the patient is talking about some topic of interest. For example, the patient discusses going hunting over the weekend. After a few sentences of esophageal speech about the hunting experience, the tape recorder is stopped and rewound to the beginning. The SLP then writes on a piece of paper or chalkboard the patient's actual language and marks the junctures used in esophageal loading. Whether the juncturing occurred appropriately then can be determined. If it did not, a predetermined pattern of more appropriate juncturing is practiced:

Key: / = Patient's first juncturing.
/ / = Suggested target of juncturing.

Terry/ took the/ truck/ up the/ road/
to/ the camp/site/. We wan/ted a/
truck/ as/ soon as/ possible.
Terry/ /took the truck/ /up the road/ /
to the campsite/ /. We wanted/ /
the truck/ / as soon as/ / possible.

Most of the time, patients can improve their speech flow by consciously attending to juncturing. There are no hard rules on this for the esophageal speaker. Rather, juncturing should occur at natural breaks in the flow of the speech. It is best, for example, not to juncture between an article and its noun. By emphasizing the noun and deemphasizing the article, the patient usually can put them together with the same load of esophageal air. Careful attention to appropriate juncturing facilitates better intelligibility in the patient's speech by providing context cues.

Avoidance of Poor Speech Habits

Many aspects of a laryngectomized person's esophageal voice, such as articulation, speech rhythm, and resonance, remain relatively unaffected by the surgery. However, the structural changes resulting from the surgery can have a negative effect on general speech habits and processes. The SLP must be aware of any potential bad habits that might become distracting and affect intelligibility. The patient should be helped to eliminate them. The following are common areas of concern.

Facial Distortion

The patient should practice speech tasks in front of a mirror in order to minimize abnormal facial tics and distortions that often are part of esophageal speaking. Eye blinks and lip grimaces during esophageal loading occur often and should be avoided from the beginning of training. This also is true of head jerks as air is taken into the esophagus. Some patients have had radical neck dissection as part of their laryngeal surgery that can have an effect on head position during speaking. The SLP should help the patient become aware of these facial, lip, head, and neck positions and determine whether adjustment during speech training can help eliminate them.

Stoma Management and Speech Noise

Breathing through the stoma presents many problems to the laryngectomized person. Mucus accumulates at the orifice and must be wiped away constantly. Tissues crust and become dried by the breathing process, often resulting in coughing when pieces fall into the trachea.

Most patients are psychologically concerned about the appearance of the stoma and wear articles of neckwear to cover it. An excellent reference for such items is Kelley and Welborn (1980). Patients become excessively "stoma conscious." This is understandable since difficulties are so common.

One of the primary concerns of stoma control involves excessive noise during breathing and speaking. The size of the stoma varies from patient to patient. Some stomas are so small that breathing is impeded to the degree that air rushing into the esophagus produces excessive noise. This sound is distracting to the quality of speech. If a patient is to experience difficulty with this injection noise, it will be apparent from the first few utterances. The SLP should help the individual become aware of the noise and attempt to reduce it. This can be done by teaching the person to inject more slowly and with less abruptness and to be more relaxed in the neck and throat area so injection requires less force. The combination of these three factors usually helps solve this problem. Once again, it is important that the SLP be aware of this noise from the first moment it occurs so it will not develop into a bad speech habit.

Reduced Loudness of Voice

One of the most perplexing problems a laryngectomized person experiences when using esophageal speech is the reduced loudness potential of the voice. It is difficult to communicate in noisy places such as stores, restaurants, nightclubs, sporting events, and cocktail parties. Counselling is necessary to help the patient recognize the loudness limitation of esophageal voice. It usually is impossible to compete with the noise of society.

To attempt to do so results in reduced articulation control, intelligibility, stoma noise, injection noise, and general speech effectiveness.

Increasing the loudness of esophageal voice should not be attempted until functional and proficient esophageal speech has been achieved. It is not an early priority in the therapy process. After speech proficiency has been attained, the patient can work to facilitate louder speech by shortening the utterance, loading the esophagus more often, and pushing harder with the abdominal muscles as voice is attempted. However, these adjustments should occur only in unique circumstances. The laryngectomee should be aware that these adjustments for greater loudness diminish quality control.

Another technique that has helped some patients to increase loudness of the voice is to apply slight digital pressure (one or two fingers) on the tissue of the neck where esophageal vibration can be felt. This slight pressure can add constriction and tonicity to the vibrating tissue and help increase the loudness of vibration. The SLP can experiment with the digital pressure to determine whether the technique is helpful.

A patient also can increase loudness by using an artificial device when going into a social situation with an expected high noise level. A Western Electric, Aurex Neovox, or similar device can be more effective than an esophageal voice in competing with the noise level. If a patient has been trained properly to use all possible methods of alaryngeal communication, and has no bias against artificial devices, a difficult communication situation can be improved.

GOAL OF FUNCTIONAL ESOPHAGEAL SPEECH

When has the goal of proficient and functional esophageal speech been reached? The SLP and the patient together must evaluate such a goal to determine when it has been attained, but Aronson (1980) lists several criteria that can be used as a guide:

- reliable phonation on demand
- rapid air intake
- short latency between air intake and phonation
- four to nine syllables per air charge
- two to three seconds of voice duration per air intake
- eighty-five to 129 words per minute
- fundamental frequency of 52 to 82 Hz
- average intensity of six to seven decibels below normal
- good intelligibility

These criteria ably represent the goal of communication rehabilitation in laryngectomees when esophageal speech is the chosen form of alaryngeal voice.

CASE EXAMPLE OF ALARYNGEAL PHONATION

The following case example illustrates the frustration as well as the satisfaction of working with laryngectomized patients:

L.W., a 49-year-old male, was laryngectomized as a result of cancer of the upper esophagus. His surgery was rather atypical in that both his esophagus and larynx were removed. This required reconstruction of a pseudoesophagus by displacing stomach tissue upward to connect it to his pharynx. He also had extensive radiation to his jaw and neck area.

After an extended stay in the hospital, L.W. was released with little clinical help in restoring communication ability, because he lived far from the hospital where his surgery was performed. He went for several weeks attempting to communicate by writing on a pad. He was an executive with the Bell Telephone Company and was aware of the electrolarynx but rejected it. On his own, he developed a pharyngeal voice by squeezing air between his tongue and the pharynx and became quite intelligible except on the telephone. He reported that working with the telephone company required extensive long distance communication and operators and clients constantly hung up on him, thinking he was a crank caller.

Six months after his surgery, with pharyngeal speech his only means of communication, L.W. was seen by the author of this chapter. Because of his extensive surgery and radiation, the prognosis for learning any other means of communication besides his present method was unclear. He was introduced to several artificial devices, which he rejected. It was decided to attempt "esophageal" speech to determine whether his displaced stomach tissue could be vibrated in the typical sense.

After three weeks of this therapy, L.W. could produce short and rather choppy utterances with the locus of vibration in the pseudoesophagus. Although he was not satisfied with the quality of his voice, it seemed to him better than his pharyngeal voice. He was loading his pseudoesophagus primarily by means of consonant and glossopress injection.

On one occasion, L.W. was speaking with a group of student SLPs about his experiences with throat cancer, using esophageal voice in a rather slow and choppy manner but with complete intelligibility. In the course of his speech, he put his hand up to press gently on the necktie he was wearing as he attempted to produce voice. A dramatic change in voice quality occurred. Rather than choppy and low in pitch, he produced voice with smoother quality and with less effort. The pitch also was higher.

After his speech, an analysis of the bases of change in his voice indicated that L.W. had begun to take air into his esophagus by inhalation and that the digital pressure, evenly dispursed by the tie, applied just enough pressure to the vibrating site (P-E junction) to allow quality phonation. The goal immediately became to improve this newly found technique of alaryngeal phonation. After two weeks of therapy, he had developed a superior voice quality with the following characteristics: $F_o = 120$ Hz (B_3); 15 syllables per inhalation maximum with a mean of 10 syllables; 120 words spoken per minute with 100 percent intelligibility.

Several times at work after developing his new voice quality, L.W. reported that when talking on the phone, clients who did not know him asked if he had a slight cold. He considered such remarks as great compliments. He now enjoys addressing youth groups and is in great demand as a speaker. He is a totally rehabilitated person and an inspiration to people who meet him (Case, 1981).

RADIATION WITHOUT SURGERY

A laryngeal cancer may be isolated enough so that radiation rather than surgery is recommended as the treatment. This often is the case in glottic cancers staged as T_1 or T_2 (Clinical Staging System). Glottic T_1 occurs when the tumor is confined to one vocal cord and the cord's mobility remains intact; T_2 occurs when the tumor involves both cords with normal or fixed mobility. In either case, no evidence of metastasis of the disease is present.

Perez, Mill, Ogura, and Powers (1971) report a five-year cure rate of 82 percent in T_1 lesions and 77 percent in T_2 lesions, which compares favorably with surgical treatment (hemilaryngectomy). One of the complications of radiation without surgery is hoarseness. This results from tissue dryness, edema, and erythema of the vocal folds and can persist for several months. It is difficult to distinguish the effect of the primary tumor in the hoarseness. However, the SLP should be aware that hoarseness is a consequence of radiation on the larynx in these localized tumors. Harwood, Hawkins, Keane, Cummings, Beale, Rider, and Bryce (1980) provide excellent references on the effects of radiotherapy on the vocal folds in early glottic cancers.

PHONATION FROM SHUNT RECONSTRUCTION

A number of surgeons have developed reconstruction techniques designed to provide alaryngeal phonation for laryngectomized persons

(Taub, 1975; Conley, De Amesti, & Pierce, 1958; Arslan & Serafini, 1972). Most of these procedures involve creating a shunt that connects the tracheostoma to the pharynx or esophagus. Through this connection, air can be shunted into the structures of the vocal tract to vibrate tissue and generate voice. These procedures often have been successful in restoring voice to laryngectomees. However, they have some potential for difficulty in the form of aspiration and spontaneous closure.

Singer and Blom (1980) report an endoscopic technique for restoring voice after laryngectomy. Following the total laryngectomy, a midline tracheoesophageal puncture is created and later fitted with a voice prosthesis that functions as a one-way valve stent. Once it is in place, the patient must place a thumb or finger over the prosthesis to shunt the exhaled air into the esophagus to vibrate the tissues of the P-E junction. Sixty patients have been treated with this prosthesis following laryngectomy, with 90 percent of them achieving fluent voice.

The SLP has a critical role in the Singer-Blom procedure. The prognosis for successful use of the procedure in voice restoration can be established by an insufflation test in which the SLP blows air through a catheter that has been placed through the nose into the esophagus. As the SLP blows gently, the patient attempts to produce sounds and words. The insufflation test determines whether alaryngeal voicing is possible with gentle air pressure forced through the P-E junction.

No operative complications of infection, wound breakdown, hemorrhage, or aspiration have been reported. The six failure patients experienced spontaneous closure of the puncture shortly after the prosthesis had been removed. One complication reported is the tendency for some patients to dislodge the prosthesis inadvertently, but Singer and Blom feel dislodgment occurred because of improper placement.

Several reconstructive techniques developed to restore voice to the laryngectomee have produced inconsistent results but the Singer-Blom procedure seems to have great promise for rehabilitation of these patients.

SUMMARY

This chapter was designed to provide practical techniques for the SLP working with laryngectomized persons. While the emphasis has been on teaching esophageal phonation, several alaryngeal alternatives have been considered. It is hoped that the SLP will become familiar with all such alternative techniques for voice restoration and provide therapeutic support to the patient regardless of the method chosen. The successful rehabilitation of a laryngectomee requires the support of several professional individuals, and the SLP is an important member of that team. It is recommended that any SLP who desires to work with laryngectomized individuals seek sufficient experience and training to be listed in the directory of instructors of alaryngeal voice published by the International Association of Laryngectomees.

REFERENCES

Aronson, A. E. *Clinical voice disorders*. New York: Thieme-Stratton, Inc., 1980.

Arslan, M., & Serafini, I. Reconstructive laryngectomy: Report of the first 35 cases. *Annals of Otology, Rhinology, and Laryngology*, 1972, *81*, 497–486.

Boone, O. *The voice and voice therapy*. Englewood Cliffs, N.J.: Prentice-Hall, Inc., 1977.

Case, J. L. Excellent pharyngeal to superior pseudoesophageal phonation after laryngoesophagectomy. A case study. Paper presented at the convention of the American Speech-Language-Hearing Association, Los Angeles, 1981.

Case, J. L., & Holen, D. *A survey of attitudes of Arizona laryngologists regarding alaryngeal rehabilitation*. Unpublished paper presented at the Arizona Speech and Hearing Association state convention, Tucson, 1976.

Conley, J. J., DeAmesti, F., & Pierce, M. K. A new surgical technique for the vocal rehabilitation of the laryngectomized patient. *Annals of Otology, Rhinology, and Laryngology*, 1958, *67*, 655–664.

Diedrich, W. M., & Youngstrom, K. A. *Alaryngeal speech*. Springfield, Ill.: Charles C Thomas, Publisher, 1966.

Duguay, M., & Shanks, J. In S. Dickson, (Ed.). *Communication disorders: Remedial principles and practices*. Glenview, Ill.: Scott, Foresman and Co., 1974.

English, G. M. *Otolaryngology: A textbook*. Hagerstown, Md.: Harper & Row Publishers, Inc., 1976.

Harwood, A. R., Hawkins, N. V., Keane, T., Cummings, B., Beale, F., Rider, W. D., & Bryce, D. P. Radiotherapy of early glottic cancer. *Laryngoscope*, 1980, *3*, 465–470.

Hinchcliffe, R., & Harrison, D. *Scientific foundations of otolaryngology*. Chicago, Ill.: Year Book Medical Publishers, Inc., 1976.

Keith, R. L., & Darley, F. L. (Eds.). *Laryngectomee rehabilitation*. Houston, Texas: College-Hill Press, Inc., 1979.

Kelley, D. H., & Welborn, P. *The cover-up:neckwear for the laryngectomee and other neckbreathers*. Houston, Texas: College-Hill Press, 1980.

Lauder, E. *Self-help for the laryngectomee*. San Antonio: Author, 1978.

Maccomb, W. S., & Fletcher, G. H. *Cancer of the head and neck*. Baltimore: The Williams & Wilkins Co., 1967.

Perez, C. A., Mill, W. B., Ogura, J. H., & Powers, W. E. Irradiation of early carcinoma of the larynx. *Archives of Otolaryngology*, 1971, *93*, 465–472.

Rosenstein, A. *Esophageal speech with health concepts and tips for laryngectomees*. Long Beach, Calif.: ELOJ Publishing Company, 1977.

Salmon, S. J., & Goldstein, L. *The artificial larynx handbook*. New York: Grune & Stratton, Inc., 1978.

Singer, M. I., & Blom, E. D. An endoscopic technique for restoration of voice after laryngectomy. *Annals of Otology, Rhinology, and Laryngology*, 1980, *90*, 529–533.

Taub, S. Air bypass voice prosthesis for vocal rehabilitation of laryngectomees. *Annals of Otology, Rhinology, and Laryngology,* 1975, *84,* 45–48.

Weinberg, B., & Riekena, A. Speech produced with the Tokyo artificial larynx. *Journal of Speech and Hearing Disorders,* 1973, *38*(4), 383–389.

NOTE

Following are the electronic speech aid devices discussed and where they may be obtained:

Cooper-Rand Electronic Speech Aid
Luminard
P.O. Box 257
7670 Acacia Avenue
Mentor, Ohio 44060

Tokyo Artificial Larynx
Red Woodward
3132 Waits Avenue
Fort Worth, Texas 76109

Western Electric 5A and 5B Electronic Larynges
Bell Telephone Company

Aurex Neovox Electronic Larynx
Aurex Corporation
844 West Adams Street
Chicago, Illinois 60607

The address of the International Association of Laryngectomees (IAL):
c/o The American Cancer Society
777 Third Avenue
New York, N.Y. 10017

The IAL Laryngectomees Directory (1981) lists officers, committee members, sources of supply of various items, club membership by geographical location. Obtained at above address.

The IAL Directory of Instructors of Alaryngeal Speech provides a listing of trained persons who have met the IAL standards. It can be obtained at the above address.

Section III
Fluency Disorders

Chapter 8

Defining and Assessing Stuttering Behavior

A graduate student asked one of her professors if he could provide her the names of ten stutterers she could contact. She needed subjects to participate in a study she planned.

"What are your criteria for selecting subjects for your study?" the professor asked.

"I just need some bona fide stutterers," she replied.

Her only criterion was that her subjects were to be labeled as stutterers. But does merely labeling individuals as stutterers make them stutterers? Will they share all the same characteristics as others who have been labeled as stutterers? What are the characteristics of stuttering and how is it defined? The student must find answers to these questions before she can hope to select a homogeneous group of subjects for her study. This section demonstrates how difficult this task is. First, a look at some definitions of stuttering.

DEFINING STUTTERING

The student in this example certainly is not the first person to be confronted with the problem of defining stuttering. This has perplexed authorities for years; even today, few can reach agreement on a standard definition, yet even the lay person has little difficulty discriminating between individuals who stutter and those who do not. Some have said stuttering is tautological, that is, the behavior is obvious as the observer confronts it and therefore needs no definition (Emerick & Hamre, 1972). West, Ansberry, and Carr (1957) state: "Everyone but the expert knows what stuttering is" (p. 15).

When people define stuttering, they usually do so in behavioral terms, namely, they identify specific behaviors they see or how the individual speaks, or what the individual does. These behaviors occur only when the person attempts to speak. They consist of sound or syllable repetitions, hesitations, and prolongations. They usually are accompanied by facial or bodily movements such as eye blinking, head shaking, lip puckering, arm or hand movements and so on. A person who communicates in this way is said to be stuttering.

Some experts prefer not to define stuttering in terms of overt behaviors but consider it an act of avoidance or a fear reaction. Johnson prefers not to consider the speech dysfluencies as part of stuttering (Johnson, Brown, Curtis, Edney, & Keaster, 1967, Ch. 5). For him, the anticipatory avoidance reaction is the key to the definition. Sheehan (1970), on the other hand, defines stuttering as a disorder of the social presentation of the self. Stuttering is not considered a speech disorder at all but simply a symptom of a deeper identity problem. This position, of course, is extremely difficult to define in objective or measurable terms.

If it is desired to define stuttering in objective terms, the behaviors the person exhibits in attempting to speak must be described accurately. Only then do the symptoms of stuttering appear in an observable form. Wingate (1964) presents a thorough description of stuttering behaviors in terms of three features:

1. Speech disruptions, or what happens to the speech signal, involve audible or silent repetitions or prolongations of sounds, syllables, or words that are not readily controllable.
2. Accessory body activities involving the speech apparatus or other body parts may accompany these speech disruptions. These activities may include arm swinging, lip protrusion, eye blinking, head jerking, and the like.
3. A state of emotional tension often characterized by fear, irritation, embarrassment, or guilt may be indicated.

These three features—speech disruption, accessory activity, and emotional reaction—usually are present when a person stutters.

Description of Speech Dysfluencies

First for consideration are the speech behaviors exhibited by people who stutter. The speech dysfluencies can be described under five categories. The first three also can be used to describe dysfluencies that occur frequently in the speech of nonstutterers. They usually are more pronounced or more frequent in the speech of stutterers.

Interjections

Interjections are additions such as *ah, oh well, you know, you see,* and *er* that add no meaning to the utterance. They may be sounds, words, or phrases and generally are used to fill silent gaps between words. Individuals who stutter may repeat these interjections several times or use several in serial order.

Pausing

Most speakers frequently pause or hesitate between phrases and sentences. However, those who stutter tend to pause at unexpected times in a manner quite unlike normal speakers. Sometimes the pauses are quite long, lasting for several seconds. Long pauses are called "blocks" because the stutterer seems unable to speak. The term "broken word" is used to describe an inaudible pause between sounds within a word.

Revisions

Individuals often revise certain phrases or sentences as they talk. They may begin with one thought and change to another or choose a different grammatical structure. Often stutterers use revision for different reasons. They may revise a sentence because they wish to avoid saying a certain word, or they may block on the first attempt and use a revision to help them to begin talking again.

Repetitions

Many speakers repeat words or even short phrases. They may repeat interjections when unsure or confused. They may say, "Uh-uh-uh, what's his name?" But they rarely repeat one sound in the way many stutterers do. Frequent sound and syllable repetitions are common among stutterers, who repeat whole words and phrases.

Prolongations

Prolongations are unique speech behaviors; they are seldom found in the speech of normal speakers, but are often exhibited by stutterers. The prolongation of a sound may be auditory or silent. A stutterer may simply exhale before uttering a sound or word. This constitutes an inaudible prolongation. Both consonants and vowels may be prolonged. Sometimes these prolongations occur within a word, as in the case of *constitu-u-u-u-ution,* in which the "u" sound is prolonged.

In summary, the two principal speech dysfluencies that act as signals to the listener that a person is stuttering are: (1) an inaudible or audible prolongation of a sound and (2) a repetition of a sound or syllable. Inappropriate or prolonged pausing and frequent use of interjections or revisions also may indicate the speaker is stuttering.

Dissatisfaction with Definitions of Stuttering

No matter what definition of stuttering is chosen, some will disagree with it. Hegde (1978), in a provocative article discussing several definitions of stuttering, writes that fluency cannot be defined in positive terms so he feels it also is virtually impossible to describe stuttering adequately. Hegde identifies five classes of definitions of stuttering and declares that none provides an adequate basis for defining fluency. This may result from the fact that so many definitions of stuttering are tied to several different theoretical positions, none of which can be proved. He feels the majority of definitions are either too restrictive or irrelevant.

Where does this leave the reader? Culatta (1978), in his response to Hegde's article, argues that the basic research necessary to define fluency and stuttering adequately must be carried out. For the present, the only solution is to be content with a description of the behaviors people tend to attribute to those who stutter. When someone exhibits these behaviors, it is said that that person stutters. This is not exactly a scientific definition but it is the best available for the present.

CAUSES OF STUTTERING

One thing can be said with certainty regarding the original cause of stuttering: it has not been identified. It has been suggested that there may be no single cause but that the same symptoms may develop from one or a combination of many factors. But this explanation does not help identify any specific cause. There must exist a set of circumstances that, when present, will lead to the development of stuttering but, for the time being, it is possible only to guess what those circumstances might be.

Although even the experts are at a loss to explain the original cause of stuttering, stimuli that trigger this behavior can be identified easily. Numerous studies show how stuttering can be increased or decreased by manipulation of certain environmental stimuli (Bloodstein, 1969; Goldiamond, 1965; Van Riper, 1971). Before these trigger stimuli are discussed, three types of theories that attempt to explain the cause of stuttering should be reviewed briefly.

The Primary Cause of Stuttering

Numerous theories have been proposed to explain how and why stuttering develops. None of these theories has been put to clinical test. No one has experimentally created a stutterer in order to prove a theory correct. It is doubtful that anyone will. Perhaps the causal factors are so unique to each situation that it is impossible to devise a single theory to explain all cases of stuttering. Theorists attempt to identify commonalities among all those who stutter, hoping this might help them to identify some of the prerequisite conditions that might indicate a common cause. Most theories of causation can be classified under one of several types of theories: neurophysiological, environmental, and multicausal.

Theories Prior to the 20th Century

References to stuttering can be found in clay tablets from Mesopotamia that date centuries before the time of Christ (Van Riper, 1966, p. 306). Even an Egyptian hieroglyphic represented by the word "nit-nit" was used as early as the 20th century B.C. to refer to stuttering (Clark & Murray, 1965). Stuttering was considered to be a bad habit. Those who stuttered were ridiculed because of their unusual speech. They were thought to be possessed by some evil spirit.

Aristotle felt stuttering resulted from a defect within the tongue. Some prescribed treatments such as drinking hot wine or vinegar, bloodletting, and even surgical removal of parts of the tongue. Little attention was given to the psychological aspects of the person who stuttered.

Theories Based on Neurophysiological Factors

For centuries it was believed that stuttering was caused by a malfunction of some part of the physiological or neurological structure. During the 1920s, stuttering was attributed to a lack of cerebral dominance (Orton, 1927; Travis, 1931). It seemed to result from forcing left-handed children to become right-handed. However, studies of handedness failed to prove that cerebral dominance was a factor. Since then there has been renewed interest in the cerebral dominance theory. In a few cases, it was reported that stuttering was eliminated as a result of brain surgery. The results of competitive dichotic listening technique studies also indicate stutterers may lack cerebral dominance (Jones, 1967; Kimura, 1961).

Van Riper (1971) reviews a number of studies that suggest stuttering is linked to some organisity factor. He points out that there is a strong likelihood that the cause of stuttering may be linked directly to a neurophysiological factor. There are many who agree.

It has been suggested that since stuttering seems to occur frequently among members of successive generations of the same family, some hereditary factor may be an explanation (Wepman, 1939; Andrews & Harris, 1964). Gray (1940) attempts to explain this finding on the basis of attitudes prevalent in certain families that might foster the development of stuttering, rather than a genetic factor. In view of studies of the higher incidence of stuttering among twins, this does not support Gray's hypothesis (Nelson, Hunter, & Walter, 1945). More recently, Kidd (1977) suggests that there is evidence to support the theory that certain genetic factors may be responsible for susceptibility to stuttering. He points out that there also may be many environmental elements that could contribute.

The theory that stuttering is caused by some type of deficiency in the neurophysiological structure gains credibility from results of a large number of research studies. It may be that some children are much more susceptible to speech fluency breakdowns under certain conditions and this predisposition may set the stage for the initial development of stuttering. Whether this susceptibility is caused by a genetic factor, a faulty feedback system, or a cerebral integration problem has not been determined. Unfortunately, many of the studies designed to pinpoint organic differences between stutterers and nonstutterers have been poorly constructed and seldom provide consistent results (Hill, 1944).

More recent evidence indicates stuttering may be caused by a malfunction of the laryngeal structure. Preliminary work by Freeman and Ushijima (1975) shows that when a person stutters, abnormal respiratory, laryngeal, and articulatory events occur that place such individuals outside the realm of normality. Stutterers exhibit improper timing, sequencing, air pressure, and airflow, resulting in a disruption of fluency. Adams (1974), discussing the effects of deviant respiratory and laryngeal behaviors upon speech, holds that stuttering is the direct result of these deviant behaviors and suggests they are its physiological cause. There also may be genetic and organic factors that could account for these behaviors (Adams, 1978).

Schwartz (1974) also suggests that the cause of stuttering rests with certain physiologic and aerodynamic events that occur in the vocal tract. He describes stuttering as an uninhibited airway dilation reflex.

It cannot be denied that these persons do engage in deviant laryngeal and respiratory behaviors during the act of stuttering, yet no one can say with certainty that they do so because of a malfunction of the physiological mechanism. Those who ascribe to learning theories argue that these inappropriate behaviors are learned and do not result from a deviant structure.

Theories Based on Environmental Factors

Several theories identify factors in the environment as causes of stuttering but they differ substantially on which specific factors contribute most to its development. These theories can be grouped into three divisions: parental diagnosis, psychoanalytic interpretations, and conditioning. Each is discussed separately next.

Parental Diagnosis. Probably the best known proponent of a theory that suggests stuttering is caused by environmental factors is Johnson, who propounds the diagnostogenic concept (Johnson, 1959). As a result of Johnson's numerous studies conducted with several associates, he contends there is no neurophysiological difference between the child who is destined to become a stutterer and the one who will become a normal speaker. Both children exhibit dysfluent speech at an early age as a normal process of acquiring language. Most children repeat syllables or words at the age of 2 or 3 as they attempt to construct more complex sentences. According to Johnson's theory, an adult (usually one or both parents), interprets or diagnoses the child's early dysfluencies as stuttering. They become anxious and concerned.

In their attempt to help prevent dysfluencies, they actually cause the child to become anxious about them. They offer suggestions that the child should speak slowly, take a deep breath before speaking, stop, and start over, all of which may actually add to the problem. When the child fails in attempts to be the fluent speaker the parents expect, this heightens the youngster's awareness and anxiety about talking at all. The resulting stress and tension disrupts fluency. In an effort to prevent dysfluent speech, the child may adopt mannerisms such as blinking eyes, pursing lips, etc. These mannerisms, known as accessory or secondary features, soon are incorporated into the child's speech pattern.

However, to make this theory tenable, Johnson has to explain away many of the known facts about stuttering that seem to conflict with his views of parental influence as the sole cause of stuttering. For example, he has to explain why the ratio of male to female stutterers is 4 to 1 no matter what the culture. This finding adds strong support to those theories supporting genetic causes. Boys who have inherited physical deformities outnumber girls at this same ratio of 4 to 1. Johnson attempts to explain why more boys stutter than girls by pointing out that since parents expect boys to speak equally as well as girls, they impose demands that boys cannot meet. These unrealistic expectations cause boys to become tense, resulting in dysfluent speech.

Another fact about stuttering is that it occurs among many family members in some families while almost never in other families. It has been suggested that it may be inherited; a genetic factor may be responsible (Wepman, 1939; Kidd, 1977). Johnson's explanation of the hereditary trait centers not on genetic factors but rather on an attitude characteristic of family members which include stutterers. He reasons that a "climate of anxiety" is prevalent in each generation. This is a learned anxiety pattern that has nothing to do with genetics.

Johnson's theory suffers from one major fault—there is no way of proving the child who develops stuttering is identical to the one who develops normal speech. There is no way of knowing how many parents create a climate of anxiety but whose children do not develop stuttering. The parents' diagnosis and subsequent behaviors may be totally unrelated to the stuttering.

Psychoanalytic Interpretations. Another theory based chiefly upon parents' reactions to their children is offered by several psychiatrists and psychologists. Viewing from a Freudian viewpoint, Glauber (1954) and Barbara (1954) assert that stuttering is caused by inadequate interpersonal relationships that arise from parental mishandling of childhood upbringing practices. They suggest the child has certain basic sociosexual needs that are unsatisfied as a result of the mother's inadequacies in providing a good love relationship. This may occur during nursing as the mother may alternately wish to feed and to withhold food from the infant.

The stutterer is viewed as a neurotic individual who cannot acquire fluent speech until the frustrations of early deprivation states are removed and the individual achieves an inner balance. A state of inner balance is achieved when an individual is fully adjusted to the environment. Seligman (1966) contends there is insufficient evidence to support the theory that parents are indeed responsible for the development of their child's stuttering. It also must be recognized that treatment programs based on the theory that stuttering is purely a psychological problem tied with psychosexual frustrations have yielded poor results (Brill, 1923). Several studies fail to show that persons who stutter are in any way more neurotic than normal speakers (Van Riper, 1971).

Conditioning. A number of theories consider stuttering a conditioned behavior, developing from certain motivational factors, stimulus variables, and reinforcing conditions.

One theory that considers conditioning an important etiological factor is advanced by Sheehan (1958). He views stuttering as the symptom of an approach-avoidance conflict: when the drive to speak and the drive to avoid speaking are equal, stuttering occurs. If the urge to speak is stronger, the person can speak fluently. If avoidance is greater, a block occurs, preventing the person from speaking. Sheehan holds that stuttering has its origin in learning situations in which speech anxieties are acquired.

Wischner (1950) also considers avoidance a chief contributory factor. He likens stuttering to an instrumental avoidance act and considers it nothing more than the individual's own effort to avoid the dysfluency. Wischner describes this sequence of events: the stutterer learns to fear the speech act, builds up anxiety before speaking, stutters because of this anxiety, and is reinforced immediately by anxiety reduction. Stuttering is learned and maintained by such consequences as the avoidance of painful unconditioned stimuli and the pleasure of reducing the anxiety level developed because of these painful stimuli.

Brutten and Shoemaker (1967) propose a two-factor theory. They hypothesize that stuttering first appears because of classical conditioning that accounts for the acquisition of conditioned negative emotional responses. They contend that this conditioned negative emotion causes involuntary disruption of fluency in the form of part-word repetitions and sound prolongations. Instrumental conditioning then plays a role in the development of secondary features, according to their concept.

Theories based solely on instrumental or operant conditioning models are best illustrated by the research of Shames and Sherrick (1963) and by Goldiamond (1965). They feel stuttering is an operant behavior that is increased or decreased merely by the consequences derived from the behavior. They hypothesize that when dysfluent responses are punished, the child may respond by silence or struggling with the speech attempt. These behaviors are reinforced by termination of listeners' aversive stimuli (negative reinforcement). Soon stutterers become their own listeners and, hence, evaluators. Stuttering also can be reinforced positively by the fact that it may gain attention from the listener or may become an excuse for inadequacy. Numerous experiments strongly indicate that stuttering is a behavior that is similar to any other learned operant behavior (Goldiamond, 1965).

Theories Based on Multicausality

One simple explanation to solve the dilemma of whether stuttering is caused by a neuropsychological anomaly or by environmental problems is to postulate that several factors are the causes (Bloodstein, 1969). While this position might seem to satisfy everyone, it does not help pinpoint the cause. Yet, what is called stuttering may not be a single disorder. There may be many different types, each resulting from a different set of circumstances. Perhaps it is folly to search for a single cause for this speech disorder. One set of circumstances could lead to its development in one individual but the same set might not cause another person to stutter.

Much of the quandary may result from the fact that it is necessary to work from such a limited definition. The symptoms can only be described. This is as hopeless as a doctor who attempts to diagnose the cause of symptoms indicating a respiratory infection without an x-ray, knowledge of bodily function, body temperature, and so on. For example, a breathy voice quality, although the symptom is the same, may stem from a variety of causes: a vocal nodule, inflammation, viral infection, cancer, muscle paralysis, or some similar condition. As is clear, the physician must identify the cause of the symptom correctly before treatment can be prescribed. Obviously, the wrong diagnosis can lead to the wrong treatment and possible prolongation of the symptom.

In the case of stuttering, its symptoms in terms of speech dysfluencies are recognized easily, but so far, as noted, no one has been successful in identifying their causes, so effective treatment cannot be prescribed. This explains why there has been so much effort devoted toward discovering the cause of stuttering. Up to now, a cause or causes remain unknown.

A Practical Point of View

If a stutterer expresses a desire to speak more fluently, the expert cannot reply, "Well, I can't do anything for you until we discover the cause of stuttering." That would be like the firefighter who rushes to the scene of a burning house only to say to the frantic homeowners, "Sorry, before I can put out the fire we must find what caused it."

If treatment must be provided for the stutterer, certain assumptions must be made about its cause, with treatment proceeding from there. Many reports of successful treatment procedures for stuttering have been published (Schwartz, 1974; Ryan, 1974; Brutten & Shoemaker, 1967; Van Riper, 1973). On the other hand, some treatment methods have proved to be utter failures (Van Riper, 1973). In view of the report by Andrews, Guitar, and Howie (1980) concerning the success of certain treatment methods, there is reason to be optimistic about the prognosis for achieving and maintaining fluent speech when certain methods are used. They found techniques using the gentle onset to initiate syllables to be the most successful technique.

It may be that stuttering is caused by some neurophysiological deviation but there is little that speech/language pathologists can do to correct such a condition. It is more practical to assume stuttering is a learned behavior since experts can do something about what a person learns. This is not to say there need be no concern about finding the cause of stuttering. The prospects of prevention lie chiefly in the discovery of the cause. This discovery currently does not appear to be forthcoming. Those who treat stuttering must turn their attention to factors that maintain stuttering behaviors. These factors are discussed in Chapter 9. Before a treatment program can begin, the stuttering behavior must be evaluated. The following section is devoted to that subject.

ASSESSING STUTTERING BEHAVIORS

As stated earlier, some feel stuttering is so obvious as to require no definition. Others feel it cannot be defined. But in spite of the lack of a specific definition, pathologists are asked to change certain speech behaviors during the treatment. It is important to describe accurately the behaviors constituting stuttering and the speaking situations that may evoke it. An individual may exhibit few if any such behaviors in some situations, yet may stutter severely in others. The authors have seen children whose mothers complained they stuttered severely, yet the youngsters speak fluently when brought into the speech clinic for diagnosis. One sure characteristic is that stuttering varies considerably in severity from time to time and from situation to situation.

Mild, Moderate, and Severe Classification System

One of the most reliable classification systems that will generate agreement among listeners is to rate the severity of stuttering heard as mild, moderate, or severe. Research studies that have used this classification system to describe their sample are published frequently.
Unfortunately this classification system is of little clinical value to speech pathologists because it tells them nothing about specific speech behaviors and provides no information about how specific situations affect the individual's fluency. The experts cannot detect small gains during treatment nor discriminate among various speakers classified in each of the three categories.
A more detailed system of rating stuttering on a seven-point scale is found in Johnson, Darley, and Spreistersbach (1963). They call it the *Scale for Rating the Severity of Stuttering*. It consists of brief criteria or descriptions of stuttering behaviors so that a speaker can be classified in any one of the seven categories. It is a more detailed version of the simple, mild, moderate, severe classification but still suffers from the subjective manner in which the speaker is rated.
This method may be useful when it is desired to convey a general impression about stuttering severity. For example, it might be said that the individual was a severe stutterer until after treatment and now is

considered a mild stutterer. However, the speech pathologist must consider many other factors when evaluating stuttering.

Describing Specific Speech Behaviors

What is heard when a stutterer speaks? The behaviors classified as stuttering have been identified, namely, (1) pauses between or within words, (2) prolongations of sounds, (3) repetitions of sounds, syllables, words, or phrases, (4) use of interjections such as sounds, words, or phrases, and (5) sentence or phrase revisions. Some stutterers may exhibit only one of these behaviors, others may (and often do) use more than one.

Counting Stuttering Behaviors

A decision must be made about how to count these behaviors. It is important to understand there is no one correct counting method. What is counted depends upon what the SLP thinks is important to report or describe. For example, what if a stutterer says, "Can I shu-shu-shu-shu-show you something?" This can be counted as four occurrences of stuttering or as one; that is, there are five words in the sentence, but only one was dysfluent.

The authors tested an adult who stuttered severely when asked to say his name. He said, "OK, uh, um, well, it's ah, lemme see, uh, OK, ah M————Mike." His statement consisted of a series of different interjections plus a sound prolongation. To say he stuttered once doesn't describe his behavior accurately. Another person who said, "F———Fred" also would receive a count of one but on the basis of this count alone it was not possible to differentiate between the severity of the two speakers.

One procedure for overcoming the limitation of counting a word as stuttered or fluent is to compute the average number of behaviors exhibited before and/or during word production. Mike, the severe stutterer, was found to average 5.2 disruptions per stuttered word while Fred, the mild stutterer, averaged only 1.5. Even though both may have stuttered on the same number of words in reading the same passage, their average number of dysfluencies provides information to help decide which speaker's case is considered the more severe.

Duration of Stuttering

Another variable to be considered is the length of time the speech dysfluency is maintained. For example, one stutterer closes his eyes, puffs out his cheeks, purses his lips, and holds his breath for as long as 30 seconds before saying any word beginning with /p/. Another stutterer may hesitate half a second on the same word. In this case, both stutterers exhibited only one behavior—a silent prolongation or pause. What is needed to enable the SLP to distinguish between the severity of the two speakers' problems is the average length of the prolongation. But as might be guessed, this is difficult to compute if pauses average only a second or two. Riley (1972), in her test of stuttering, estimates the duration of the three longest blocks from a "fleeting" (less than 1/2 second) category to one lasting 60 seconds or more. This evaluation method provides only a rough approximation of duration.

Van Riper (1971, p. 231) feels it is easier to count the individual durations of the moments of stuttering than it is to count their frequencies. Sheehan (1946) reports the average duration of the blocks of the subjects he studied is 1.6 seconds and the average prolongation .87 seconds. A block or prolongation lasting two to three seconds is considered severe stuttering.

Rate of Speaking and Stuttering

A simple answer to these problems of distinguishing among various types of severity is to record the time required for the person to read a passage or speak on a topic. Most people speak 140 to 160 words per minute (Fairbanks, 1960). If a stutterer uses many repetitions, interjections, and prolongations, the rate of speech will be slow. For example, one severe stutterer, a junior high school boy, spoke an average of only 17 words per minute and stuttered on an average of 15 of those. It is all too easy to imagine the difficulty he was experiencing while attempting to speak. Those who viewed videotapes thought this boy had cerebral palsy.

Ryan (1974) advises computing both the number of words stuttered per minute and the number of words spoken per minute as measures of severity. Rate of stuttering is calculated simply by dividing the number of minutes the person spoke into the number of stuttered words. Ryan considers a word as either stuttered or fluent no matter how many times the person repeats it or how long the prolongation. For example, if the examiner counts 24 stuttered words in 6 minutes, the rate of stuttering is 4. If, in the same sample, 720 words are spoken during that same 6 minutes, then 120 words per minute are spoken.

Rather than counting the number of words spoken per minute, it is more accurate to count syllables per minute. Most people speak at a rate of five syllables per second (Miller, 1951). Using syllables as units for counting negates differences between long and short words. For example, the word *constitution* is counted as four syllables and the word *come* as one syllable.

Sample Size

How many words should be included in a sample of speech? Here again there is no ideal number. Some examiners use a 100-word sample of each speaking situation. Van Riper (1971, p. 228) suggests 400 words as a minimum sample. Still others pay little attention to the number of words but specify a time period such as three or five minutes. If all that is wanted is a sample of a serial type speaking situation, counting to 10 may suffice. Again, the size of the speech sample will depend upon what the SLP is trying to find out about the person's speech. A 100-word sample probably is the smallest for assessing stuttering in a reading or conversational speech situation.

Criteria for Diagnosing Stuttering in Children

One interesting test, developed by Adams (1977), is designed to help the pathologist differentiate between young children who are less likely to become stutterers and those who are more likely to do so. The basic criteria involve counting and classifying the number of dysfluencies per 100 words in a 300-to-500 word sample of the child's speech. Adams suggests counting the number of dysfluencies per 100 words, then the number of part-word repetitions and prolongations among all dysfluencies, and determining the percent of occurrence of these two types. He also counts the number of times each part-word is repeated and determines the average number of repetitions. The percent of part-word repetitions that contain the schwa vowel as a substitute for the intended vowel is computed next. Finally, the number of part-word repetitions and prolongations that are marked by abnormal termination of voice or airflow (a voiceless sound) is determined.

From an analysis of these computations, Adams suggests the following criteria be used to identify children who are more likely to develop stuttering:

1. 10 or more dysfluencies per 100 words
2. 35 percent or more of the dysfluencies consist of part-word repetitions and prolongations
3. 25 or more of the part-word repetitions include the schwa sound
4. 50 percent of the part-word repetitions and prolongations are abrupt
5. 3 or more repetitions occur on the same sound or syllable

As can be seen, those who evaluate stuttering pay close attention not only to the type of specific behavior exhibited but also to how frequently those behaviors occur. A number of other factors must be considered when evaluating stuttering, as the next section demonstrates.

Describing Speaking Situations

It is well known that the nature of the speaking situation strongly influences the amount of stuttering. Information on the severity of their cases obtained from more than 200 stutterers in more than 100 different speaking situations reveals some situations in which most of these individuals report little or no stuttering. In other situations, the persons felt they would stutter severely (Bloodstein, 1950). For example, almost no one in Bloodstein's study reported they stuttered while singing. The majority said they stuttered most when called up to speak in class. In many situations, some stutterers reported their speech was highly dysfluent while others said their stuttering decreased.

Eisenson and Horowitz (1945) report that as the meaning of the message and the speaker's responsibility for communicating meanings increased, so did stuttering. Variations in the size of the audience also affect the amount of stuttering (Siegel & Haugen, 1964).

Since stuttering varies considerably from one speaking situation to another, it is important that speech be sampled in a variety of circumstances. This multiple sampling also can provide an idea of the severity of the problem. The speaker who stutters while counting to ten, an automatic type speaking situation in which little information is conveyed, is considered more severe than one who does not stutter while counting.

Ryan (1974) developed an instrument, the *Stuttering Interview*, for measuring severity of stuttering. In this test, speech is sampled in a variety of speaking situations. Form A, designed to be used with preschool and primary school children, samples speech in 17 situations:

1. delivering automatic memorized speech sequences
2. making echoic responses of single words, phrases, and sentences
3. reading (optional if child cannot read)
4. picture naming
5. speaking alone
6. speaking using a puppet
7. speaking in monologue
8. giving commands to tester
9. speaking while acting out certain activities
10. speaking simultaneously with the tester but about different subjects
11. repeating words that are difficult to pronounce
12. naming objects quickly
13. speaking while drawing
14. answering and asking questions
15. speaking using the telephone

16. conversing with the tester
17. conversing with someone other than the tester

A similar set of ten speaking situations evaluates upper elementary through adult speakers (Form B). Norms are presented as means and standard deviations for both forms.

The *Stuttering Severity Instrument* developed by Riley (1972) samples speech in only two speaking situations: (1) talking for 3 minutes about school or the person's occupation, and (2) reading a 125-word passage if the individual can read or telling a story about cartoon picture sequences if the person cannot read. The number of silent or audible prolongations or sound or syllable repetitions are counted and compared with norms to yield a measure of severity from very mild to very severe.

Describing Overt Behaviors Associated with Stuttering

So far, the specific speech behaviors classified as stuttering have been described. Next are behaviors that can be seen as well as those that can be heard. They are called associated features or secondary symptoms. They consist of one or more of a wide variety of behaviors that accompany stuttering. For example, the stutterer may blink the eyes while prolonging a sound, wrinkle the forehead, shake the head, purse the lips, rock back and forth, or stamp a foot. Most of these behaviors occur in the head and neck region and may be as slight as a movement of the nasal nares or as violent as head shaking. One young man the authors knew frequently dislocated his jaw while stuttering.

Riley (1972) includes an evaluation of what she calls four physical concomitants associated with stuttering blocks as part of her total analysis. She uses a point scale of 0 to 5, varying from absence of these behaviors to severe and painful incidents. The concomitants are: (1) distracting sounds such as coughing, clicks, snorts, etc., (2) distracting facial grimaces, (3) distracting head movements, and (4) distracting movements of the extremities. The scores of each physical concomitant are totaled and are considered as part of an overall figure used to evaluate severity.

Since stutterers vary so greatly in the number and type of their associated features, it is difficult to devise objective measurement procedures to assess these behaviors and assign specific severity ratings. The examiner's report can only describe these features as accurately as possible.

Describing Attitudes of Stutterers

There have been a number of attempts to measure the attitudes stutterers have about themselves and their speech. One of the early ones was by

Ammons and Johnson (1944) who devised the *Iowa Scale of Attitude Toward Stuttering*. This test consists of 45 statements that the testee rates on a 0-4 point scale from undecided to strongly agree but contains no norms, so its score has little meaning. Van Riper (1971, p. 241) suggests that its use is limited only to clinical exploration.

In an effort to develop a pencil-paper type test of questions to differentiate between stutterers and nonstutterers, Lanyon (1967) devised 64 items—called the SS scale (stuttering severity scale)—that can be answered true or false. These items sample the individuals' reported behaviors and attitudes about their speech. He reports his SS Scale not only discriminates between those who do and do not stutter but also among three levels of severity. Lanyon's test is concerned only minimally with attitudes; its chief focus is statements about behavior.

Another effort to assess attitudes by using an attitude inventory is that of Erickson (1969). He uses a list of 39 statements that can be answered by true or false evaluations called the S-scale (stuttering scale). He concludes that the results of his scale are related to clinician ratings of stuttering severity, self-rating of improvement following treatment, and self-rating and self-descriptions of reactions to social communication.

Andrews and Cutler (1974) use Erickson's S-scale to determine whether there are consistent changes in a stutterer's attitude before and after treatment. They report Erickson's original 39 items could be reduced to 24, resulting in a test that is a more reliable and valid way of measuring attitudes about speaking situations. They find that after treatment, when the treated stutterers experience fluency in everyday life situations, their scores on the 24 items (called the S-24 scale) are similar to scores nonstutterers attain. According to Guitar (1976) the S-24 scale has undergone appropriate development as a test of attitudes and may be positively related to treatment outcomes. The 24 items are published in the Andrews and Cutler (1974) article, should the reader wish to administer this test.

Describing Self-Knowledge of Stuttering

It is surprising to find that many people who stutter know very little about the disorder. Some are under the misconception that stuttering is caused by a birth defect, a mother who was frightened during pregnancy, or even a disease. Some have no idea of how prevalent the problem is, its universality, or the nature of its development.

Whether or not these misconceptions influence progress during treatment is not known. Yet considerable time usually is spent informing stutterers about the nature of the disorder. Crowe and Cooper (1977) developed a pencil-paper test to determine how much an individual knows about the nature of stuttering. Unfortunately, normative data are not available so it is not possible to determine what constitutes a good or poor score. If it is desired to measure knowledge about stuttering with any degree of accuracy, considerably more research must be done in this area, but at least some attempts are being made.

Describing the Case History

It is important to obtain a complete case history before treatment is begun. This information can provide valuable insight into many areas that can aid in planning therapeutic strategies.

Van Riper (1966, pp. 492–502) presents a form for taking a case history that can be used for most individuals who have communication problems. The first section is concerned with routine information such as the client's address, age, and parental information. The second section deals with birth history, including birth and prenatal conditions. This is followed by a developmental history covering age of walking, talking, diseases, accidents, physical coordination, physical condition, mental and educational development, language development, home environment, and childhood problems such as shyness, tongue sucking, fainting, and the like. A final section is designed for adult developmental history. By being selective in applying the information, the SLP can use Van Riper's guide for developing an adequate case history for stutterers.

Another general case history form can be found in the appendix of Emerick and Hatten's text, *Diagnosis and Evaluation in Speech Pathology* (1974). They also suggest specific questions in their chapter on diagnosing stuttering that can be helpful.

One important part of the case history is a section describing the person's response to a wide variety of speaking situations. It is valuable to assist the individual in establishing a hierarchy of situations. This hierarchy ranks situations from those in which the stutterer experiences the most speech difficulty to those that are easiest. Thus, when devising a treatment plan, this information can be useful in preparing specific speech assignments. These situations should include speaking environments such as using the telephone, speaking in a classroom, and speaking at home, as well as speaking to different people such as a teacher, a stranger, a child, etc.

The history of attempts to remediate the problem also is important. The SLP may wish to contact others who have worked with the individual to learn what procedures were used. Often helpful information can be acquired by talking or corresponding with pathologists who may have worked with or observed the individual.

Finally, it is important to discover the person's speech fluency goals and how they are to be obtained. Stutterers frequently hold unrealistic goals of how fluent they want to be. Some desire perfect speech devoid of dysfluencies. Of course, this is unrealistic. A normal speaker is expected to use some interjections, pauses, and word or phrase repetitions or revisions. The goal should not be to talk like a programmed machine with no dysfluencies whatever.

Many stutterers also feel they should never experience fear when speaking. This, too, is unrealistic. All speakers experience various degrees of anxiety when speaking to large groups or to important people. The term commonly used to describe their anxiety is stage fright. A certain amount of anxiety often is helpful to the speaker. Too much anxiety, of course, disrupts speech fluency. SLPs can learn a great deal about how a stutterer feels about past, present, and future speech goals by taking a thorough case history.

SUMMARY

Speech/language pathologists must make a decision as to the cause and nature of stuttering. As is all too well known, experts are unable to identify the cause. There is strong evidence to indicate neurophysiologic reasons. Certain hereditary factors also may play an important role in the early developmental stages. On the other hand, there also is strong evidence to indicate stuttering is a learned behavior and, as such, responds to conditioning in much the same manner as other learned behaviors. A combination of both neurophysiological and environmental factors could cause the disorder.

There is no doubt that by manipulating only environmental factors, SLPs can greatly reduce or eliminate stuttering. The treatment outlined in Chapter 9 is based on the premise that the pathologist can be extremely instrumental in helping the stutterer develop a more fluent way of speaking.

But before therapy is initiated, the pathologist must carefully define the behaviors to be changed and assess the degree of severity. A variety of tests, many of them self-made, are designed to assist the SLP in accomplishing these assessment tasks. Once this is done, the pathologist can concentrate on the modification of stuttering, the subject of Chapter 9.

REFERENCES

Adams, M. A physiologic and aerodynamic interpretation of fluent and stuttered speech. *Journal of Fluency Disorders*, 1974, *1*, 35–47.

Adams, M. A clinical strategy for differentiating the normally nonfluent child and the incipient stutterer. *Journal of Fluency Disorders*, 1977, *2*, 141–148.

Adams, M. Stuttering theory, research and therapy: The present and future. *Journal of Fluency Disorders*, 1978, *3*, 139-147.

Ammons, R., & Johnson, W. Studies in the psychology of stuttering: The construction and association of a test of attitude toward stuttering. *Journal of Speech Disorders*, 1944, *9*(1), 49-59.

Andrews, G., & Cutler, J. Stuttering therapy: The relation between changes in symptom level and attitudes. *Journal of Speech and Hearing Disorders*, 1974, *39*(3), 312-319.

Andrews, G., Guitar, B., & Howie, P. Meta-analysis of the effects of stuttering treatment. *Journal of Speech and Hearing Disorders*, 1980, *45*(3), 287-307.

Andrews, G., & Harris, M. *The syndrome of stuttering*. London: The Spastics Society Medical Education and Information Unit in association with William Heinemann Medical Books, 1964.

Barbara, D. A. *Stuttering: A psychodynamic approach to its understanding and treatment*. New York: Julian, 1954.

Bloodstein, O. A rating scale study of conditions under which stuttering is reduced or absent. *Journal of Speech and Hearing Disorders*, 1950, *15*(1), 29-36.

Bloodstein, O. *A handbook on stuttering*. Chicago: National Easter Seal Society for Crippled Children and Adults, 1969.

Brill, A. A. Speech disturbances in nervous and mental diseases. *Quarterly Journal of Speech Education*, 1923, *9*, 129-135.

Brutten, G., & Shoemaker, D. *The modification of stuttering*. Englewood Cliffs, N.J.: Prentice-Hall, Inc., 1967.

Clark, R. M., & Murray, F. M. Alterations in self-concept: A barometer of progress in individuals undergoing therapy for stuttering. In D. A. Barbara (Ed.). *New directions in stuttering*. Springfield, Ill.: Charles C Thomas, Publisher, 1965.

Crowe, T. A., & Cooper, E. B. Parental attitudes toward and knowledge of stuttering. *Journal of Communication Disorders*, 1977, *10*, 343-357.

Culatta, R. Some thoughts about fluency disorders: Their definition, measurement, and modification. *Journal of Fluency Disorders*, 1978, *3*, 295-296.

Eisenson, J., & Horowitz, E. The influence of propositionality on stuttering. *Journal of Speech Disorders*, 1945, *10*(3), 193-197.

Emerick, L. L., & Hamre, C. E. *An analysis of stuttering*. Danville, Ill.: Interstate Printers and Publishers, Inc., 1972.

Emerick, L. L., & Hatten, J. *Diagnosis and evaluation in speech pathology*. Englewood Cliffs, N.J.: Prentice-Hall, Inc., 1974.

Erickson, R. L. Assessing communication attitudes among stutterers. *Journal of Speech and Hearing Research*, 1969, *12*(4), 711-724.

Fairbanks, G. *Voice and articulation drillbook*. New York: Harper & Row, 1960.

Freeman, F., & Ushijima, T. Laryngeal activity accompanying the moment of stuttering: A preliminary report of EMG investigations. *Journal of Fluency Disorders*, 1975, *3*, 36-45.

Glauber, I. P. The nature of stuttering. *Social Casework*, 1954, *34*, 95-103.

Goldiamond, I. Stuttering and fluency as manipulatable operant response classes. In L. Krasner & L. P. Ullman (Eds.), *Research in behavior modification*. New York: Holt Rinehart Winston Inc., 1965.

Gray, M. The X family: A clinical and laboratory study of a stuttering family. *Journal of Speech Disorders*, 1940, *5*, 343-348.

Guitar, B. Pretreatment factors associated with the outcome of stuttering therapy. *Journal of Speech and Hearing Research,* 1976, *19*(3), 590–600.

Hegde, M. N. Fluency and fluency disorders: Their definition, measurement, and modification. *Journal of Fluency Disorders,* 1978, *3,* 51–71.

Hill, H. Stuttering: I. A critical review and evaluation of biochemical investigations. *Journal of Speech Disorders,* 1944, *9*(3), 245–261.

Johnson, W. *The onset of stuttering.* Minneapolis: University of Minnesota Press, 1959.

Johnson, W., Brown, S., Curtis, S., Edney, C., & Keaster, M. *Speech handicapped school children* (3rd ed.). New York: Harper & Row, 1967.

Johnson, W., Darley, F. L., & Spriestersbach, D. C. *Diagnostic methods in speech pathology.* New York: Harper & Row, 1963.

Jones, R. K. Dyspraxic ambiphasia: A neurophysiologic theory of stammering. *Transactions of the American Neurological Association,* 1967, *92,* 197–201.

Kidd, K. A genetic perspective on stuttering. *Journal of Fluency Disorders,* 1977, *2,* 259–270.

Kimura, D. Some effects of temporal lobe damage on auditory perception. *Canadian Journal of Psychology,* 1961, *15,* 156–165.

Lanyon, R. L. The measurement of stuttering severity. *Journal of Speech and Hearing Research,* 1967, *10*(4), 836-843.

Miller, G. A. Speech and language. In S. S. Stevens (Ed.), *Handbook of experimental psychology.* New York: John Wiley & Sons, Inc., 1951.

Nelson, S. E., Hunter, N., & Walter, M. Stuttering in twin types. *Journal of Speech Disorders,* 1945, *10*(4), 335–343.

Orton, S. T. Studies in stuttering. *Archives of Neurology and Psychiatry,* 1927, *18,* 671–672.

Riley, G. D. A stuttering severity instrument for children and adults. *Journal of Speech and Hearing Disorders,* 1972, *37*(3), 314–322.

Ryan, B. *Programmed therapy for stuttering in children and adults.* Springfield, Ill.: Charles C Thomas, Publisher, 1974.

Schwartz, M. The core of the stuttering block. *Journal of Speech and Hearing Disorders,* 1974, *39*(2), 169–177.

Seligman, J. The personality, attitudes, and behavior of parents of children who stutter: An annotated bibliography. *Journal of Ontario Speech and Hearing Association,* 1966, *2,* 35–106.

Shames, G., & Sherrick, C. A discussion of nonfluency and stuttering as operant behavior. *Journal of Speech and Hearing Disorders,* 1963, *28*(1), 3–18.

Sheehan, J. G. *A study of the phenomena of stuttering.* Unpublished master's thesis, University of Michigan, 1946.

Sheehan, J. Conflict theory of stuttering. In J. Eisenson (Ed.), *Stuttering: A symposium.* New York: Harper & Row, 1958.

Sheehan, J. *Stuttering: Research and therapy.* New York: Harper & Row, 1970.

Siegel, G. M., & Haugen, D. Audience size and variations in stuttering behavior. *Journal of Speech and Hearing Research,* 1964, *7,* 381–388.

Travis, L. E. *Speech pathology.* New York: Appleton-Century, 1931.

Van Riper, C. *Speech correction: Principles and methods* (4th ed.). Englewood Cliffs, N.J.: Prentice-Hall, Inc., 1966.

Van Riper, C. *The nature of stuttering.* Englewood Cliffs, N.J.: Prentice-Hall, Inc., 1971.

Van Riper, C. *The treatment of stuttering.* Englewood Cliffs, N.J.: Prentice-Hall, Inc., 1973.

Wepman, J. M. Familial incidence in stammering. *Journal of Speech Disorders,* 1939, *4,* 199–204.

West, R., Ansberry, M., & Carr, A. *The rehabilitation of speech* (3rd ed.). New York: Harper & Row, 1957.

Wingate, M. E. A standard definition of stuttering. *Journal of Speech and Hearing Disorders,* 1964, *29*(4), 484–489.

Wischner, G. J. Stuttering behavior and learning: A preliminary theoretical formulation. *Journal of Speech and Hearing Disorders,* 1950, *15*(4), 324–335.

Chapter 9

Treatment Procedures for Stutterers

It is difficult to know where to begin a discussion of the treatment of stuttering. Literally thousands of treatment procedures have been described, involving widely divergent techniques from surgery to psychotherapy. Many of these procedures and techniques are described by Van Riper (1973). Almost half of his textbook is devoted to brief reviews and critiques of some of the more prominent treatment procedures that have been reported in the literature. No attempt is made here to present such an extensive review; instead, only a few of the more current treatment approaches are discussed.

It might be asked: Why not just present the best approach for the treatment of stuttering? The problem is: Who decides what the best approach is among several methods? Johnson (1939, p. 170) pointed out more than four decades ago that there was no such thing as *the* method for treating stuttering. Even though most authorities agree that treatment procedures used today are greatly improved over those of the past, few are so bold as to claim the "sure cure" for stuttering.

Deciding which method is best depends upon the goals the speech/hearing pathologist wishes to attain. If the goal is to establish immediate speech fluency, there are several effective procedures such as choral reading, timing devices, or masking. If the goal is to alter the stutterer's self-concept, a different set of procedures employs counselling or psychotherapy. Perhaps the goal is to teach the stutterer to relax. The SLP can select one of any number of relaxation procedures from biofeedback to Jacobson's (1938) progressive relaxation. The best method for accomplishing a goal is the one that can demonstrate a high degree of success in reaching the prescribed objective.

Some procedures contain certain constraints that may prohibit the pathologist from selecting a goal. For example, a successful method may require the use of expensive equipment such as a Delayed Auditory Feedback (DAF) instrument used in the therapy program developed by Shames & Florance (1980). Special training may be required to deliver a program, and such training may not be available in many geographic areas. These represent only a few of the constraints that prohibit the pathologist from using certain procedures even though they may be shown to be more successful than others. This section reviews several current therapy techniques that have proved successful in the hope that one or more may be suitable to the goals chosen for therapy.

OVERVIEW OF THERAPY GOALS

It is necessary first to identify some of the goal options available. Gregory (1980), in his discussion of current issues in stuttering therapy, identifies two major goals embraced by those who advocate certain procedures. The first typifies the major objective of traditional approaches to stuttering therapy, the stutter-more-fluently goal. This approach, illustrated in procedures recommended by Van Riper (1973), Johnson (1967), and Bloodstein (1975), seeks to modify the moment of stuttering, thus enabling the person to stutter more easily. The focus is on the moment of stuttering. The techniques teach the individual how to overcome a block or struggle associated with stuttering by using some special technique such as pausing, repeating the syllable or word, prolonging the first sound, and the like. The person should not seek to avoid stuttering, for this only heightens anxiety and increases stuttering.

The chief criticism of this approach is that the end product is a "happy stutterer" who, although the stuttering is greatly reduced, probably will never achieve normal, fluent speech. The fact that several speech/language pathologists who use this approach continue to stutter themselves, although their disorder often is minimal, points up the truth of this criticism. Of course, those who ascribe to the stutter-more-fluently goal do not regard easy stuttering as undesirable or objectionable to the speaker or the listener. The important point is that this concept holds that such stutterers should feel good about their speech, should be in control of their fluency, and should not exhibit behaviors that interfere with communication.

A second goal Gregory (1980) identifies is to teach the stutterer to speak more fluently. Obviously this is not new. Numerous corrective schools at the turn of the 20th century offered guaranteed cures for stuttering. These schools used techniques that focused on breathing exercises, rhythm and timing activities, mechanical gadgets, and so forth. Their focus was on establishing normal fluency, usually the faster the better. Van Riper (1973) reports having attended a residential school for stutterers that ascribed to these procedures but the rigors of the activities were so intense that he left in disgust. The turn-of-the-century distraction devices have since been abandoned by professionals.

More recently, considerable interest has been shown in developing new procedures to help stutterers speak fluently. Goldiamond (1965) reports success teaching stutterers to speak fluently in a relatively short time using Delayed Auditory Feedback (DAF). The principle of DAF involves delaying one's speech feedback by 250 milliseconds. Only by prolonging the vowels can one overcome the confusion caused by this 250 millisecond echo effect. When speaking by prolonging vowels, all traces of stuttering disappear. Shames & Florance (1980) also use the DAF technique in their treatment program. Perkins (1973) also incorporated the DAF technique but focused more on teaching breath management skills by helping the stutterer control procedures. Webster (1974, 1975, 1980) advocates reconstructing specific speech event targets to generate a normal sounding fluent speech. Ryan (1974) and Ryan and Van Kirk (1971) also seek fluent speech as a goal of their treatment approach which is based upon operant conditioning strategies.

Rather than teach a new way of talking, Mowrer (1975a, 1979) feels that since stutterers already can speak fluently in some situations, there is no need to teach them some unique way of speaking. By structuring the situation so that fluent speech is produced and gradually increasing the difficulty of the speaking, long periods of fluency can be generated. Again, the goal is to establish fluent speech.

In summary, two different goals can be identified and treatment programs can be classified as pursuing one or the other. One goal is focused on procedures designed to modify the moment of stuttering. The result is a modified form of the dysfunction that is more acceptable and better controlled than previous speech. The second goal seeks to establish fluent speech and thereby eliminate stuttering.

The next question is how to proceed in achieving a selected goal. Three procedures are discussed. First, the Van Riper (1973) method best typifies a therapy program focusing on attempts to modify the moment of stuttering. The goal is to reduce anxiety associated with speaking by teaching the individual how to stutter more acceptably. The two other procedures represent ways of establishing a fluent speech pattern. Webster's (1974, 1980) attends to minute details of the speech act in building fluent speech patterns. Mowrer's (1975a, 1979) builds upon the fluent speech already present in the stutterer's repertoire. The goal of both programs, of course, is to help the stutterer develop and maintain a fluent way of speaking that cannot be differentiated from that of nonstutterers. It should be borne in mind that there are many other treatment procedures designed to accomplish these goals. The authors have selected only three programs because they are representative of many others; this is not to imply they are the best ones.

ATTENDING TO MOMENT OF STUTTERING

Treatment procedures that focus on the moment of stuttering teach the stutterer how to modify and control dysfluent speech behaviors. The fear reaction and resulting tension experienced by stutterers when anticipating or experiencing a dysfluency only serve to increase stuttering. If the stutterer learns to reduce the fear associated with the stuttering act by modifying the behaviors associated with stuttering, then stuttering should be reduced in severity and frequency.

The goal of these treatment programs is not to establish normal speech fluency, but rather teach the stutterer how to cope with the speech problem more effectively. The chief concern is how the stutterer feels about speaking, not the fluency. It is assumed that the individual's chief problem is the strong desire to avoid stuttering. Treatment is aimed at reducing or eliminating these avoidance tendencies. Said in another way, the stutterer must learn to accept stuttering and modify ways of approaching speaking situations. When apprehension subsides, the severity of stuttering will be greatly reduced.

Description of Van Riper's Procedures

Although Van Riper (1973) recommends an eclectic approach to the treatment of stuttering, considerable attention is given to modifying the moment of stuttering. Stutterers must unlearn their old stuttering response patterns by substituting more adaptive ones. Stutterers also must learn how to monitor their speech by concentrating on proprioceptive stimuli, that is, feedback from oral sensations, rather than acoustic stimuli. Finally, he feels it is important to help stutterers alter their attitudes about speaking situations and their ability to deal with these situations. This may involve extensive counselling or even psychotherapy.

Van Riper draws from various areas of learning theory, servosystems, and counselling to formulate his treatment procedures. Each stutterer receives therapy that is tailored to the individual's needs. No two people receive the same treatment.

He feels intensive therapy for three hours daily, five times a week over three to four months is required to effect positive speech changes. This amounts to about 200 hours of therapy followed by another 20 to 30 hours of less intensive work over three to four months. A major effort is required in committing that much time over a six-month period. If a stutterer sought help from a speech/language pathologist in the private sector whose fees were $40 per hour, the treatment program would cost more than $9,000.

Description of Van Riper's Four Steps

Van Riper's treatment program consists of four steps that usually are taught in this sequence: identification, desensitization, modification, and stabilization.

Identification. It is at this initial stage of therapy that the stutterer is helped to analyze specific overt and covert behaviors. This step is most helpful because the individual learns to identify and describe each of the deviant behaviors that must be modified. The speech/language pathologist also creates a warm and accepting atmosphere, unlike the emotionally charged situations to which stutterers usually are accustomed. The pathologist assists the stutterer in breaking down dysfluent speech responses into small units of behavior.

Van Riper suggests moving from the least difficult task to more difficult ones. Since identifying fluent words is the easiest task, this is where treatment begins. The next step consists of identifying short dysfluencies. This is followed by identifying avoidance behaviors such as starters, postponements, repetitions, facial and body tension, reluctance to speak in certain situations, etc. Videotapes showing the stutterer speaking are shown next. The individual learns to identify all acts of stuttering. A mirror is used to provide immediate feedback on the behaviors exhibited.

Desensitization. This second stage has as a chief goal the reduction of the anxiety associated with speaking situations. Since it is felt certain stimuli trigger anxiety reactions, the stutterer must be taught to disassociate those stimuli from the resulting reactions. Desensitization is the process of presenting the trigger stimuli in an accepting, secure environment so the stutterer can experience a different reaction in the presence of another person—a reaction devoid of anxiety. The SLP's job is to create that atmosphere of acceptance. A hierarchy of trigger stimulus conditions is presented, starting with the one that evokes the least anxiety reaction. If this situation involves reading single words, the stutterer does so from lists in the nonthreatening environment. When the person feels comfortable reading the single words, the next task in the hierarchy is presented, also in the accepting environment. This process is continued until the individual can cope with what once were threatening speaking situations.

Thus, by presenting a progressive sequence of anxiety-provoking stimuli in the nonthreatening confines of the clinic, it is anticipated that the person will become desensitized to problem stimuli so they no longer trigger the stuttering response. Anxiety is decreased greatly.

Van Riper also suggests using counterconditioning by substituting a nonfeared response following a fear-producing stimulus. For example, the individual is encouraged to imitate or fake stuttering when in the relaxed atmosphere of the clinic. Feared words are repeated many times in this accepting environment until the dread subsides. The purpose is to help the client learn a new way of stuttering that will not evoke the penalties associated with the former ways.

In summary, desensitization involves the individual speaking in various situations, beginning with those that are nonthreatening. The consequences of speaking are pleasant and accepting and hence desensitize anxiety. Counterconditioning is the process of practicing the act of stuttering as an imitation of stuttering and following this with an accepting environment instead of the emotional reaction that ensues. In this way, a new anxiety-free response is substituted for the old emotional reaction.

Modification. This third stage of Van Riper's therapy requires considerable time since it is at this point that attempts are made to break old thinking habits and speech behaviors by substituting new ones.

How does the SLP go about changing what people think about themselves? Van Riper suggests five steps the SLP should take:

1. Help them analyze their attitudes about themselves.
2. Discuss their daily habits, appearance, life style, concepts, and factors that affect self-concept; help them find ways to break old habit patterns; substitute new habits and life styles by encouraging them to create new hair styles, wear different clothing, select different foods, or change any other features that might affect self-concept.
3. Help them adopt new roles so they can become more pleasant and outgoing or can join groups or clubs and engage in different activities with the stress on breaking behavioral rigidity.
4. Encourage them to realize that they can change their attitudes and improve their self-concept by thinking and acting differently.
5. Show them how they can vary their patterns of stuttering by speaking in different ways to confirm that they have the ability to change their speech.

Up to this point in therapy, the individual has learned to: (1) identify specific behaviors associated with stuttering, (2) become desensitized to threatening situations, (3) demonstrate ability to change stuttering patterns, and (4) trust and like the speech/language pathologist. Once these advances have been accomplished, direct work on the stuttering act itself is initiated. Van Riper suggests the next goal is to help the stutterer concentrate on a different process—proprioceptive monitoring. This type of monitoring requires that the stutterer focus upon motor sequencing rather than auditory features of speech. Van Riper feels that the auditory features of the speech act are instrumental in triggering stuttering behavior. It is well known that when these auditory feedback factors are removed or altered using masking, DAF, choral speaking, or whispering, stuttering is reduced greatly. Procedures designed to change proprioceptive monitoring help the stutterer get the feel of fluent speech and learn to concentrate on sensing as opposed to listening to the speech act. Van Riper also suggests using an electrolarynx (Chapter 7) to help the individual become accustomed to the sensation of feeling speech movements more accurately.

The reason stutterers must develop a keener proprioceptive awareness of the speech act is to minimize the old habits developed when they attended to their auditory feedback. Therefore, a different monitoring system is substituted for the old way of attending to speech signals. When individuals sense stuttering, they can take deliberate counteractions. Van Riper reports this is difficult when the stutterer is apprehensive about a speaking situation. In such stressful situations, Van Riper declares the person must be taught to stutter in a more fluent way so as not to disrupt the communication process.

Stutterers learn two procedures to use when they feel the dysfunction will occur: cancellation and pull-out. When a person stutters on a word, cancellation is used by pausing momentarily (about three seconds) and repeating the word fluently. In this way the person learns to use a new response in the presence of old stimuli that used to evoke the stuttering.

Van Riper feels the use of this pause period is important. Usually after an occasion of stuttering, fear subsides and fluency follows. This consequence actually can serve as a reinforcer for stuttering. Pausing interrupts these reinforcing consequences and provides the stutterer time to get control of the speech act and think about how to modify the previous speech attempt. It provides time to pantomime short versions of the behavior during the act of stuttering and also permits pantomiming a modified version of the act. In this way, the person becomes highly aware of what occurs during the act of stuttering. Since the act has been completed, anxiety is reduced during the pause period, thus allowing the person to be more objective about the behavior and to plan an alternate response.

After the pause, the stuttered word is repeated aloud but this time the person concentrates on the motoric aspects of speech, not the acoustic feedback. First, there is slow, deliberate articulation of the word by keeping the breath stream uninterrupted. Vowels can be prolonged to keep a constant flow of breath. In this way, the stutterer learns a new way to attack the word. This fluent way of stuttering requires a greater degree of control during the act of speaking. Thus, the new behavior is reinforced since fluent words follow this second attempt rather than the first stuttered attempt.

What can be done to lessen the act of stuttering when a person experiences great difficulty saying a certain word? Here, Van Riper suggests using a procedure he calls the pull-out. This technique is called a pull-out because it helps the individual pull out of the stuttering act itself. A pull-out procedure is used to terminate the stuttering. It may be used in instances of excessive repetitions. In such a case, the individual attempts to prolong the repetitions. During tremors, the person uses slower speech to reduce them. Laryngeal closure (blocks) and vocal fry are two other severe forms of stuttering that must be modified.

Van Riper is not as explicit when explaining the use of pull-out procedures as he is in the use of the cancellation process. He describes learning to use pull-outs as the knack of altering the usual speech attempt. Motor planning can help greatly in modifying abnormal positions. Prolonging the vowel seems to be especially helpful. As stutterers learn to modify the stuttering pattern, they gain confidence in their ability to change the habitual dysfunctional forms.

Stabilization. The fourth or stabilization phase of therapy is used to help stutterers make permanent changes in speech behavior. It is what some call a maintenance program. When stutterers reach this stage, they should be fluent and able to cope with speaking fears. They have changed many of their attitudes and feel better about themselves. If treatment stops at this point, it is likely these persons gradually will revert to stuttering. They need to continue practicing the integration of new speech patterns.

The SLP must explain why the stabilization process is necessary, then make a number of assignments to be practiced. Some of this practice can be done during the weekly visits to the clinic, some in outside situations. Smoothing out speech in an effort to keep the airflow moving should be practiced. Prosodic features of speech are learned best by reading aloud with another person and repeating what the other has said. Cancellation is performed after phrases and sentences and not merely following single words.

Undoubtedly stutterers will experience anxiety about saying certain words. One way to deal with this is for the SLP to prepare short passages containing these feared words and have them practice saying these passages many times, even to the point of memorizing them. The stutterers can prepare for feared speaking situations in advance and plan what they should say, and how. It is wise for them to seek out difficult speaking situations and apply the newly learned procedures that are designed to evoke more fluent stuttering.

Finally, they should try to develop an attitude of expecting fluent speech rather than stuttering. Practice in giving themselves positive suggestions before speaking in difficult situations is helpful. It is during the stabilization stage that stutterers go through a period when self-concept changes are most apparent. Although they may vacillate between stutterer and non-stutterer attitudes, they should begin to behave more like normal speakers.

The therapy procedures Van Riper advocates require that the pathologist be familiar with counselling techniques. These skills are not learned easily. The therapy, although it follows some general guidelines, differs greatly from person to person. Each person receives unique treatment based upon individual needs. Van Riper feels no single treatment procedure can be a panacea to all stutterers.

Data Regarding Van Riper's Program

Unfortunately, Van Riper did not publish data concerning the number of persons who successfully completed his course of treatment. He has written many anecdotal reports about his successes and failures but has provided little information on pretest and posttest measures or long-term results.

Van Riper (1973) notes in his text that a few individuals stop stuttering completely but most of his clients continue to do so to some degree. He feels they are greatly improved compared with the way they spoke before treatment. Considering Van Riper's goal, SLPs would not expect stuttering to disappear. He tries to help the stutterer achieve a comfortable level of dysfluency that does not interfere with communication. The goal is not to attain fluent speech but to reduce anxiety. This is difficult to measure by objective means.

ATTENDING TO FLUENT SPEECH

Webster's Speech Reconstruction Therapy

The treatment program developed by Webster (1974) focuses on rebuilding fluent speech patterns. It is one of the few programs that has been documented with a large number of stutterers. Webster reports data are available for more than 1,000 persons who have been treated by his procedures.

Webster is not concerned with the cause of the dysfunctions, although he suggests children who begin to stutter may differ in some neurological aspect from so-called normal speaking children. He makes three assumptions:
1. that stuttering is a learned behavior, although he concedes this is not a necessary assumption
2. that fluent speech can be taught using a behavior-shaping process in much the same way many other motor skills can be taught
3. that once fluent speech is established, it will be reinforced in the environment so there is no need for transfer program steps

He maintains that if the SLP teaches the new speech behaviors well enough, there will be no problem in transferring them to other environments or in maintaining the fluent speech habits.

Webster is critical of traditional treatment that focuses on reducing anxiety, confronting stutterers with the problem, teaching them to cope better in social situations, speaking with less struggle behavior, and the like. He views many of the current treatment procedures as an art form rather than as a scientific approach. He feels a standardized procedure based on principles of operant conditioning will be successful with most stutterers.

In summary, his procedures deal directly with teaching the stutterer a new way of speaking. He gives little or no direct attention to the moment of stuttering, changing attitudes, or transfer type activities.

Description of Webster's Program

The Webster program results from modifying several of his earlier programs, each of which was more successful in establishing fluency than the previous ones. He identifies certain target behaviors, each of which is taught in a series of carefully defined steps. He points out the act of speaking is extremely complex, requiring at least 600 vocal shapes per minute. The SLP who wishes to modify how a person speaks must simplify this act into a series of specific behaviors that can be taught. These behaviors are divided into three major classes: respiration, voicing, and articulation.

First, a small unit of behavior is isolated from one of the three major classes. This unit or element is called a target. A target behavior might be velocity or duration and is expressed in terms of a physical movement that can be measured accurately. Each target has a physical referent that can be measured. There are no subjective behavioral evaluations.

Target behaviors must be overlearned and exaggerated. They must be made highly discriminable when first taught so that their execution is understood clearly.

Once one target behavior is learned to a specified criterion level, another is taught and added to the first. This establishes complex behaviors that result from the careful execution of a sequence of target actions.

Immediate feedback is provided as to the adequacy of each target response. Decisions about that adequacy are determined by well-defined criteria using precision instruments: a stopwatch to measure duration of speech and an instrument Webster developed—the Voice Monitor—which measures voice onset time accurately. Pathologists do not depend upon subjective evaluations when evaluating specific aspects of the speech response.

Stutterers must perform target behaviors according to exact standards. For example, the SLP sets precise tolerance limits. If the stutterer's target behavior is the prolongation of a vowel, the vowel must be prolonged for two seconds, then one second, and finally for half a second. In this way the client progresses from exaggerated to normal movement.

What about the role of the pathologist who administers this program? Webster compares the pathologist to a guide who shows the hiker the path up the mountain. The hiker must do the climbing. The guide must not carry the hiker. Thus, the pathologist serves as an instructor whose only job is to teach a motor skill. Pathologists in this program perform no counselling nor do they deliberately attempt to change attitudes of clients. Webster feels attitudes change as a result of learning a fluent way of speaking. The SLP must follow the program schedule exactly, with no variation. There is no room for inaccuracy, deviation from the program, or innovation. All target behaviors must be learned in the specified order and to specified criteria. There is no exception. Webster finds that when the scheduled procedures are not followed as written, success in establishing and maintaining fluent speech does not result.

A stutterer who elects to attend Webster's program in Roanoke, Va., must reside there during the three weeks of intensive training. Participants attend day-long therapy sessions to learn five target behaviors—the stretched syllable, syllable transition, slow change, full breath, and gentle onset:

1. The stretched syllable involves the client's prolonging vowel and consonant syllables for two seconds (one second for the vowel and one for the consonant, a continuant). In the syllable *on*, both the / ɔ / and the /n/ are prolonged for one second each in a continuous vocalization. The stutterers learn to discriminate between correct and incorrect prolongation times when they are demonstrated by the pathologist. The clients then attempt to match correct prolongation times as they prolong syllables. Then two- and three-syllable words are added. This is done the first day. Stutterers then use the stretched

syllable approach when saying words in conversational speech in the clinic. Gradually, the "stretching" is reduced to a kind of slow-motion speech.
2. The syllable transition target behavior consists of putting two syllables together and is performed by joining two syllables of a two-syllable word like *window* or *housefly*.
3. The slow change target behavior focuses on the articulatory movements or motor planning. For example, articulatory gestures from /m/ to /aI/ are planned to result in the slowed production of the word *my*.
4. The full breath target involves teaching improved breathing habits.
5. The gentle onset target behavior is taught using the Voice Monitor, an electronic instrument that accurately measures initial voice amplitude. If voice amplitude is above the setting on the instrument, no signal is given; if voice amplitude falls within specified limits, a green light is presented. First, the client produces vowels beginning with long voice onset times. The objective is to reduce voice onset time gradually in a series of progressive steps. Next, voiced continuants are prolonged using several voice onset times each reduced in length. Then, other sound classes (sonorants, voiceless fricatives) are practiced in the same manner. In this way, the client learns to plan articulatory gestures with great precision. The exaggerated voice onset time is practiced for one week. Shorter onset times are practiced the second week. At the end of the second week, syllable duration is reduced to one-half second. This new speech pattern is used immediately in speaking environments outside the clinic such as talking to people on the phone, in shopping centers, and other places. At this point, the speaker is deliberately using a slowed form of speech. It is not yet automatic.

There is a final check of speech mastery at the end of the third week and if satisfactory, the client returns home to use the newly learned speech pattern. Follow-up is maintained by periodic phone calls and reports the client sends to the clinic.

All target behaviors are taught to all clients regardless of individual differences. Transfer activities are also the same for all. About 100 hours are required to complete the program over the three-week period.

Data Reported on Webster's Program

Webster (1980) discusses the progress of 200 subjects selected randomly from more than 1,000 stutterers who had completed his program. The mean percent of dysfluent words taken from reading and spontaneous speaking samples was 15.2 during pretreatment and 1.3 during posttreatment 19 days later. The percentage of dysfluent speech had risen to only 3.2 ten months later when follow-up speech samples were taken from the same individuals.

The *Perceptions of Stuttering Inventory* (PSI), a self-report inventory developed by Woolf (1967), also was administered during these same test periods. The PSI purportedly measures how satisfied individuals are with their speech. The mean pretreatment score was 3.4, mean posttreatment was 5.7, and ten months later was 9.2. Scores of 10 or under are obtained by nonstuttering speakers. Scores obtained by clients 10 months after therapy indicate they hold attitudes of satisfaction with their speech similar to attitudes of nonstutterers.

According to one of Webster's subjective rating questionnaires administered to the stutterers after treatment, most reported they did not stutter except for an occasional repetition and 83 percent felt their fluency was adequate.

For those few who show little or no change in fluency as a result of attending Webster's program, he explains that some people are not skilled in obtaining new motor skills, the social environment may reinforce their stuttering, some of the pathologists may fail to deliver the program with the required precision, and the technology of program procedures has not been perfected. Nevertheless, the data Webster reports are impressive.

A variation of this program was designed by Schwartz and L. M. Webster (1977a, 1977b). Instead of intensive therapy, clients were seen three times a week for two hours each session over three months. The total hours of therapy amounted to about the same as R. L. Webster's Roanoke clinic program. These experts report that 97 percent of the 29 subjects studied showed a positive degree of change in fluency. About 70 percent of them attained fluency levels of 94 percent or better compared with R. L. Webster's (1975) report that 80 percent achieved a fluency level of 97 percent or better. Schwartz and L. M. Webster conclude that although their results are not quite as impressive as R. L. Webster's, their program is less expensive and does not require that the client travel a long distance or leave school or work for several weeks.

The important feature about Schwartz and L. M. Webster's data is that they attest that they replicated R. L. Webster's program with comparable results. None of the programs that employ extensive counselling techniques can be replicated.

Dissemination of Webster's Program

As noted, speech/language pathologists must attend Webster's training course in Roanoke to qualify to administer the program as he feels it should be. His observation of those who deliver his program is that there is a great deal of variability in how people define and attach consequent events to target behaviors. He feels it is extremely important to the success of the program that instructors receive thorough training in the use of his procedures. There are many skills that cannot be acquired simply by listening to someone talk about procedures or observing as someone administers the program. Webster feels no amount of loving and concern toward those who stutter can take the place of precision skills necessary to operate this program. For these reasons, Webster prefers to train instructors at the center where he developed the program rather than distribute a description in printed form.

Summary

The contrasts between the distinctive features of Webster's program and some of the traditional ones include the following:

WEBSTER'S PROGRAM	TRADITIONAL APPROACH
Pathologist is an instructor.	Pathologist is a counselor.
Evaluation is empirical.	Evaluation is subjective.
Focus is on details of behavior.	Focus is on global aspects of behavior.
Emphasis is on technical competence in speaking.	Emphasis is on understanding the problem.
Focus is on teaching fluent speech patterns.	Focus is on teaching modification of the moment of stuttering.
Reliance on self is stressed.	Reliance on pathologist is stressed.
Pathologist receives highly specialized training.	Pathologist receives generalized training.

Thus, Webster views stuttering as a problem that can be solved best by rebuilding fluent speech patterns. This is accomplished by teaching very specific types of speech acts that lead to the reconstruction of new speech habits. He pays no attention to the modification of the moment of stuttering.

Mowrer's Fluency Program

The last treatment program to be discussed is one developed by Mowrer (1975a, 1975b, 1979). The basic approach is to increase the length of fluent utterances gradually. It is based on the results reported by Rickard and

Mundy (1965) and Leach (1969), later modified by Ryan (1974). Rickard and Mundy (1965) observed that stutterers can read aloud a list of single words with considerable fluency following several trials. Once a pre-established fluency criterion is met, stutterers are asked to read two words at a time, then three-word phrases, to prescribed fluency levels. Longer word strings are added until the individual can read longer passages fluently. Positive consequences in the form of encouraging verbal statements as well as money are used.

The logic of this strategy is simple: create a speaking situation that is likely to result in fluent speech, ask the individual to respond, and follow each fluent response with pleasurable consequences. According to the learning theory set forth by Skinner (1953), behavior is controlled by its consequences. If it is desired to increase the frequency of a behavior, it should be followed with pleasurable consequences immediately and frequently. When undesired behavior is followed by aversive stimuli (punishment) or no positive consequences (extinction), the behavior should decrease.

Stuttering and fluent speech responses are viewed as operant behaviors that can be increased or decreased simply by controlling their consequences. There is no need to teach stutterers a new way of speaking since the desired behavior (fluent speech) is present as a response class. There is no need to modify stuttering behaviors since they will be reduced greatly, or eliminated, as fluent speech behaviors increase in frequency as a result of being reinforced.

Description of Mowrer's Program

The program Mowrer (1975a) developed, called the *S-1 Treatment Program*, is divided into nine instructional parts designed to accomplish three goals: (1) the first five parts, programs A through E, are designed as the Establishment Phase and are intended to evoke fluent speech in a controlled instructional setting, (2) programs F and G, the Transfer Phase, deal with transferring fluent speech to other speaking situations, and (3) programs H and I, the Maintenance Phase, seek to maintain fluent speech in several situations.

Each program contains several steps, each consisting of a different task. These tasks are arranged from speaking situations in which only one word is read, on up to reading textual material. The stutterer advances from one step to another as specific criterion standards are reached. If that standard is not met within a specific time limit, branch steps are administered until it is reached. Specific steps are not written for Programs F through I.

The Establishment Phase. To establish fluency in Program A, Step 1 requires that the speaker read any monosyllabic word from a list immediately following the sound of a half-second 1000 Hz tone. The stutterer is instructed to say only those words that can be read fluently. If the stutterer reads the word fluently, the pathologist says, "Good;" if the individual stutters, the pathologist says, "Stop." Tones are presented at five-second intervals during a ten-minute period. The purpose of the tones is to decrease the rate of speech so consequences can follow each utterance. The stutterer is required to complete three consecutive ten-minute readings with 95 percent fluency in each before proceeding to the next step.

Step 2 is identical to Step 1 except that the stutterer is required to read the words from a list in the order presented. When the individual meets the criterion standard of three consecutive ten-minute readings at 95 percent fluency, Step 3 is presented.

Step 3 eliminates the tone cue and the stutterer is asked to read the words in order, slowly and without the aid of cue signals.

Step 4 calls for two words to be read in any order from a list. The tone signal is reintroduced and used as it was during Step 1.

Step 5 requires the words be read in order again, using the tone signal.

Step 6 removes the tone cue so that the reading is at the stutterer's own selected rate.

The same procedure is followed in Steps 7, 8, and 9 using three-word combinations. By the conclusion of Step 9, the objective of Program A will have been reached, i.e., to read 120 three-word phrases with 95 percent fluency within a ten-minute period without the aid of tone cues.

Program B is presented next. Its objective is to read selections from a story at a rate of 100 or more words per minute during a five-minute period while maintaining 95 percent fluency. Program B contains seven steps.

Step 1 requires that the stutterer read a short sentence each time a tone is sounded at five-second intervals. As in Program A, sentences read fluently are followed by the word "Good" and those containing a dysfluent word are followed by "Stop."

Steps 2 and 3 eliminate the tone. A sentence list containing two to four words is used in Step 2 and sentences of two to seven words in Step 3.

Step 4 asks the individual to read a paragraph that has been divided into three- to five-word segments. The tone is used to signal when to read each segment.

Step 5 removes the tone signal while reading the same material.

Step 6 deletes the spaces between word groups.

Step 7 consists of the objective for Program B, i.e., reading selections from a story at a rate of 100 or more words per minute with 95 percent fluency.

If Program B is completed satisfactorily, the stutterer proceeds to Program C. Its objective is for the individual to be able to talk to the pathologist at a rate of 100 or more words per minute for five minutes with 95 percent fluency. Up to this point, the client has been looking at textual material while speaking.

Step 1 seeks to establish eye contact between speaker and listener, so the stutterer is asked to look at a written phrase, then look at the pathologist and repeat the phrase to the latter from memory. The five-second interval tone is used as a signal to respond.

Step 2 omits the tone cue and the task remains the same.

Step 3 requires the speaker to read sentences, then say them while looking at the pathologist.

Step 4 calls for the stutterer to tell the pathologist as much of a short story as can be remembered.

Step 5 asks the stutterer to look at a picture, then tell the pathologist one sentence about it.

Step 6 requires two sentences.

Step 7 advances the individual to three sentences.

Step 8 asks the stutterer to make up stories about pictures, talking for half-minute periods.

Step 9 also calls for the person to make up stories about pictures but this time talking to the pathologist for one-minute periods while looking directly at the SLP.

The objective of Program D is to converse with the pathologist during a five-minute period about selected topics while maintaining 95 percent fluency. This program contains four steps.

Step 1 provides for the stutterer to answer questions asked by the pathologist.

Step 2 has the stutterer role-play certain situations while talking to the pathologist.

Step 3 directs the pathologist to ask about things the stutterer does and where the individual lives.

Step 4 asks the stutterer to talk about selected topics for five-minute periods.

Statements of "Good" occur three to four times per minute during fluent periods. The stutterer again is told, "Stop," immediately following a dysfluent utterance.

If the stutterer's speaking rate falls below 100 words per minute during Step 4 of Program D, Program E is used to increase the rate of speaking. If speaking rate is above 100 words per minute, this program is omitted. Program E consists of 14 steps designed to increase oral reading rate from 60 to 120 words per minute. At the completion of this program, the stutterer should be able to converse with the pathologist at or above the 95 percent fluency level while speaking at more than 100 words per minute.

The Transfer Phase. Transferring fluent speech learned during the establishment phase to other speaking situations requires careful manipulation of stimulus conditions. Most speaking situations do not resemble the stimulus conditions present in the establishment phase. An effort is made to maximize generalization of fluent speech by incorporating in other speaking situations some of the stimuli present in the establishment phase. For example, Program G, a six-step program, is designed to help school-aged children transfer fluent speech learned in the clinic to speaking situations in the school. The discriminative stimuli consist of word lists and reading passages used in Programs A through C. Classmates apply consequences following fluent or dysfluent utterances in much the same way as did the pathologist. At the completion of Step 6 in this phase, the stutterer should be able to read aloud to the class at a rate of more than 100 words per minute with 98 percent fluency.

A home transfer program also is put into effect with school-aged children. Speech is monitored during meal time in the following manner: after the child says two to three fluent sentences, the father or mother says, "Good," and marks an X on a score sheet similar to the one used in the clinic. If stuttering occurs, the child is told to wait five seconds and begin again. An 0 is placed on the score sheet following each dysfluent utterance. Score sheets are turned in each week to the pathologist.

For adults, Program H consists of conversing with college students on campus, ordering food in restaurants, asking directions, and engaging strangers in various speaking situations on and around the campus. The pathologist accompanies the stutterer on these assignments to monitor speech. Cues such as "Wait" or "Watch out" are provided, contingent upon dysfluencies. Words spoken are tabulated using a hand counter.

The Maintenance Phase. Program I is aimed at providing a means of maintaining the fluency achieved in a variety of speaking situations outside the clinic. Half-hour bimonthly visits are scheduled at the clinic to converse with the SLP about fluency in various speaking situations. One to two phone calls are placed weekly to maintain fluency in such situations.

Conferences are held with others who frequently engage in conversations with the stutterer. Suggestions are offered regarding cues that should be provided when dysfluencies occur. The Maintenance Program is tailored to the individual stutterer and to the types of speaking situations occurring in that person's environment.

Data Reported about Mowrer's Program

Mowrer (1975a) reports data from 20 stutterers who completed some or all of the programs. The ages of the stutterers ranged from 8 to 43 years, with a mean of 22.1. Before beginning Program A, a test of speech fluency developed by Ryan (1971) was administered to each subject. This test consisted of evoking speech samples in ten different speaking situations: repeating after the examiner, counting, singing, conversing, reciting a monologue, telephoning, speaking alone, answering questions, reading loud, and finally, speaking with the instruction, "Read as fluently as you can." This test was administered again when the program was terminated.

Stuttering was defined as any partial or whole-word repetition, any pause, or any hesitation lasting two seconds or more and occurring before or during utterance of a word, and/or any prolongation of a sound. A stuttering incident was counted only once regardless of the severity or number of hesitations, repetitions, or length of prolongation per occasion. If, for example, the stutterer paused for three seconds before saying a word, then repeated the first syllable several times before saying the word, this was counted as only one dysfluency.

Fifteen persons were scheduled daily for four to six hours of therapy. The remaining five were seen daily for two hours. Run time or time clients spent in the program was considered as actual subject speaking time during program administration.

Each word spoken was evaluated as either fluent or dysfluent and recorded as such on a data sheet. Speaking times were recorded using a stopwatch.

The programs were administered to each subject by two or more individuals. For example, four undergraduate students majoring in speech pathology and one graduate student supervisor was assigned to one stutterer. Student A administered the program during the first hour, student B the second hour, and so on. The supervisor administered the pretests and posttests as well as some parts of the therapy. A total of 58 instructors participated. Their professional training ranged from a minimum of two years of college to training beyond a master's degree.

Six stutterers completed one or more of the programs in the Establishment Phase but not all of them. Nine of the 20 subjects completed all programs in the Establishment Phase, two the Transfer Phase, and three the Maintenance Phase.

A tabulation of the total words spoken during administration of the program, words stuttered, words fluent, percent of words fluent, program and step completed, program run time, and pretest and posttest results are presented in Table 9-1. The occurrence of stuttering on words spoken during program administration was extremely low as compared with the

Table 9-1 Data Analysis From 20 Stutterers Who Completed Part or All of the S-1 Program

Subject	Age	Total Words Spoken	Total Words Stuttered	Total Words Fluent	Percent Fluent	Step Completed	Run Time (Minutes)	Pretest Stuttered Words	Posttest Stuttered Words
N.C.	32	7,841	283	7,558	96.4	B-6	6 3/4	11	6.1
V.T.	16	21,720	225	21,495	98.9	C-4	5 3/4	18	5
M.T.	24	10,253	244	10,099	97.6	C-7	5 1/4	9	3.5
S.M.	43	9,598	185	9,413	98.1	C-9	4 1/2	21	2
J.W.	28	17,857	37	17,820	99.8	C-9	6 3/4	4.4	1
J.A.	28	9,954	54	9,905	99.5	D-2	6	18	1
R.P.	29	36,880	1,214	35,666	96.7	D-4	16 1/3	18	6
K.J.	8	29,266	511	28,755	98.3	D-4	13	2	.5
J.P.	27	10,728	44	10,584	99.6	D-4	3 1/2	23	4
M.R.	12	30,162	281	29,881	99.1	F	9 1/4	3	1.5
R.L.	13	85,845	1,263	85,582	98.5	F	20	17.7	6.9
T.H.	8	38,750	413	38,337	98.9	F	13	8.4	.3
D.D.	32	29,368	184	29,184	99.4	F	7 2/3	9.2	2.5
M.P.	26	5,302	184	5,218	98.4	F	4 1/2	16	2
S.S.	15	56,896	2,120	54,776	96.3	F	46 1/2	14	3.2
C.N.	14	33,683	114	33,569	99.7	G	7	8	.9
K.T.	24	16,530	175	16,355	98.9	H	10	12	.2
V.B.	10	26,920	55	26,865	99.8	I	10	10.3	0.0
G.M.	31	121,843	219	121,624	99.8	I	19 1/2	3.2	.3
D.P.	23	21,142	63	21,079	99.7	I	10	7	.4

Source: Reprinted from *Technical Research Report S-1: Reduction of Stuttering Behaviors* by Donald E. Mowrer by permission of IDEAS, © 1975.

number of words spoken fluently. In no case was the level of stuttered words over 3.7 percent of the total words spoken.

The greatest reduction in mean stuttered words per minute was evidenced in the speech of the five stutterers who completed at least one or more of the transfer and/or maintenance programs, namely, G, H, and I. The mean number of stuttered words per minute on their pretest was 8.1, on the posttest, .36, a 99.6 percent reduction. Those who completed either of the Programs A through F achieved a mean pretest score of 13.5 stuttered words per minute and a mean posttest score of 3.0, a 78 percent drop.

The reduction in the number of dysfluencies as shown by pretest and posttest scores adds further support to the findings reported by Rickard and Mundy (1965), Curlee and Perkins (1969), and Ryan (1971). Dysfluencies not only decreased dramatically in most cases during posttesting, they also occurred but rarely during program administration. Considering the age spread of the subjects (from 8 to 43) and the wide range of dysfluency rates of the pretests (from 2 to 23 per minute), more variance might have been expected with respect to their percent during program administration. The procedure appears to offer powerful controls over dysfluent speech.

One of a combination of several factors could account for high fluency rates noted during program administration: the controlled gradual increase in mean length of the utterance, social reward contingent upon fluent utterances, criterion fluency levels that had to be met before advancement was permitted, and the stop contingency following disfluent utterances.

One distinct variable was program run time. Some of the subjects required much more time to complete program steps than did others. This variable does not appear to be related to any measurable factors identified in this study. There seems to be no way of predicting how much time each person will need to reach criterion levels at each of the program steps. Some severe stutterers went through the program steps rapidly with few dysfluencies while some mild stutterers required longer to meet each of the criterion standards.

The students experienced no difficulty in conducting the program in spite of the fact that many had received little or no formal training in such administration. The written instructions appeared to include sufficient information to allow students to administer the program with little difficulty.

Important Features of Mowrer's Program

The success of the Mowrer program depends chiefly upon the careful arrangement of stimuli designed to evoke verbal responses from the stutterer plus the systematic management of consequent events. Some other variables that may be equally important seldom are reported in experimental studies.

One important variable is the relationship between the speech/language pathologist and the stutterer. For example, the subject R.L. (Table 9-1) was a 13-year-old boy whose clinician was a young male graduate student. R.L. was seen in therapy two hours daily for three weeks. At the end of that time, he spoke fluently when discussing selected topics in the clinic. Visits were reduced to three times per week as transfer activities were initiated. During this time, the graduate student accompanied R.L. in a wide variety of speaking situations and visited his home and classroom on several occasions. Needless to say, R.L. and the graduate student became very good friends. The client depended upon and respected his teacher. By the same token, the graduate student was intensely involved in R.L.'s progress not only with respect to speech but also as a maturing young person. They made frequent telephone calls to one another, the student visited R.L.'s home occasionally, and they shared several common activities. For the first time, the youth began to participate in classroom speech activities, called his friends on the telephone, and was fluent in many speaking situations, although there were times when he was dysfluent.

This relationship ended abruptly at the end of the spring semester when the graduate student returned to his home in the East. A female graduate student was assigned to work with R.L. during the summer session. Another female student scheduled R.L. twice weekly during the fall semester but after two months the youth requested treatment be terminated because he did not like it.

His mother was contacted four months later and again eight months later. She reported he was becoming increasingly dysfluent in many speaking situations. Perhaps R.L. had become too dependent upon the first student and did not take responsibility for his speech behavior. Also, his subsequent students did not appear to be successful in motivating him to practice fluent speech patterns. None of the students were as experienced as was the first and none took a particular liking to or interest in R.L. Planned transfer speaking activities were not carried out to completion and he still had not attained the desired and anticipated high fluency rates in all speaking situations.

A second factor that could have contributed to lack of progress was R.L.'s lack of motivation to work with the female students. He was not fond of females. Once the strong motivating force (the male student) was removed, R.L. seemed to lose the desire to improve. Had the male student remained six months longer until fluent speech patterns could be firmly established and could gradually have reduced contact time, R.L. may have retained a fluent way of talking.

The point here is that in addition to administration of the treatment program, other variables may be as important as, or even more important than, the program itself. One important variable may be the relationship between client and pathologist. It is difficult to describe in research reports the subtle personal interactions that occur between client and pathologist. These personal feelings and relationships could be a key motivating factor needed to assist the stutterer in overcoming the speech problem.

The successes reported of so many different types of treatment programs Van Riper (1973) describes may result largely from the unreported personal relationship factors that are an inevitable part of the treatment process. It is possible that when these relationships are not established, treatment is not successful. There is insufficient evidence to support possible importance of personal relationships, so it remains in the realm of a clinical hunch.

SUMMARY

The three treatment procedures presented in this chapter, each reporting a degree of success in helping the stutterer speak more fluently, represent different treatment approaches. Of course, there are many other procedures. For the most part these procedures have certain commonalities that may help explain why so many different methods are helpful.

The authors believe that stuttering as seen in most adolescents and adults is a problem of attitudes individuals hold regarding speaking situations. Obviously, attitude is a poor choice as a word to describe a characteristic of a person because it cannot be measured objectively. Its existence can only be assumed on the basis of the behavior that can be measured. It is circular reasoning to say that a person stutters because of a poor attitude because when the person becomes fluent, it is said that the attitude changed. How is it known that the attitude changed? Because the person stopped stuttering. But why did the person stop stuttering? Because the attitude changed. The circular reasoning of this argument is obvious. Other concepts attributed to changes in fluency such as self-concept, feelings, beliefs, and so forth are equally difficult to define and cannot be subjected to objective measurement.

Today's learning theorists in the behavioral school favor using words to describe behavior that can be measured or observed objectively. One of the reasons why Freud's theories were abandoned was because many of the concepts he used such as the ego, id, superego, and the like, could not be observed. Pathologists all are well aware of the many concepts in metaphysics that fall in the same category. When words are used to represent vague and immeasurable concepts, they signify a departure from the scientific method. Those who approach the treatment of stuttering as a science must abide by the rigors of the scientific method. Consequently, the use of vague concepts such as attitudes that can be measured only by crude paper-pencil questionnaires to describe the cause of a behavior is highly questionable.

Van Riper (1973) is quite definite in his position regarding the importance of changing attitudes and devotes most of his therapy toward that goal. Cooper (1977) also stresses the importance of attending to the stutterer's attitudes and feelings. He states, "Any stuttering program that does not at some time assist the individual in assessing and clarifying his feelings and attitudes about stuttering and fluency control is, in my opinion, inadequate" (p. 77).

To illustrate how an attitude can affect speech, the authors are reminded of a young woman who stuttered severely. She was asked to say her address. "W-W-W-White Street," she replied. She was asked to say white paint, which she did with ease. She was able to repeat fluently several two-word combinations beginning with the word "white" until she was asked to say "White Street," when she stuttered as before. The question is, why would she stutter on the word "white" only when followed by "street?" Perhaps it could be argued that she was conditioned to stutter on that particular two-word combination or it reminded her of home, a place where she felt anxious. Incidentally, the next day she came to the clinic, she walked up to the SLP and said, "White Street" without a moment's hesitation. Evidently, her attitude concerning her ability to say "White Street" fluently had changed.

Every speech/language pathologist who has worked with stutterers is well aware of the effects of using suggestion as a means of effecting change in speech patterns. Simply by telling the individual to read more fluently can result in decreased stuttering. The tendency to stutter often operates like a self-fulfilling prophecy. If stutterers expect to stutter, then they usually will.

Most treatments are designed to change this self-fulfilling prophecy, or expectancy to stutter. There are numerous ways this can be done. Van Riper deals with attitude in a direct manner. He shows stutterers how to change their attitudes by changing the method of stuttering. Conversely, Webster focuses upon rebuilding speech patterns to modify dysfluent speech. Individuals are convinced they will not stutter when using the newly learned speech patterns. Mowrer shows stutterers they are able to speak fluently by beginning with short fluent utterances and gradually lengthening them into longer conversational speech units. No matter what type of therapy the pathologist chooses to use, success seems to hinge upon whether or not attitudes about speaking situations are changed.

At present, the authors cannot determine which type of procedure best achieves this goal. The documentation reported by Webster regarding the success of his program is impressive, but those who enroll in his program do not represent a random sample of stutterers. They represent only individuals who can afford the program and who are highly motivated to speak fluently. Van Riper (1973), in his review of reports of those who have treated stuttering during the last hundred years, points out that regardless of the type of treatment used, most report high success rates with at least some of their clients. By the same token, there are many ineffective treatment programs that provide little or no help to the stutterer. The authors can only conclude that there is no program that can guarantee success in the treatment of all who stutter.

REFERENCES

Bloodstein, O. *A handbook on stuttering*. Chicago: National Easter Seal Society for Crippled Children and Adults, 1975.

Cooper, E. B. Controversies about stuttering. *Journal of Fluency Disorders*, 1977, *2*, 75–86.

Curlee, R., & Perkins, W. Conversational rate control therapy for stuttering. *Journal of Speech and Hearing Disorders*, 1969, *34*(3), 245–250.

Goldiamond, I. Stuttering and fluency as manipulatable operant response classes. In L. P. Krasner & L. Ullman (Eds.), *Case studies in behavior modification*. New York: Holt Rinehart Winston Inc., 1965.

Gregory, H. Contemporary issues in stuttering therapy. *Journal of Fluency Disorders*, 1980, *5*, 291–302.

Jacobson, E. *Progressive relaxation*. Chicago: University of Chicago, 1938.

Johnson, W. The treatment of stuttering. *Journal of Speech Disorders*, 1939, *3*, 170–171.

Johnson, W. Stuttering. In W. Johnson & D. Moeller (Eds.), *Speech handicapped school children*. New York: Harper & Row, 1967.

Leach, E. Stuttering: Clinical application of response-contingent procedures. In B. Gray & G. England (Eds.), *Stuttering and the conditioning therapies*. Monterey, Calif.: Monterey Institute for Speech and Hearing, 1969.

Mowrer, D. E. *Technical research report S-1: Reduction of stuttering behavior*. Tempe, Ariz.: IDEAS, 1975a.

Mowrer, D. E. An instructional program to increase fluent speech of stutterers. *Journal of Fluency Disorders*, 1975b, *1*, 25–35.

Mowrer, D. E. *A program to establish fluent speech*. Columbus, Ohio: The Charles E. Merrill Publishing Co., Inc., 1979.

Perkins, W. Replacement of stuttering with normal speech: II. Clinical procedures. *Journal of Speech and Hearing Disorders*, 1973, *38*(3), 295–303.

Rickard, H., & Mundy, M. Direct manipulation of stuttering behavior: An experimental-clinical approach. In L. P. Ullman & L. Krasner (Eds.), *Case studies in behavior modification*. New York: Holt Rinehart Winston Inc., 1965.

Ryan, B. *Programmed therapy for stuttering in children and adults.* Springfield, Ill.: Charles C Thomas, Publisher, 1974.

Ryan, B., & Van Kirk, B. *Programmed conditioning for fluency: Program book.* Monterey, Calif.: Monterey Learning Systems, 1971.

Schwartz, D., & Webster, L. M. A clinical adaptation of Hollins Precision Fluency Shaping Program through deintensification. *Journal of Fluency Disorders,* 1977a, *2,* 3-10.

Schwartz, D., & Webster, L. M. More on the efficacy of a protracted precision fluency shaping program. *Journal of Fluency Disorders,* 1977b, *2,* 205-216.

Shames, G., & Florance, C. L. *Stutter-free speech: A goal for therapy.* Columbus, Ohio: The Charles E. Merrill Publishing Co., Inc., 1980.

Skinner, B. F. *Science and human behavior.* New York: The Macmillan Company, 1953.

Van Riper, C. *The treatment of stuttering.* Englewood Cliffs, N.J.: Prentice-Hall, Inc., 1973.

Webster, R. L. *The precision fluency shaping program: Speech reconstruction for stutterers.* Roanoke, Va.: Communication Development, Ltd., 1974.

Webster, R. L. *Hollins Communication Research Institute Report.* Roanoke, Virginia: Hollins College, 1975, *2*(1), 4.

Webster, R. L. Evolution of a target-based behavioral therapy for stuttering. *Journal of Fluency Disorders,* 1980, *5,* 303-320.

Woolf, G. The assessment of stuttering as struggle, avoidance, and expectancy. *The British Journal of Disorders of Communication,* 1967, *2,* 158-171.

Index

A

Adams, M., 244, 252
Alaryngeal phonation
  extrinsic methods, 213–215
  intrinsic methods, 216–219
Allergies, 201
Allophones, 12
  definition, 12
American Cancer Society, 222, 236
Amonons, R., 255
Aminoff, M.J., 170, 171
Amyotrophic lateral sclerosis (ALS), 181
Anderson, V., 52
Andrews, G., 244, 248, 255
Ansberry, M., 239
Aphonia, 163
Aronson, A.E., 119, 132, 137, 143, 158, 160, 171, 174, 176, 178, 182, 186, 216, 217, 231
Arslan, M., 234
Articulation
  automatic speech, 77
  development of, 17
    babbling, 18
    cooing, 18
    connected speech, 77
    reflexive, 17
    word approximations, 19
  location of, 9
  procedures for evoking sounds, 59
  prevalence, 3
  selection of sounds for correction, 54
  syllable production, 74
  therapy method, 86
Articulation tests
  reliability, 36
  types of, 31
  validity, 36
Articulation therapy, 51–99
  automatic speech, 77
  connected speech, 77
  fill-in procedures, 78
  hypernasality, 149
  syllable production, 74
  use of stories, 78, 79, 80
Articulators, 10
  function of, 10
Assimilation, 16, 24
  sound changes, 16
  syllable change, 16
Auditory discrimination. *See* discrimination
Auditory memory span
  test of, 47
Aurex Neovox electronic larynx, 214–215

B

Bailey, C.W., 137
Baker, R., 53, 79, 93
Barbara, D., 246

Barnes, M., 147, 148
Basal pitch, 187–188
Beale, F., 233
Beebe, H., 48
Behavioral objectives, 84
Bernholtz, N., 20
Biofeedback, 166
Blom, E.D., 234
Bloodstein, O., 242, 247, 253, 262
Boone, D., 124, 131, 133, 137, 161, 165–166, 167, 169, 174, 180, 219, 225
Bradbury, D., 23
Bradley, D., 59, 149
Breath support, 202–203
Brill, A., 246
Brown, R., 17
Brown, J.R., 176, 182
Brown, S., 240
Brutten, E., 247, 248
Bryce, D.P., 233
Buccal speech, 216
Buck, M., 44
Byrne, M., 3
Bzoch, K., 40, 142, 144, 145, 147, 148, 152

C

Calcaterra, T.C., 137, 200
Cancellation procedure, 267
Cancer-laryngeal, 209
Carter, E., 44
Carr, A., 239
Carrow, E., 42
Case, I., 23
Case, J.L., 128, 178, 209, 223, 233
Chen, H., 18
Changing pitch, 190–192
Cheerleading, 127–128
Chir, B., 143
Chomsky, N., 12
Clark, R., 243
Cleary, K., 178
Cleft palate, 142
Coarticulation, 15
Compton, A., 40
Conley, J.J., 234

Consonants
 classification of, 4, 5
 development of, 28
 evoking procedures, 59
 error type, 56
 frequency of use, 57
 place of articulation, 6
 manner of articulation, 7
 obstruents, 7
  affrication, 7
  fricatives, 7
  sibilants, 7
  stop, 7
 sonorants, 7
  glide, 7
  liquid, 7
  nasal, 7
 unvoiced, 7, 9
 voiced, 7, 9
Consonant clusters, 19, 24
Consonant injection, 217
Contact ulcers
 case example, 192–194
 defined, 185
 etiology, 185–186
 evaluation, 186–189
 symptoms, 186
 therapy, 189–192
Cooper, E., 255, 284
Cooper, H.K., 144
Cooper, M., 103, 128, 167, 174, 201
Cooper-Rand electronic speech aid, 213–214
Coughing and throat clearing, 199
Coup de glotte, 185, 190, 198
Crocker, J., 29, 58, 90, 93
Crowe, T., 255
Crozier, P., 147
Cullata, R., 148, 242
Curlee, R., 281
Cul-de-sac resonance, 145
Cummings, B., 233
Curtis, 240
Cutler, J., 255

D

Damste, P.H., 202
Daniloff, R., 108

Darley, F., 19, 33, 35, 36, 37, 38, 43, 176, 182, 217, 220, 225, 249
DeAmestic, F., 234
Dedo, H.H., 170, 171, 179
Delack, J., 18
Delayed auditory feedback, 263
Diagnostic tests, 32, 8
  Arizona Articulation Proficiency Scale, 41
  Austin Spanish Articulation Test, 42
  Bzoch Error Pattern Diagnostic Articulation Test, 40
  Compton-Hutton Phonological Assessment Test, 40
  A Deep Test of Articulation, 39
  Developmental Articulation Test, 42
  Fisher-Logemann Test of Articulation Competence, 39
  Goldman-Fristoe Test of Articulation, 38, 86
  Integrated Articulation Test, 43
  Iowa Pressure Articulation Test, 43
  Ohio Tests of Articulation and Perception of Sounds, 42
  Phonological Process Analysis, 41
  Photo Articulation Test, 42
  purpose of, 32
  Southwestern Spanish Articulation Test, 43
  Templin-Darley Test of Articulation, 38, 43
  types of, 38
Diedrich, W.M., 217, 220, 224, 225
Dickey, S., 42
Dickson, S., 33, 35
Discrimination, auditory, 52
  importance of, 52
  interdiscrimination, 53
  intradiscrimination, 53
  tests of, 48
Distinctive features, 12
  definition, 12
  development of, 26, 27
Doyle, W., 18
Drumwright, A., 37
Dugvay, M., 219, 220, 225
Dworkin, J.P., 148
Dysarthria, 176, 179, 181

E

Ease of production, 21
Echolalia, 20
Edney, C., 240
Eimas, P., 18
Erickson, R., 44, 255
Eisenson, J., 253
Emerick, L., 32, 239, 256
English, G.M., 211
Esophageal speech methods, 217–220
Establishment of fluent speech, 275
Evoking consonant sounds, 59
  /f/, 64
  frontal lisp, 60
  /k/, 65
  lateral lisp, 61
  /l/, 66
  /r, ɝ, ɚ/, 67
  /s/, 59
  /ʃ/, 62
  /θ/, 64
  /ts/, 63

F

Fairbanks, G., 251
Farwell, C., 22
Ferguson, C., 22
Feth, L., 108
Finnie, N.R., 203
Fisher, H., 37, 39
Fletcher, G.H., 201
Fletcher, S., 144
Florance, C., 262, 263
Fourcin, A., 17, 18
Fowlow, P., 18
Frazier, D., 137
Freeman, F., 244
Fristoe, M., 38, 86
Fudala, J., 41

G

Game activities in articulation therapy, 83
Gentle onset, 272
Gillespie, S.K., 103
Glassel, W.L., 129

Glauber, I., 246
Glossopalatal or glossopharyngeal press, 218
Goldiamond, I., 242, 247, 263
Goldman, R., 38, 86
Goldstein, L., 215, 220, 223
Gould, W.J., 202
Gray, M., 244
Gregory, H., 262
Grunting, 200
Guitar, B., 248, 255

H

Habitual pitch, 110, 187
Halle, M., 12
Hard glottal attack. See coup de glotte
Hamre, 239
Harding, R.L., 144
Harris, M., 244
Harrison, D., 211
Harwood, A.R., 233
Hawkins, N.V., 233
Hatten, J., 32, 256
Haugen, D., 253
Hegde, M., 242
Hejna, R., 42
Hierarchy analysis, 205–206
Hinchcliffe, R., 211
Hill, H., 244
Hixon, T.J., 108, 203
Holbrook, A., 137
Holen, D., 223
Horowitz, E., 253
Howie, P., 248
Hedrick, D., 23, 54
Hunter, N., 244
Huston, K., 13, 58
Hutton, J., 40
Hypernasality, 117, 140–142, 144, 148, 149, 150–152
Hyponasality, 116, 140, 144, 148

I

IAL. See International Association of Laryngectomees
Inhalation, alaryngeal, 218
Ingram, D., 23

Interjections, 241
International Association of Laryngectomees (IAL), 220, 236
Irwin, J., 37, 44
Irwin, O.C., 17, 18, 42
Irwin, R., 42
Isshiki, N., 179
Izdebski, K., 170, 171

J

Jacobson, E., 165, 261
Jargon, 20
Jex, J., 37
Johns, D.F., 182, 203
Johnson, T., 127, 134, 137
Jones, J., 37
Jones, R., 243
Johnson, 33, 34, 37, 240, 245, 246, 249, 255, 261, 262
Jusczyk, R., 18

K

Keane, T., 233
Keaster, M., 240
Keith, R.L., 217, 220, 225
Kern, C., 23, 54
Kidd, K., 244, 246
Kimura, D., 243
Klatt, D., 150
Kohler, S., 128
Kohn, J., 52
Krogman, W.M., 144
Kuehn, J., 43

L

Lalling, 20
Lamb, M.M., 129
Lanyon, R., 255
Laryngectomy, 211–212
Laryngectomy rehabilitation
 artificial larynx, 223–224
 case example, 232
 formal alaryngeal therapy, 224–228
 goals, 231
 phrasing, 228–229

Index 291

poor speech habits, 229–230
presurgery visit, 220–223
problems, 230–231
role of SLP, 213
Lauder, E., 217, 220, 222, 225, 228
Laughing abusively, 204
Leach, E., 275
Lieberman, P., 17
Lisping
frontal, 60
lateral, 61
Logemann, J., 37, 39

M

Maccomb, W.S., 201
Mager, R., 84
Masaki, S., 179
Mason, R., 148
Massehiro, T., 179
Mattson, P.J., 129
Mazaheri, M., 144
McCabe, R., 59
McCall, G.N., 147, 148
McDonald, E., 34, 38, 39, 56
McNeill, D., 17
McReynolds, E., 13, 52, 53
McWilliams, B.J., 147
Mecham, M., 37
Medical evaluation and referral
processes, 104
Mengert, I., 23
Menstrual cycle, 202
Menyuk, P., 20
Mill, W.B., 233
Millard, R.T., 144
Miller, G., 251
Minifie, F.D., 108
Montgomery, A., 166
Moore, P., 137
Morris, H., 43
Mosby, D., 129
Moses, P.J., 159
Motivation, 82, 93
Mowrer, D., 53, 79, 84, 93, 263, 274,
275, 279, 281, 284
Mowrer, O.H., 19
Mueller, K., 172
Mundy, M., 275, 281
Munro, I.R., 143

Murai, J., 17
Murphy, A.T., 170
Murry, F., 243
Musgrave, R., 147
Muselman, B., 42
Mutational falsetto (puberphonia),
117–123
Myasthenia gravis, 182
Myklebust, H., 19

N

Nasal listening tube, 146
Neck breather, 212
Nelson, S., 244
Neurogenic voice disorder
case example, 177, 180
central nervous system lesions, 179
laryngeal innervation, 174
medical treatment, 179
superior laryngeal lesions, 178
therapy, 180
vagus nerve lesions, 176–177

O

Ogura, J.H., 233
Oldring, D.J., 172
Optimal pitch, 110, 188
Oral examination, 46
hard palate, 47
jaws and teeth, 47
tongue, 47
velum, 47
Oral motor coordination
test of, 48
Oller, D., 18
Orton, S., 243

P

Palate
neurological abnormalities, 143
postadenoidectomy, 143
structural abnormalities, 143

Palatopharyngeal closure. *See* velopharyngeal closure
Papillomatosis (juvenile), 107
Parameters of voice
  aphonia, 113
  breathiness, 114
  excessive tension, 115
  hoarseness, 115
  hyperfunctional, 113
  hypofunctional, 113
  normal, 114
  pitch, 108
  quality, 112
  resonance, 116
  spasticity, 115
  whisper, 113
P-E junction, 212, 217, 233
Perez, C.A., 233
Pendergast, K., 42
Perkins, W., 18, 263, 281
Pharyngeal speech, 216
Phonemes, segmental, 11
  definition, 11
Phones, 11
  definition, 11
Pierce, M.K., 234
Pitch evaluation, 109
Pitch (inappropriate), 200
Poole, E., 23, 54
Powers, W.E., 233
Prather, E., 23, 54
Predictive tests, 33, 43
  The Predictive Screening Test of Articulation, 44
Prognostic tests. *See* prediction
Progressive relaxation, 165–166
Prolongations, 241
Prosek, R., 166
Pseudoswallowing (alaryngeal), 219
Psychogenic voice disorder
  biofeedback, 166
  case example, 158, 163, 168
  defined, 158
  digital manipulation, 167
  evaluation, 160
  progressive relaxation, 165–166
  symptoms, 159
  therapy, 161–165
Puberphonia. *See* mutational falsetto
Pull-out procedure, 267

R

Radiation without surgery, 233
Rapport, 52
Rate of speaking, 251
Repetitions, 241
Revisions, 241
Rice, M., 105, 106, 134, 137, 205
Rickard, H., 275, 281
Rider, W.D., 233
Riley, G., 251, 254
Riekena, A., 215
Rolnick, M.I., 137
Rosenstein, A., 228
Ross, C., 18
Ryan, B., 248, 251, 253, 263, 275, 279, 281

S

S-1 Treatment Model, 275
Salmon, S.J., 215, 220, 223
S-PACK, 93
Saxman, J.H., 203
Schuckers, G., 108
Schwartz, D., 273
Schwartz, M., 244, 248
Screening tests, 32, 36
  Denver Articulation Screening Examination, 37
  Fisher-Logemann Test of Articulation Competence, 37
  purpose of, 32
  A Screening Deep Test of Articulation, 38
  The Screening Speech Articulation Test, 37
  Templin-Darley Screening Test of Articulation, 37
  The Triota Ten Word Test, 37
  types of, 36
Schutz, R., 53, 79, 93
Segmental phonemes, 11
Seligman, J., 246
Selmar, J., 42
Senturia, B.H., 103, 123, 127
Serafini, I., 234
Shames, G., 247, 262, 263
Shanks, J., 219, 220, 225

Sheehan, J., 240, 246, 251
Sherrick, C., 247
Shervanian, C., 3
Shipp, T., 171
Shoemaker, D., 247, 248
Shriberg, L.D., 203
Shunt reconstruction (alaryngeal), 233–234
Shvachkin, N., 22
Siegel, G., 253
Sigueland, E., 18
Silent cough, 200
Silverman, F.H., 103, 182
Singer, M.I., 234
Singing (abusive), 198
Skinner, B., 275
Skolnick, L.M., 147, 148
Slow change, 272
Smith, F.M., 202
Smoking, 201
Soder, A., 42
Sound simplification process, 23
　liquid replacement, 25
　substitution, 24
　syllable structure, 23
　velar preference, 25
Spasmodic (spastic) dysphonia
　case example, 172–174
　described, 170
　surgery, 171
　symptoms, 171
　therapy, 172
Speech production mechanism, 9
　alveolar ridge, 9
　hard palate, 9
　larynx, 9, 10
　location of important parts, 9, 10
　mandible, 10
　pharynx, 9
　resonator, 11
　tongue, 9
　velum, 9
Speech reconstruction, 269
Spriestersbach, W., 33, 43, 249
Stetson, R., 34
Stimulability, 34, 54
　selecting target sounds, 54
Stoma. See tracheostoma
Stretched syllable, 271
Strong, M.S., 195

Stuttering, 239
　amount of in different speaking situations, 253
　assessment of, 249
　　sample size, 252
　case history, 256
　classes of, 249
　classical conditioning, 247
　criteria used for diagnosing in children, 252
　definition of, 239
　description of, 250
　desensitization, 265
　duration of, 250
　counting stuttering behaviors, 250
　etiology, 242
　　environmental, 245
　　multicausality, 247
　　neurological, 243
　　psychological, 246
　goals in therapy, 262
　　speak more fluently, 262
　　stutter more fluently, 262
　identification, 265
　instrumental conditioning, 247
　measurement of, 250
　tests of stuttering
　　Iowa Scale of Attitude toward Stuttering, 255
　　Perceptions of Stuttering Inventory, 273
　　Scale for Rating Severity of Stuttering, 249
　　S-Scale, 255
　　SS Scale of Attitudes toward Stuttering, 255
　　Stuttering Interview, 253
　　Stuttering Severity Instrument, 254
　rate of, 251
　treatment models of stuttering
　　Mowrer's method, 274
　　Van Riper's method, 264
　　Webster's method, 269
　types of, 240
Stabilization of fluent speech, 268
Submucous cleft, 142
Suprasegmental phonemes, 13, 14, 15
　juncture, 13, 15
　pitch, 13, 15
　stress, 13

Syllable transition, 272
s/z ratio, 131

T

Taub, S., 234
Templin, M., 23, 37, 38, 48, 54
Tetter, D.L., 198
Therapy progress tests, 33, 44
    purpose of, 33
Thome, J., 128
Thorp, R., 43
Tokyo artificial larynx, 214, 215
Toohill, R.J., 129
Toronto, A., 43
Townsend, J.J., 171
Tracheostoma, 212
Transfer of fluent speech, 278
Travis, L., 243

U

Upper respiratory infections (URI), 201
Ushijima, T., 244

V

Van Demark, D., 43
Van Kirk, B., 263
Van Riper, C., 37, 44, 48, 51, 52, 82, 242, 243, 246, 248, 251, 252, 255, 256, 261, 262, 263, 264, 265, 266, 267, 269, 283, 284, 285
Vaughan, C.W., 195
Velopharyngeal closure, 116, 117, 140, 141, 142, 143, 144, 146, 147, 148, 152, 176
Vigorito, J., 18
Voice characteristics analysis form, 131
Voice monitor, 271
Voice screening, 106
Vocal abuse, children and adults. *See* vocal nodules

Vocal nodules, adults
    case examples, 195, 208
    described, 194
    etiology, 196–204
    evaluation, 196–197
    pitch, 204
    quality, 205
    surgery, 195
    therapy, 207
Vocal nodules, children
    case example, 137
    described, 123
    etiology, 126–129
    pitch, 124
    quality, 126
    therapy, 132–137
Von Leden, H., 137
Vowels, 8
    age of mastery, 8
    classification of, 8
    diphthong, 9

W

Walden, B.E., 166
Walter, M., 244
Webster, L., 273
Webster, R., 263, 269, 270, 271, 272, 273, 274
Weiman, L., 18
Weinberg, B., 215
Weiner, F., 41
Weiner, P., 53
Wellman, B., 23, 54
Wepman, J., 48, 244, 246
Western Electric Electronic Larynges, 214–215
West, R., 239
Weston, A., 44
Williams, F., 108
Williams, G., 52, 53
Wilson, F.B., 103, 105, 106, 123, 127, 129, 134, 172, 205
Wingate, M., 240
Winitz, H., 19, 23, 36
Wischner, G., 247
Witzel, M.A., 143
Woolf, G., 273
Wright, V., 45

Y

Yelling and screaming, 127, 198
Youngstrom, K.A., 217, 220, 224, 225

Z

Zemlin, W.R., 175
Zimmer, C.H., 103
Zwitman, D., 137, 200

About the Authors

Dr. Donald E. Mowrer and *Dr. James L. Case* are professors in the Department of Speech and Hearing Science at the Arizona State University, Tempe. Professor Mowrer teaches classes in articulation, stuttering, and behavior therapy. He has published extensively in these areas. His Ph.D. was earned at Arizona State University in 1964. Dr. Mowrer is a Fellow of the American Speech and Hearing Association.

Dr. Case, an associate professor, obtained his Ph.D. from the University of Utah. His specialty areas are voice and neurological disorders associated with communication dysfunctions. He is an active practicing speech/language pathologist, which accounts for his in-depth knowledge of the clinical management of clients. He was chosen as outstanding teacher of the year in 1981 by the College of Liberal Arts at Arizona State.

About the Authors

NO LONGER THE PROPERTY OF THE UNIVERSITY OF R. I. LIBRARY